T0179873

DSM-5-TR®

Handbook
of
Differential
Diagnosis

DSM-5-TR®
Handbook
of
Differential
Diagnosis

Michael B. First, M.D.

Professor of Clinical Psychiatry, Columbia University
New York, New York

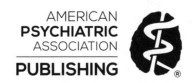

AMERICAN
PSYCHIATRIC
ASSOCIATION
PUBLISHING

Note: The author has worked to ensure that all information in this book is accurate at the time of publication and consistent with general psychiatric and medical standards, and that information concerning drug dosages, schedules, and routes of administration is accurate at the time of publication and consistent with standards set by the U.S. Food and Drug Administration and the general medical community. As medical research and practice continue to advance, however, therapeutic standards may change. Moreover, specific situations may require a specific therapeutic response not included in this book. For these reasons and because human and mechanical errors sometimes occur, we recommend that readers follow the advice of physicians directly involved in their care or the care of a member of their family.

Books published by American Psychiatric Association Publishing represent the findings, conclusions, and views of the individual authors and do not necessarily represent the policies and opinions of American Psychiatric Association Publishing or the American Psychiatric Association.

DSM, DSM-5, and DSM-5-TR are registered trademarks of the American Psychiatric Association (APA). Use of these terms is prohibited without permission of the APA.

If you wish to buy 50 or more copies of the same title, please go to www.appi.org/specialdiscounts for more information.

The author, Michael B. First, M.D., has no competing interests to disclose.

Copyright © 2024 American Psychiatric Association
ALL RIGHTS RESERVED

Manufactured in the United States of America on acid-free paper
27   26   25   24   23   5   4   3   2   1
First Edition

Typeset in Palatino LT Std and HelveticaNeue LT Std.

American Psychiatric Association Publishing
800 Maine Ave., SW
Suite 900
Washington, DC 20024-2812
www.appi.org

Library of Congress Cataloging-in-Publication Data
Names: First, Michael B., 1956– author. | American Psychiatric Association, issuing body.
Title: DSM-5-TR handbook of differential diagnosis / by Michael B. First.
Description: First edition. | Washington, DC : American Psychiatric Association Publishing, [2024] | Includes index.
Identifiers: LCCN 2023026279 (print) | LCCN 2023026280 (ebook) | ISBN 9781615373598 (paperback) | ISBN 9781615373604 (ebook)
Subjects: MESH: Diagnostic and statistical manual of mental disorders (Fifth edition, text revision) | Mental Disorders—diagnosis | Diagnosis, Differential
Classification: LCC RC473.D54 (print) | LCC RC473.D54 (ebook) | NLM WM 141 | DDC 616.89/075—dc23/eng/20230727
LC record available at https://lccn.loc.gov/2023026279
LC ebook record available at https://lccn.loc.gov/2023026280

British Library Cataloguing in Publication Data
A CIP record is available from the British Library.

To Leslee,
my bashert, for all the love and support
that made this book possible.

Contents

Bipolar and Related Disorders

Depressive Disorders

Anxiety Disorders

Obsessive-Compulsive and Related Disorders

Trauma- and Stressor-Related Disorders

Dissociative Disorders

Somatic Symptom and Related Disorders

Feeding and Eating Disorders

Sleep-Wake Disorders

Sexual Dysfunctions

Gender Dysphoria

Disruptive, Impulse-Control, and Conduct Disorders

Substance-Related and Addictive Disorders

Neurocognitive Disorders

Personality Disorders

Paraphilic Disorders

Preface

Differential diagnosis is the bread and butter of our task as clinicians. Most patients do not come to the office saying, "I have major depressive disorder…give me an antidepressant" (although some do!). More typically, the patient consults us seeking some relief from particular symptoms such as depressed mood and fatigue (the "chief complaints" in the parlance of medicine) that are the source of clinically significant distress or impairment. When we are confronted with these presenting symptoms, our job is to cull from all of the myriad conditions included in DSM-5-TR those that could possibly account for them (e.g., for depressed mood and fatigue, the possibilities include Major Depressive Disorder, Persistent Depressive Disorder, Bipolar I Disorder, Bipolar II Disorder, Schizoaffective Disorder, Depressive Disorder Due to Another Medical Condition, Substance/Medication-Induced Depressive Disorder, Adjustment Disorders). Once we have determined a list of candidates, our next job is to collect additional information—from personal history, other informants, treatment records, mental status examination, and laboratory investigations—that will allow a winnowing down of this differential diagnosis list to a single most likely contender, which becomes the initial diagnosis leading to an initial treatment plan. We must still keep an open mind, however, for the possibility that additional information that becomes available after the initial assessment is completed might justify a change in the diagnosis and possibly the treatment plan. For example, an initial diagnosis of recurrent Major Depressive Disorder might be changed to Bipolar I Disorder after a requested copy of the medical record for a past hospitalization reveals that what was reported by a patient as a past Major Depressive Episode was in fact a Manic Episode With Mixed Features.

This handbook should improve your skill in formulating a comprehensive differential diagnosis by presenting the problem from a number of different perspectives. Chapter 1, "Differential Diagnosis Step by Step," explores the differential diagnostic issues that must be considered in each and every patient being evaluated by providing a six-step diagnostic framework. In Chapter 2, "Differential Diagnosis by the Trees," the differential diagnosis is approached from the bottom up—that is, from a point of origin that begins with the patient's presenting symptom(s) such as depressed mood, delusions, and insomnia. Each of the 30 decision trees indicates which DSM-5-TR diagnoses must be considered in the differential diagnosis of that particular symptom, and offers decision points reflecting the thinking process involved in choosing from among the possible contenders. In Chapter 3, "Differential Diagnosis by the Tables," the differential diagnosis is approached from a later point in the diagnostic assessment process—that is, after you have reached a tentative diagnosis and want to ensure that all reasonable alternatives have received adequate consideration. The chapter contains 67 differential diagnosis tables, one for each of the most important DSM-5-TR disorders. To facilitate the linkage between the decision trees in Chapter 2 and the differential diagnosis tables in Chapter 3, each of the disorders included in the terminal branches of the decision trees indicates the corresponding differential diagnosis table. Additionally, appendixes to this handbook include the DSM-5-TR Classification, which has been included to facilitate coding and to provide an overview of all the DSM-5-TR diagnoses that must be considered in formulating a differential diagnosis, as well as alphabetical indexes of the decision trees and differential diagnosis tables, which provide an alternate way to locate a particular decision tree or differential diagnostic table that may be of interest.

The information provided in the decision trees and the differential diagnosis tables is somewhat overlapping, but each format has its own strengths and may be more or less useful, depending on the situation. The decision trees highlight the overall algorithmic rules that govern the classification of a particular symptom. Differential diagnosis tables are provided for most of the disorders in DSM-5-TR and indicate those disorders that share important features and thus should be considered and ruled out. The tables have the advantage of providing a head-to-head comparison of each disorder, highlighting both the points of similarity and the points of differentiation. Various readers will have different purposes for and different methods of using this handbook. Some individuals will be interested in a comprehensive overview of the process of making DSM-5-TR diagnoses and will find it rewarding to review the handbook cover to cover. Others will use the handbook more as a reference guide to assist in the differential diagnosis of a particular patient.

The art and science of psychiatric diagnosis is both impeded and blessed by the fact that individuals are so much more complex than the diagnostic rules laid out in any set of decision trees or tables. On the one hand, clinicians must always guard the temptation to apply the DSM-5-TR criteria or the decision trees and differential diagnosis tables in this handbook in a rote or cookbook fashion. The approaches outlined here are meant to enhance and not to replace the central role of clinical judgment and the wisdom of accumulated experience. On the other hand, clinicians who are not aware of the guidelines for differential diagnosis included in DSM-5-TR may become idiosyncratic in their diagnostic habits, undermining one of the central functions of DSM-5-TR, which is to facilitate communication of diagnostic information among clinicians and between clinicians and their patients and family members. It is useful to know and take advantage of the precision afforded by following the DSM-5-TR rules but not to be enslaved by them.

Acknowledgments

I would like to thank Jared W. Keeley, Ph.D.; Cary Kogan, Ph.D.; Richard J. Loewenstein, M.D.; Andrew E. Skodol, M.D.; and Dan J., Stein, M.D., Ph.D., for their assistance with the development of the Repetitive Pathological Behaviors Tree (2.16) and the Depersonalization/Derealization Tree (2.18). I would also like to thank Allen Frances, M.D., and Harold Alan Pincus, M.D., my coauthors on the DSM-IV and DSM-IV-TR editions of the

Handbook of Differential Diagnosis, for helping to provide a solid foundation for this book. Finally, I would like to thank those at American Psychiatric Association Publishing who assisted in the production of this book: Rick Prather, Production Manager, who expertly redrew and typeset all the decision trees; Rebecca Richters, Senior Editor, for her skillful editorial review; and especially Ann M. Eng, DSM Managing Editor, whose meticulous editing of the decision trees, chapter text, and differential diagnosis tables has helped to ensure that I got all of the details right.

Differential Diagnosis Step by Step

The process of DSM-5-TR differential diagnosis can be broken down into six basic steps: 1) ruling out Malingering and Factitious Disorder; 2) ruling out a substance etiology; 3) ruling out an etiological medical condition; 4) determining the specific independent mental disorder(s) (i.e., nonsubstance-induced and not due to another medical condition); 5) differentiating Adjustment Disorders from the residual Other Specified and Unspecified conditions; and 6) establishing the boundary with no mental disorder. A thorough review of this chapter provides a useful framework for understanding and applying the decision trees presented in the next chapter.

Step 1: Rule Out Malingering and Factitious Disorder

The first step is to rule out Malingering and Factitious Disorder (which involve the intentional production of false or grossly exaggerated physical or psychological symptoms), because if the patient is not being honest regarding the nature or severity of their symptoms, all bets are off regarding the clinician's ability to arrive at an accurate psychiatric diagnosis. Most psychiatric work depends on a good-faith collaborative effort between the clinician and the patient to uncover the nature and cause of the presenting symptoms. There are times, however, when everything may not be as it seems. Some patients may elect to deceive the clinician by producing or feigning the presenting symptoms. Two conditions in DSM-5-TR are characterized by feigning: Malingering and

Factitious Disorder. These two conditions are differentiated based on the motivation for the deception. When the motivation is the achievement of a clearly recognizable goal (e.g., insurance compensation, avoiding legal or military responsibilities, obtaining drugs), the patient is considered to be Malingering. When the deceptive behavior is present even in the absence of obvious external rewards, the diagnosis is Factitious Disorder. Although the motivation for many individuals with Factitious Disorder is to assume the sick role, this requirement was dropped in DSM-5 because of the inherent difficulty in determining an individual's underlying motivation for their observed behavior.

The intent is certainly not to advocate that every patient be treated as a hostile witness nor that every clinician become a cynical district attorney. Rather, the clinician's index of suspicion should be raised 1) when there are clear external incentives to the patient for a psychiatric diagnosis (e.g., disability determinations, forensic evaluations in criminal or civil cases, prison settings), 2) when the patient presents with a cluster of psychiatric symptoms that conforms more to a lay perception of mental illness than to a recognized clinical entity, 3) when the nature of the symptoms shifts radically from one clinical encounter to another, 4) when the patient has a presentation that mimics that of a role model (e.g., another patient on the unit, a mentally ill close family member), and 5) when the patient is characteristically manipulative or suggestible. Finally, it is useful for clinicians to become mindful of tendencies they might have toward being either excessively skeptical or excessively gullible.

Step 2: Rule Out Substance Etiology (Including Drugs of Abuse, Medications)

The first question that should always be considered in the differential diagnosis is whether the presenting symptoms arise from a substance that is exerting a direct effect on the central nervous system (CNS). Virtually any presentation encountered in a mental health setting can be caused by substance use. Missing a substance etiology is probably the single most common diagnostic error made in clinical practice. This error is particularly unfortunate because making a correct diagnosis has immediate treatment implications. For example, if the clinician determines that psychotic symptoms are due to Cocaine Intoxication, it usually does not make sense for the patient to immediately start taking an antipsychotic medication unless the psychotic symptoms are putting the patient (or others) in immediate danger. The determination of whether psychopathology is due to substance use often can be difficult because although substance use is fairly ubiquitous and a wide variety of different symptoms can be caused by substances, the fact that substance use and psychopathology occur together does not necessarily imply a cause-and-effect relationship between them.

Obviously, the first task is to determine whether the person has been using a substance. This entails careful history taking and physical examination for signs of Substance Intoxication or Substance Withdrawal. Because substance-abusing individuals are notorious for underestimating their intake, it is usually wise to consult with family members and obtain a laboratory analysis of body fluids to ascertain recent usage of particular substances. It should be remembered that patients who use or are exposed to any of a variety of substances (not only drugs of abuse) can and often do present with psychiatric symptoms. Medication-induced psychopathology is common and very often missed, especially as the population ages and many individuals are taking multiple medications. Although it is less common, toxin exposure should be considered, especially for people whose occupations bring them into contact with potential toxins.

Once substance use has been established, the next task is to determine whether there is an etiological relationship with the psychiatric symptomatology. This requires distinguishing among three possible relationships between the substance use and the psychopathology: 1) the psychiatric symptoms result from the direct effects of the substance on the CNS (resulting in a diagnosis of Substance/Medication-Induced Mental Disorder in DSM-5-TR; e.g., Cocaine-Induced Psychotic Disorder, Reserpine-Induced Depressive Disorder); 2) the substance use is a consequence (or associated feature) of having a primary psychiatric disorder (e.g., self-medication); and 3) the psychiatric symptoms and the substance use are independent. Each of these relationships is discussed in turn.

1. **In diagnosing a Substance/Medication-Induced Mental Disorder, there are three considerations in determining whether there is a causal relationship between the substance use and the psychiatric symptomatology.** First, you must determine whether there is a close temporal relationship between the substance or medication use and the psychiatric symptoms. Then, you must consider the likelihood that the particular pattern of substance/medication use could result in the observed psychiatric symptoms. Finally, you should consider whether there are better alternative explanations (i.e., a non-substance/medication-induced cause) for the clinical picture.

   - **Consider whether a temporal relationship exists between the substance/medication use and the onset or maintenance of the psychopathology.**
     The determination of whether there was a period of time when the psychiatric symptoms were present outside the context of substance/medication use is probably the best (although still fallible) method for evaluating the etiological relationship between substance/medication use and psychiatric symptoms. At the extremes, this is relatively straightforward. If the onset of the psychopathology clearly precedes the onset of the substance/medication use, then it is likely that a non-substance/medication-induced psychiatric condition is primary and the substance/medication use is secondary (e.g., as a form of self-medication) or is unrelated. Conversely, if the onset of the substance/medication use clearly and closely precedes the psychopathology, it lends greater credence to the likelihood of a Substance/Medication-Induced Mental Disorder. Unfortunately, in practice this seemingly simple determination can be quite difficult to discern because the onsets of the substance/medication use and the psychopathology may be more or less simultaneous or impossible to reconstruct retrospectively. In such situations, you will need to rely on the course of the psychiatric symptoms when the person is no longer taking the substance or medication.
     Psychiatric symptoms that develop during or soon after Substance Intoxication, Substance Withdrawal, and medication use result from the effects of the substance or medication on neurotransmitter systems. Once these effects have been removed (by a period of abstinence after the withdrawal phase), the psychiatric symptoms should spontaneously resolve. Persistence of the psychiatric symptomatology for

a significant period of time after the cessation of acute withdrawal or severe intoxication or after stopping a medication suggests that the psychopathology is primary and not due to substance/medication use. The exceptions are the Persistent type of Substance/Medication-Induced Major or Mild Neurocognitive Disorder, in which by definition the neurocognitive impairment continues to be significant after an extended period of abstinence; and Hallucinogen Persisting Perception Disorder, in which following cessation of hallucinogen use, one or more of the perceptual symptoms that the individual experienced with Hallucinogen Intoxication (e.g., geometric hallucinations, flashes of color, trails of images of moving objects, halos around objects) are reexperienced.

The DSM-5-TR criteria for substance/medication-induced mental disorder presentations suggest that psychiatric symptoms be attributed to substance use if they remit within 1 month of the cessation of acute intoxication, withdrawal, or medication use. It should be noted, however, that the need to wait 1 full month before making a diagnosis of an independent psychiatric disorder is only a guideline that must be applied with clinical judgment; depending on the setting, it might make sense to use a more extended duration or a shorter duration, depending on your concern for avoiding false positives versus false negatives with respect to detecting a substance/medication-induced mental disorder presentation. On the one hand, some clinicians, particularly those who work in substance use treatment settings, are most concerned about the possibility of misdiagnosing a substance/medication-induced mental disorder presentation as an independent mental disorder that is not caused by substance use and might prefer allowing 6–8 weeks of abstinence before considering the diagnosis to be an independent mental disorder. On the other hand, clinicians who work primarily in psychiatric settings may be more concerned that given the wide use of substances among patients seen in clinical settings, such a long waiting period is impractical and might result in an overdiagnosis of Substance/Medication-Induced Mental Disorders and an underdiagnosis of independent mental disorders. Moreover, it must be recognized that the one-size-fits-all 1-month time frame applies to a wide variety of substances and medications with very different pharmacokinetic properties and a wide variety of possible consequent psychopathologies. Therefore, the time frame must be applied flexibly, considering the extent, duration, and nature of the substance/medication use.

Sometimes it is simply not possible to determine whether there was a period of time when the psychiatric symptoms occurred outside of periods of substance/medication use. This may occur in the often-encountered situation in which the patient is too poor a historian to allow a careful determination of past temporal relationships. In addition, substance use and psychiatric symptoms can have their onset around the same time (often in adolescence), and both can be more or less chronic and continuous. In these situations, it may be necessary to assess the patient during a current period of abstinence from substance use or, in the case of a suspected medication-induced psychiatric disorder, to stop the medication suspected of causing the psychiatric symptoms. If the psychiatric symptoms persist in the absence of substance/medication use, then the psychiatric disorder can be considered to be independent. If the symptoms remit during periods of abstinence, then the substance use is probably primary. It is important to realize that this judgment can only be made after waiting for enough time to elapse so as to be confident that the psychiatric symptoms are not a consequence of withdrawal. Ideally, the best setting for making this determination is in a facility where the patient's access to substances can be controlled and the patient's psychiatric symptomatology can be serially assessed. Of course, it is often impossible to observe a patient for as long as 4 weeks in a tightly controlled setting. Consequently, these judgments must be based on less controlled observation, and the clinician's confidence in the accuracy of the diagnosis should be more guarded.

- **In determining the likelihood that the pattern of substance/medication use can account for the symptoms, consider whether the nature, amount, and duration of substance/medication use are consistent with the development of the observed psychiatric symptoms.**

  Only certain substances and medications are known to be causally related to particular psychiatric symptoms. Moreover, the amount of substance or medication taken and the duration of use must be above a certain threshold to reasonably be considered the cause of the psychiatric symptomatology. For example, a severe and persisting depressed mood following the isolated use of a small amount of cocaine should probably not be considered to be attributed to the cocaine use, even though depressed mood is sometimes associated with Cocaine Withdrawal. For individuals who are regular substance users, a significant change in the amount used (either a large increase or a decrease in amount sufficient to trigger withdrawal symptoms) may in some cases cause the development of psychiatric symptoms.

- **Consider other factors in the presentation that suggest causes other than a substance or medication.**

  These factors include a history of many similar episodes not related to substance/medication use, a strong family history of the particular independent psychiatric disorder, or the presence of physical examination or laboratory findings suggesting that a nonpsychiatric medical condition might be involved. Considering factors other than substance/medication use as a cause for the presentation of psychiatric symptoms requires fine clinical judgment (and often waiting and seeing) to weigh the relative probabilities in these situations. For example, an individual may have a significant family history of Anxiety Disorders and still have a cocaine-induced panic attack that does not necessarily presage the development of an independent Panic Disorder.

2. **In some cases, the substance use can be the consequence or an associated feature (rather than the cause) of the psychiatric symptomatology.** Not uncommonly, the substance-taking behavior can be considered a form of self-medication for the psychiatric condition. For example, an individual with an independent Anxiety Disorder might use alcohol excessively for its sedative and antianxiety effects. One interesting implication of using a substance to self-medicate is that individuals with particular psychiatric disorders often preferentially choose certain classes of substances. For example, patients with negative symptoms of Schizophrenia often prefer stimulants, whereas patients with Anxiety Disorders often prefer CNS depressants.

The hallmark of an independent psychiatric disorder with secondary substance use is that the independent psychiatric disorder occurs first and/or exists at times during the person's lifetime when they are not using any substance. In the most classic situation, the period of comorbid psychiatric symptomatology and substance use is immediately preceded by a period of time in which the person had the psychiatric symptomatology but was abstinent from the substance. For example, an individual currently with 5 months of heavy alcohol use and depressive symptomatology might report that the alcohol use started in the midst of a Major Depressive Episode, perhaps as a way of counteracting insomnia. Clearly the validity of this judgment depends on the accuracy of the patient's retrospective reporting. Because such information is sometimes suspect, it may be useful to confer with other informants (e.g., family members) or review past records to document the presence of psychiatric symptoms occurring in the absence of substance use.

3. **In other cases, both the psychiatric disorder and the substance use can be initially unrelated and relatively independent of each other.** The high prevalence rates of both psychiatric disorders and Substance Use Disorders mean that by chance alone, some patients would be expected to have two apparently independent illnesses (although there may be some common underlying factor predisposing to the development of both the Substance Use Disorder and the psychiatric disorder). Of course, even if initially independent, the two disorders may interact to exacerbate each other and complicate the overall treatment. This independent relationship is essentially a diagnosis made by exclusion. When confronted with a patient having both psychiatric symptomatology and substance use, you should first rule out that one is causing the other. A lack of a causal relationship in either direction is more likely if there are periods when the psychiatric symptoms occur in the absence of substance use and if the substance use occurs at times unrelated to the psychiatric symptomatology.

After deciding that a presentation is due to the direct effects of a substance or medication, determine which DSM-5-TR Substance/Medication-Induced Mental Disorder best describes the presentation. DSM-5-TR includes a number of specific Substance/Medication-Induced Mental Disorders, along with Substance Intoxication and Substance Withdrawal. Refer to the Excessive or Problematic Substance Use Tree (2.28) in Chapter 2, "Differential Diagnosis by the Trees," for a presentation of the steps involved in making this determination. See also the DSM-5-TR Classification, "Substance-Related and Addictive Disorders" section in the Appendix to this book, for the specific substance/medication-induced mental disorders by substance class.

Step 3: Rule Out a Disorder Due to Another Medical Condition

After ruling out a substance/medication-induced etiology, the clinician next determines whether the psychiatric symptoms are due to the direct effects of a nonpsychiatric medical condition. This and the previous step of the differential diagnosis make up what was traditionally considered the "organic rule-outs" in psychiatry, in which the clinician is asked to first consider and rule out "physical" causes of the psychiatric symptomatology. Although DSM no longer uses words such as *organic* or *physical*, to avoid the anachronistic mind-body dualism implicit in such terms, the need to first rule out substances and nonpsychiatric medical conditions as specific causes of the psychiatric symptomatology remains crucial. For similar reasons, the phrase "due to a medical condition" is avoided in DSM because of the potential implication that psychiatric symptomatology and mental disorders are separate and distinct from the concept of "medical conditions." In fact, from a disease classification perspective, psychiatric disorders are but one chapter of the International Classification of Diseases (ICD), as are infectious diseases, neurological conditions, and so forth. Thus, when the phrase "due to another medical condition" is used in DSM-5-TR disorder names, what is really meant is that the symptoms are due to a medical condition that is classified outside the ICD mental disorders chapter—that is, a nonpsychiatric medical condition. In DSM-5-TR text, the phrase "medical condition" is modified with adjectives such as *another, other,* or *general* to clarify that the etiological condition, like a mental disorder, is a medical condition—but is differentiated from psychiatric medical conditions by virtue of being nonpsychiatric.

From a differential diagnostic perspective, ruling out a nonpsychiatric medical etiology is one of the most important and difficult distinctions in psychiatric diagnosis. It is important because many individuals with nonpsychiatric medical conditions have resulting psychiatric symptoms as a complication of the medical condition and because many individuals with psychiatric symptoms have an underlying medical condition. The treatment implications of this differential diagnostic step are also profound. Appropriate identification and treatment of the underlying nonpsychiatric medical condition can be crucial in both avoiding medical complications and reducing the psychiatric symptomatology.

This differential diagnosis can be difficult for four reasons: 1) symptoms of some psychiatric disorders and of many nonpsychiatric medical conditions can be identical (e.g., symptoms of weight loss and fatigue can be attributable to a Depressive or Anxiety Disorder or to a nonpsychiatric medical condition); 2) sometimes the first presenting symptoms of a medical condition are psychiatric (e.g., depression preceding other symptoms in pancreatic cancer or a brain tumor); 3) the relationship between the nonpsychiatric medical condition and the psychiatric symptoms may be complicated (e.g., depression or anxiety as a psychological reaction to having the nonpsychiatric medical condition vs. the medical condition being a cause of the depression or anxiety via its direct physiological effect on the CNS); and 4) psychiatric patients are often seen in settings primarily geared toward the identification and treatment of mental disorders in which there may be a lower expectation for, and familiarity with, the diagnosis of medical conditions.

Virtually any psychiatric presentation can be caused by the direct physiological effects of a nonpsychiatric medical condition, and these presentations are diagnosed in DSM-5-TR as one of the Mental Disorders Due to Another Medical Condition (e.g., Depressive Disorder Due to Hypothyroidism). It is no great trick to suspect the possible etiological role of a nonpsychiatric medical condition if the patient is encountered in a general hospital or primary care outpatient setting. The real diagnostic challenge occurs in mental health settings in which the base rate of nonpsychiatric medical conditions is much lower but nonetheless consequential. While it is not feasible (nor cost-effective) to order every conceivable screening test on every patient, it is important to direct the history, physical examination, and laboratory tests toward the diagnosis of those nonpsychiatric medical conditions that are most commonly encountered and most likely to account for the presenting psychiatric symptoms (e.g., thyroid function tests for depression, brain imaging for late-onset psychotic symptoms).

Once a nonpsychiatric medical condition is established, the next task is to determine its etiological relationship, if any, to the psychiatric symptoms. There are five possible relationships: 1) the nonpsychiatric medical condition causes the psychiatric symptoms through a direct physiological effect on the brain; 2) the nonpsychiatric medical condition causes the psychiatric symptoms through a psychological mechanism (e.g., depressive symptoms in response to being diagnosed with cancer—diagnosed as Major Depressive Disorder or Adjustment Disorder); 3) medication taken for the nonpsychiatric medical condition causes the psychiatric symptoms, in which case the diagnosis is a Medication-Induced Mental Disorder (see "Step 2: Rule Out Substance Etiology" in this chapter); 4) the psychiatric symptoms cause or adversely affect the nonpsychiatric medical condition (e.g., in which case Psychological Factors Affecting Other Medical Conditions may be indicated); and 5) the psychiatric symptoms and the nonpsychiatric medical condition are coincidental (e.g., hypertension and Schizophrenia). In the real clinical world, however, several of these relationships may occur simultaneously with a multifactorial etiology (e.g., a patient treated with an antihypertensive medication who has a stroke may develop depression due to a combination of the direct effects of the stroke on the brain, the psychological reaction to the resultant paralysis, and a side effect of the antihypertensive medication).

There are two clues suggesting that psychopathology is caused by the direct physiological effect of a nonpsychiatric medical condition. Unfortunately, neither of these is infallible, and clinical judgment is always necessary.

- **The first clue involves the nature of the temporal relationship and requires consideration of whether the psychiatric symptoms a) begin following the onset of the nonpsychiatric medical condition, b) vary in severity with the severity of the medical condition, and c) remit when the medical condition resolves.** When all of these relationships can be demonstrated, a fairly compelling case can be made that the nonpsychiatric medical condition has caused the psychiatric symptoms; however, such a clue does not establish that the relationship is physiological (the temporal covariation could also be due to a psychological reaction to the nonpsychiatric medical condition). Also, sometimes the temporal relationship is not a good indicator of underlying etiology. For instance, psychiatric symptoms may be the first harbinger of the nonpsychiatric medical condition and may precede by months or years any other manifestations. Conversely, psychiatric symptoms may be a relatively late manifestation occurring months or years after the nonpsychiatric medical condition has been well established (e.g., depression in Parkinson's disease).
- **The second clue that a nonpsychiatric medical condition should be considered in the differential diagnosis is whether the psychiatric presentation is atypical in symptom pattern, age at onset, or course.** For example, the presentation cries out for a medical workup when severe memory or weight loss accompanies a relatively mild depression or when severe disorientation accompanies psychotic symptoms. Similarly, the first onset of a manic episode in an elderly patient may suggest that a non-

psychiatric medical condition is involved in its etiology. However, atypicality does not in and of itself indicate a nonpsychiatric medical etiology because the heterogeneity of independent psychiatric disorders leads to many "atypical" presentations.

Nonetheless, the most important bottom line with regard to this task in the differential diagnosis is not to miss possibly important underlying nonpsychiatric medical conditions. Establishing the nature of the causal relationship often requires careful evaluation, longitudinal follow-up, and trials of treatment.

Finally, if the clinician concludes that a nonpsychiatric medical condition is responsible for the psychiatric symptoms, they must determine which of the DSM-5-TR Mental Disorders Due to Another Medical Condition best describes the presentation. DSM-5-TR includes a number of such disorders, each differentiated by the predominant symptom presentation. These disorders are included across the various decision trees in this book and are as follows: Psychotic Disorder Due to Another Medical Condition, Bipolar and Related Disorder Due to Another Medical Condition, Depressive Disorder Due to Another Medical Condition, Anxiety Disorder Due to Another Medical Condition, Obsessive-Compulsive and Related Disorder Due to Another Medical Condition, Delirium Due to Another Medical Condition, Major or Mild Neurocognitive Disorder Due to Another Medical Condition, Personality Change Due to Another Medical Condition, and Other Specified/Unspecified Mental Disorder Due to Another Medical Condition. See also the DSM-5-TR Classification in the Appendix to this book for the specific disorders.

Step 4: Determine the Specific Independent Mental Disorder(s)

Once substance use and nonpsychiatric medical conditions have been ruled out as etiologies, the next step is to determine which among the independent DSM-5-TR mental disorders best accounts for the presenting symptomatology. Many of the diagnostic groupings in DSM-5-TR (e.g., Schizophrenia Spectrum and Other Psychotic Disorders, Anxiety Disorders, Dissociative Disorders) are organized around common presenting symptoms precisely to facilitate this differential diagnosis. The decision trees in Chapter 2 provide the decision points needed for choosing among the independent mental disorders that might account for each presenting symptom. Once the clinician has selected what appears to be the most likely disorder, they may wish to review the pertinent differential diagnosis table in Chapter 3, "Differential Diagnosis by the Tables," to ensure that all other possible contenders in the differential diagnosis have been considered and ruled out.

Step 5: Differentiate Adjustment Disorders From the Residual Other Specified or Unspecified Mental Disorders

Many clinical presentations of mental disorders (particularly in outpatient and primary care settings) do not conform to the particular symptom patterns in DSM-5-TR diagnostic criteria, or they fall below the established severity or duration thresholds to qualify for one of the specific DSM-5-TR diagnoses. In such situations, if the symptomatic presentation is severe enough to cause clinically significant impairment or distress and reflects a dysfunction in the psychological, biological, or developmental processes underlying mental functioning in the individual (part of the DSM-5-TR definition of a mental disorder, p. 14), a diagnosis of a mental disorder is still warranted, and the differential comes down to either an Adjustment Disorder or one of the residual Other Specified or Unspecified categories. If the clinical judgment is made that the symptoms have developed as a maladaptive response to a psychosocial stressor, the diagnosis would be an Adjustment Disorder. If it is judged that a stressor is not responsible for the development of the clinically significant symptoms, then the relevant Other Specified or Unspecified category may be diagnosed, with the choice of the appropriate residual category depending on which DSM-5-TR diagnostic grouping best covers the symptomatic presentation. For example, if the patient's presentation is characterized by depressive symptoms that do not meet the criteria for any of the disorders included in the DSM-5-TR chapter "Depressive Disorders," then Other Specified Depressive Disorder or Unspecified Depressive Disorder is diagnosed (rules regarding which of these two categories to use are provided in the next paragraph). Because stressful situations are a daily feature of most people's lives, the judgment in this step is centered more on whether a stressor is the cause of the symptoms rather than on whether a stressor is present.

DSM-5-TR offers two versions of residual categories: Other Specified [Mental Disorder] and Unspecified [Mental Disorder]. As these names suggest, the differentiation between the two depends on whether the clinician chooses to specify the reason that the symptomatic presentation does not meet the criteria for any specific category in that diagnostic grouping. If the clinician wants to indicate the specific reason, the name of the disorder ("Other Specified [Mental Disorder]") is followed by the reason why the presentation does not conform to any of the specific disorder definitions. In some cases, the specific reason may already be listed as one of the examples of presentations that do not meet the diagnostic criteria for any of the specific categories in the diagnostic grouping. For example, if a patient has a clinically significant symptomatic presentation characterized by 4 weeks of depressed mood, most of the day nearly every day, which is accompanied by only two additional depressive symptoms (e.g., insomnia and fatigue), the clinician could record Other Specified Depressive Disorder, Depressive Episode With Insufficient Symptoms, which is listed as the third example in Other Specified Depressive Disorder. In other cases, the clinician can record their own description of the clinical presentation (e.g., Other Specified Disruptive, Impulse-Control, and Conduct Disorder; compulsive sexual behavior). If the clinician chooses not to indicate the specific reason why the presentation does not conform to any of the specific diagnostic criteria, the Unspecified [Mental Disorder] designation is used. For example, if the clinician declines to indicate the reason why the depressive presentation does not fit any of the specified categories, the diagnosis Unspecified Depressive Disorder is made instead. The clinician might also choose the unspecified option if there is insufficient information to make a more specific diagnosis and the clinician expects that additional information may be forthcoming, or if the clinician decides it is in the patient's best interest not to be specific about the reason (e.g., to avoid offering potentially stigmatizing information about the patient). Because the Other Specified [Mental Disorder] and Unspecified [Mental Disorder] residual categories differ only with regard to whether the clinician chooses to indicate the reason that the criteria for a specific disorder are not met, throughout this book, the Other Specified [Mental Disorder] and Unspecified [Mental Disorder] categories are combined into a single category for ease of reference, as "Other/Unspecified [Mental Disorder]."

Step 6: Establish the Boundary With No Mental Disorder

Generally, the last step in each of the decision trees is to establish the boundary between a disorder and no mental disorder. This decision is by no means the least important or easiest to make. Taken individually, many of the symptoms included in DSM-5-TR are fairly ubiquitous and are not by themselves indicative of the presence of a mental disorder. During the course of their lives, most people may experience periods of anxiety, depression, sleeplessness, or sexual dysfunction that may be considered as no more than an expected part of the human condition. To be explicit that not every such individual qualifies for a diagnosis of a mental disorder, DSM-5-TR includes with most criteria sets a criterion that is usually worded more or less as follows: "The disturbance causes clinically significant distress or impairment in social, occupational, or other important areas of functioning." This criterion requires that any psychopathology must lead to clinically significant problems in order to warrant a mental disorder diagnosis. For example, a diagnosis of Male Hypoactive Sexual Desire Disorder, which includes the requirement that the low sexual desire causes clinically significant distress in the individual, would not be made in a man with low sexual desire who is not currently in a relationship and who is not particularly bothered by the low desire.

Unfortunately, but necessarily, DSM-5-TR makes no attempt to define the term *clinically significant*. The boundary between disorder and normality can be set only by clinical judgment and not by any hard-and-fast rules. What may seem clinically significant is undoubtedly influenced by the cultural context, the setting in which the individual is seen, clinician bias, patient bias, and the availability of resources. "Minor" depression may seem much more clinically significant in a primary care setting than in a psychiatric emergency room or state hospital where the emphasis is on the identification and treatment of far more impairing conditions.

In clinical mental health settings, the judgment regarding whether a presentation is clinically significant is often a nonissue; the fact that the individual has sought help automatically makes it "clinically significant." More challenging are situations in which the symptomatic picture is discovered in the course of treating another mental disorder or a nonpsychiatric medical condition, which, given the high comorbidity among mental disorders and between mental disorders and nonpsychiatric medical conditions, is not an uncommon occurrence. Generally, as a rule of thumb, if the comorbid psychiatric presentation warrants clinical attention and treatment, it is considered to be clinically significant.

Finally, some conditions that can impair functioning, such as Uncomplicated Bereavement, may still not qualify for the use of an Other Specified or Unspecified Mental Disorder category because they do not represent an internal psychological or biological dysfunction in the individual, as is required in the DSM-5-TR definition of a mental disorder. Such "normal" but impairing symptomatic presentations may be worthy of clinical attention, but they do not qualify as mental disorders and should be given a code, if available (usually an ICD-10-CM Z code), from the DSM-5-TR chapter "Other Conditions That May Be a Focus of Clinical Attention," which concludes Section II.

Differential Diagnosis and Comorbidity

Differential diagnosis is generally based on the notion that the clinician is choosing a single diagnosis from among a group of competing, mutually exclusive diagnoses to best explain a given symptom presentation. For example, in a patient who presents with delusions, hallucinations, and manic symptoms, the question is whether the best diagnosis is Schizophrenia, Schizoaffective Disorder, or Bipolar Disorder With Psychotic Features; only one of these can be given to describe the current presentation. Very often, however, DSM-5-TR diagnoses are not mutually exclusive, and the assignment of more than one DSM-5-TR diagnosis to a given patient is both allowed and necessary to adequately describe the presenting symptoms. Thus, the clinician may need to consult multiple decision trees in this book to adequately cover all of the important clinically significant aspects of the patient's presentation. For example, a patient who presents with multiple unexpected panic attacks, significant depression, binge eating, and problematic substance use would require a consideration of the following decision trees: Panic Attacks (2.14), Depressed Mood (2.10), Appetite or Weight Change or Abnormal Eating Behavior (2.20), and Excessive or Problematic Substance Use (2.28). Moreover, because of comorbidity within diagnostic groupings, multiple passes through a particular decision tree may be required to cover all possible diagnoses. For example, it is well recognized that if a patient has one Anxiety Disorder (e.g., Social Anxiety Disorder), they are more likely to have other comorbid Anxiety Disorders (e.g., Separation Anxiety Disorder, Panic Disorder). The Anxiety Tree (2.13), however, helps to differentiate among the various Anxiety Disorders, and therefore a pass through this tree will result in the diagnosis of only one of the Anxiety Disorders. Multiple passes through the Anxiety Tree, answering the key questions differently each time, depending on which anxiety symptom is the current focus, are needed to capture the comorbidity.

The use of multiple diagnoses is in itself neither good nor bad as long as the implications are understood. A naïve and mistaken view of comorbidity might assume that a patient assigned more than one descriptive diagnosis actually has multiple independent conditions. This is certainly not the only possible relationship. In fact, there are six different ways in which two so-called comorbid conditions may be related to one another:

1. Condition A may cause or predispose to condition B.
2. Condition B may cause or predispose to condition A.
3. An underlying condition C may cause or predispose to both conditions A and B.
4. Conditions A and B may, in fact, be part of a more complex unified syndrome that has been artificially split in the diagnostic system.
5. The relationship between conditions A and B may be artifactually enhanced by definitional overlap.
6. The comorbidity is the result of a chance co-occurrence that may be particularly likely for those conditions that have high base rates.

The particular nature of these relationships is often very difficult to determine. The major point to keep in mind is that a patient "having" more than one DSM-5-TR diagnosis does not mean that there is more than one underlying pathophysiological process. Instead, DSM-5-TR diagnoses should be considered descriptive building blocks that are useful for communicating diagnostic information.

How to Use the Handbook: Case Example

To demonstrate how to use the diagnostic tools provided in this handbook to determine a differential diagnosis, consider the following case, adapted from *DSM-5-TR Clinical Cases*, edited by John W. Barnhill, M.D. (pp. 36–38).[1]

> John Evans was a 25-year-old single, unemployed white man who had been seeing a psychiatrist for several years for management of psychosis, depression, anxiety, and abuse of marijuana and alcohol.
>
> After an apparently normal childhood, Mr. Evans began to show dysphoric mood, anhedonia, low energy, and social isolation by age 15 years. At about the same time, Mr. Evans began to drink alcohol and smoke marijuana every day. In addition, he developed recurrent panic attacks, marked by a sudden onset of palpitations, diaphoresis, and thoughts that he was going to die. When he was at his most depressed and panicky, he twice received a combination of sertraline 100 mg/day and psychotherapy. In both cases, his most intense depressive symptoms lifted within a few weeks, and he discontinued the sertraline after a few months. Between episodes of severe depression, he was generally seen as sad, irritable, and amotivated. His school performance declined around tenth grade and remained marginal throughout the rest of high school. He did not attend college, as his parents expected, but instead lived at home and did odd jobs in the neighborhood.
>
> Around age 20, Mr. Evans developed a psychotic episode in which he had the conviction that he had murdered people when he was 6 years old. Although he could not remember who these people were or the circumstances of the event, he was absolutely convinced that this had happened—something that was confirmed to him by continuous voices he heard accusing him of being a murderer. He also became convinced that other people would punish him for what had happened; thus, he also feared for his life. Over the next few weeks, he became guilt ridden and preoccupied with the idea that he should kill himself by slashing his wrists, which culminated in his being psychiatrically hospitalized. Although he was predominantly anxious on admission, Mr. Evans soon became very depressed with prominent anhedonia, poor sleep, and decreased appetite and concentration. With the combined use of antipsychotic and antidepressant medications, both the depression and the psychotic symptoms remitted after 4 weeks. Therefore, the total duration of the psychotic episode was approximately 7 weeks, 4 of which were also characterized by major depressive disorder. Mr. Evans had been hospitalized with the same pattern of symptoms two additional times before age 22, and each of these episodes started with several weeks of delusions and hallucinations related to his conviction that he had murdered people when he was a child, followed by severe depression lasting an additional month. Both relapses occurred while he was apparently adherent to reasonable dosages of antipsychotic and antidepressant medications. During the 3 years prior to this evaluation, Mr. Evans had been adherent to clozapine and had been without hallucinations and delusions. He had also

---

[1] Adapted with permission from Ahmed AO: "Sad and Psychotic," in *DSM-5-TR Clinical Cases*. Edited by Barnhill JW. Washington, DC, American Psychiatric Association Publishing, 2023, pp. 36–38. Copyright © 2023 American Psychiatric Association Publishing.

been adherent to his antidepressant medication and supportive psychotherapy, although his dysphoria, irritability, and amotivation never completely resolved.

Mr. Evans's history was significant for marijuana and alcohol misuse that began when he was age 15. Before the onset of psychosis at age 20, he smoked several joints of marijuana almost daily and binge drank on weekends with occasional blackouts. After the onset of the psychosis, he decreased his marijuana and alcohol use significantly, with two several-months-long periods of abstinence, yet he continued to have psychotic episodes through age 22. He started attending Alcoholics Anonymous and Narcotics Anonymous groups, achieved sobriety from marijuana and alcohol at age 23, and had remained sober for the 2 years prior to this evaluation.

This case presentation includes both prominent psychotic symptoms (delusions and hallucinations) and mood symptoms (depression). Thus, the clinician can start the differential diagnosis process with any of the following decision trees: Delusions (2.5), Hallucinations (2.6), or Depressed Mood (2.10). Given the especially prominent nature of the delusions, we first start with the Delusions Tree (2.5). The first question, whether the beliefs are a manifestation of a culturally or religiously sanctioned belief system, can be answered "no" because Mr. Evans's fixed belief that he murdered people when he was age 6 is not a manifestation of any sanctioned belief system and is thus appropriately considered to be a delusion. The next question, regarding whether his delusions are due to the direct physiological effects of a substance, must be seriously considered given the fact that his delusions first emerged at age 20 during a time when he was smoking several joints of marijuana almost daily. To answer this question, we need to consider Step 2 of the six differential diagnosis steps presented earlier in this chapter, which provides guidance on how to rule out a substance etiology. In determining whether there is a causal relationship between the marijuana use and the delusions, we need to determine whether all three of the following conditions are true: 1) that there is a close temporal relationship between marijuana use and the onset and maintenance of the delusions, 2) that the pattern of marijuana use is consistent (in terms of dosage and duration) with the development of delusions, and 3) that there is no alternative (i.e., non-substance/medication-induced) explanation for the delusions. Although it is not common for marijuana to cause florid delusions, heavy marijuana use in some vulnerable individuals can result in delusions during Marijuana Intoxication, so the second condition (i.e., substance use is heavy and/or prolonged enough to induce the symptom) is met. In evaluating the first condition, however, although the delusions emerged during heavy marijuana use, the fact that the delusions persisted in the hospital when Mr. Evans was abstinent from marijuana and then subsequently reoccurred when his marijuana use was minimal indicates that the delusions cannot be explained as a manifestation of his marijuana use. Thus, the answer to the second question in the Delusions Tree, regarding whether there is a cannabis etiology for the delusions, is "no." The absence of any reported nonpsychiatric medical conditions in Mr. Evans also rules out a medical etiology, and therefore the answer to the following question is also "no."

After ruling out cultural and religious, substance/medication-induced, and nonpsychiatric medical etiologies for Mr. Evans's delusions, we then must differentiate among the independent psychotic and mood disorders as possible explanations for the delusions. The next question, which asks whether the delusions have occurred only in the context of an episode of elevated, expansive, or irritable mood, is answered "no" because of the absence of a history of manic or hypomanic symptoms. The subsequent question, about whether the delusions have occurred only in the context of an episode of depressed mood, is also answered "no" because the delusions also occurred at times when Mr. Evans was not experiencing a depressive episode (i.e., each psychotic episode is characterized by a several-week period of delusions before the development of the severe depressive symptoms).

The next block of questions in the Delusions Tree provides the differential diagnosis of non-mood-restricted delusions. The question inquiring whether the delusions last for 1 month or more is answered "yes" (i.e., each time the delusions have occurred, they lasted for several weeks), moving us for the first time to the right in the decision tree to consider the differential between Schizophrenia, Schizophreniform Disorder, Schizoaffective Disorder, Delusional Disorder, and Other Specified Schizophrenia Spectrum and Other Psychotic Disorder. The subsequent question about whether the delusions are accompanied by other psychotic symptoms characteristic of Schizophrenia (i.e., hallucinations, disorganized speech, grossly disorganized or catatonic behavior, or negative symptoms) is also answered "yes," given that in Mr. Evans's case, the delusions of having murdered a person when he was a child are accompanied by accusatory auditory hallucinations. The next question (i.e., whether there is a history of Major Depressive or Manic Episodes) is answered "yes," given the history of recurrent Major Depressive Episodes, as is the following question (i.e., whether during an uninterrupted period of illness, the psychotic symptoms occur concurrently with the mood episodes), because the delusions and hallucinations continued to persist after the Major Depressive Episodes emerged, thus indicating a period of overlap.

The next question, which provides the crucial differential diagnostic distinction between Schizoaffective Disorder and Schizophrenia, asks whether, during an uninterrupted period of illness, the mood episodes have been present for a *majority* of the total duration of the active and residual phases of the illness. In Mr. Evans's case, each of the psychotic episodes was present for approximately 7–8 weeks, with about 4 of those weeks characterized by the simultaneous occurrence of a severe Major Depressive Episode. Therefore, it is *not* the case that the mood episodes were present for a majority of the time during an uninterrupted episode of illness, so the question is answered "yes," ruling out the diagnoses of both Schizophrenia and Schizophreniform Disorder. The next question, regarding whether delusions and hallucinations have occurred for at least 2 weeks in the absence of a Major Depressive Episode or Manic Episode, is answered "yes" (i.e., for the first 3 or 4 weeks of the psychotic episode, Mr. Evans was anxious but not suffering from significant depressed mood), bringing us to the terminal branch of the Delusions Tree (2.5) and the diagnosis of Schizoaffective Disorder. It should be noted that given the complete co-occurrence of the delusions and hallucinations during the psychotic episodes, had we started with the Hallucinations Tree (2.6) instead of the Delusions Tree (2.5), we would have gone through almost the exact same sequence of steps to arrive at the diagnosis of Schizoaffective Disorder, given the similarity of the branching structure of the Delusions and Hallucinations Trees.

Alternatively, we could have approached this case from the perspective of Mr. Evans's severe depressive symptoms and instead started with the Depressed Mood Tree (2.10).

The first question in this tree inquires about a substance etiology for the depressive symptoms. Applying the same principles discussed in previous paragraphs with regard to the relationship between Mr. Evans's marijuana use and his delusions, this question can also be answered in the negative because although the marijuana use is sufficient to cause depressed mood, the fact that Mr. Evans continued to experience episodes of severe depression after he stopped his heavy use of marijuana indicates that, like the delusions, his depression cannot be considered to have been induced by the marijuana use. The next question asks whether the depression is due to the direct physiological effects of a nonpsychiatric medical condition, and that question can also be answered "no" because of the absence of any history of medical problems. The next question asks whether the depressed mood was part of a Major Depressive Episode. The answer to that question is "yes" given that the depressive periods that developed after the onset of delusions and hallucinations were characterized by approximately 4 weeks of dysphoric mood, prominent anhedonia, poor sleep, decreased appetite, and reduced concentration, thus meeting syndromal criteria for a Major Depressive Episode. Note that the decision tree does not end at this point but that the diagnostic flow continues onward because Major Depressive Episode is not a codable diagnostic entity in DSM-5-TR but instead comprises one of the building blocks for the diagnoses of Bipolar I or Bipolar II Disorder, Major Depressive Disorder, and Schizoaffective Disorder. The next question, about the presence of clinically significant manic or hypomanic symptoms, is answered "no," bringing us to a consideration of the relationship between the Major Depressive Episodes and the psychotic symptoms. The question about whether there is a history of delusions or hallucinations is answered "yes," bringing us to the critical question as to whether the delusions or hallucinations occur exclusively during Manic or Major Depressive Episodes. In Mr. Evans's case, the psychotic symptoms have *not* occurred exclusively during the Major Depressive Episodes (i.e., the delusions and hallucinations occurred on their own for 3–4 weeks prior to the onset of the depressive episode), so the answer to this question is "no." At this point in the Depressed Mood Tree (2.10), rather than being offered additional questions, we are told that a Schizophrenia Spectrum or Other Psychotic Disorder is present and are instructed to go to the Delusions Tree (2.5) or Hallucinations Tree (2.6) for the differential diagnosis, resulting in the diagnosis of Schizoaffective Disorder.

After arriving at the diagnosis of Schizoaffective Disorder through the use of the decision trees, we can refer to the DSM-5-TR Classification in the Appendix to get the diagnostic code for Schizoaffective Disorder, and/or we can review the differential diagnosis table for Schizoaffective Disorder in Chapter 3 (Table 3.2.2) to confirm that the key contenders to a diagnosis of Schizoaffective Disorder have been appropriately ruled out. The two main diagnostic contenders in this case are Schizophrenia and Major Depressive Disorder With Psychotic Features. Accordingly, the differential diagnosis table for Schizoaffective Disorder notes that Schizophrenia is differentiated from Schizoaffective Disorder by virtue of the fact that Schizophrenia is characterized by mood episodes that "have been present for a minority of the total duration of the active and residual periods of the illness." In Mr. Evans's case, each episode of the illness was characterized by a Major Depressive Episode being present for more than half of the time (i.e., about 4 weeks) of the total duration (i.e., 7–8 weeks), thus ruling out the diagnosis of Schizophrenia. Moreover, the table also notes that Schizoaffective Disorder is differentiated from Major Depressive

Disorder With Psychotic Features by virtue of the fact that Major Depressive Disorder With Psychotic Features is characterized by psychotic symptoms that occur exclusively during Major Depressive Episodes. In Mr. Evans's case, the psychotic symptoms were not confined exclusively to the depressive episodes, ruling out the diagnosis of Major Depressive Disorder With Psychotic Features.

Differential Diagnosis
by the Trees

Differential diagnosis is at the heart of every initial clinical encounter and is the beginning of every treatment plan. The clinician must determine which disorders are possible candidates for consideration and then choose from among them the disorder (or disorders) that best accounts for the presenting symptoms. The biggest problem encountered in differential diagnosis is the tendency for premature closure in coming to a final diagnosis. Studies in cognitive science have indicated that clinicians typically decide on the diagnosis within the first 5 minutes of meeting the patient and then spend the rest of the time during their evaluation interpreting (and often misinterpreting) elicited information through this diagnostic bias. Forming initial impressions can be valuable in helping to suggest which questions need to be asked and which hypotheses need to be tested. Unfortunately, however, first impressions are sometimes wrong—particularly because the patient's current state may not be a true reflection of the longitudinal course. Accurate diagnosis requires a methodical consideration of all possible contenders in the differential diagnosis.

Perhaps the best way to avoid prematurely jumping to a diagnostic conclusion is to approach the problem from the bottom up: by generating the differential diagnosis based on the presenting symptoms. This section of the handbook, which includes 30 symptom-oriented decision trees, facilitates this process. Each decision tree starts with a particular presenting symptom and then provides decision points for determining which diagnosis may best account for it. For any given patient, several trees may (and often do) apply. In many instances, following the branches within the different pertinent decision trees will lead to the same diagnosis, suggesting that the presenting symptoms constitute a single syndrome. In other instances, more than one diagnosis may be indicated.

The first step in using these decision trees is to determine which ones apply to the clinical presentation. The listings of the decision trees included in this handbook are organized in three different ways to facilitate finding the relevant decision trees. Two lists are provided at the end of this introduction to Chapter 2. The first itemizes the decision trees in order of the DSM-5-TR diagnostic groupings (trees related to neurodevelopmental presentations are listed first, trees related to psychotic presentations second, and so forth). The second list is organized by mental status examination domain (trees related to mood/affect, trees related to behavior, and so forth). Finally, at the end of this handbook, an alphabetical index of the decision trees is included, as well as an alphabetical index of the differential diagnosis tables covered in Chapter 3.

Each decision tree is laid out in a standardized fashion. The presenting symptom for each tree is shown in bold text in a gray-shaded box at the upper left. The boxes on the far right, the diagnostic end points, are indicated by gray shading and a thick border; these show all of the disorders that need to be considered in the differential diagnosis of the presenting symptom. In these boxes (i.e., diagnostic end points), numbers in parentheses after the diagnosis or diagnoses refer to the corresponding differential diagnostic table in Chapter 3. Unshaded intermediate boxes are decision points that indicate how different disorders are ruled in or ruled out. The clinician should consider the statement in the decision box and then follow the "Y" branch if the answer is "yes" and the "N" branch if the answer is "no." Occasional intermediate boxes are not decision points per se but represent intermediate diagnostic conclusions, and thus lack the "Y" and "N" choices. For example, the Elevated or Expansive Mood Tree (2.8) includes intermediate boxes in which the presence of a Manic Episode or Hypomanic Episode is asserted, reflecting the fact that Manic Episode and Hypomanic Episode are building blocks for the diagnoses of Bipolar I and Bipolar II Disorders.

For a majority of the decision trees, the first or second decision box concerns whether the presentation is due to the direct physiological effects of a substance or medication; if so, the diagnosis is a substance/medication-induced mental disorder. In most cases, the specific classes of substance known to induce the symptomatic presentation corresponding to the entry point of the decision tree are noted, and the substance listing adopts the same format used in Table 1 ("Diagnoses associated with substance class") at the beginning of the DSM-5-TR chapter "Substance-Related and Addictive Disorders," in which "(I)" indicates that the substance-induced symptom has its onset during intoxication, "(W)" indicates that its onset occurs during withdrawal from the substance, and "(I/W)" indicates that the symptom can have its onset during intoxication or withdrawal.

Note that the separate designations in DSM-5-TR for the residual categories (e.g., Other Specified Anxiety Disorder and Unspecified Anxiety Disorder) have been combined into a single residual category (e.g., Other/Unspecified Anxiety Disorder). These diagnoses differ only with regard to whether the clinician chooses to specify the reason that the criteria are not met for a specific disorder ("Other Specified") or chooses not to specify anything ("Unspecified").

The clinician should always keep in mind that the decision trees are no more than an overview of the DSM-5-TR diagnostic system and a guide to differential diagnosis. Clinical judgment is always required in the evaluation of each decision point. Moreover, when the clinician has arrived at a diagnostic end point in a tree (i.e., a "final diagnosis"), it is important to review the actual DSM-5-TR criteria set for the disorder in question to ensure that the full criteria for that disorder have in fact been met. This confirmation is necessary for two reasons. First, the decision trees contain only summarized versions of the DSM-5-TR diagnostic criteria rather than the complete text of the criteria. Second, the decision trees only include selected criteria from the criteria sets—that is, those diagnostic criteria that differentiate between the various DSM-5-TR disorders. A review of the complete DSM-5-TR diagnostic criteria sets is needed to ensure that the case meets the full set of required diagnostic features and course requirements (e.g., persistence, minimum duration); for the most part, these are not included in the decision trees.

Many of the decision trees follow a standard format that mirrors the stepwise thought process used in making a differential diagnosis presented in Chapter 1 of this handbook. The first consideration is whether the particular symptom is the result of the direct physiological effects of substance use (including medication) or a nonpsychiatric medical condition (Steps 2 and 3 in Chapter 1). The next steps in the decision tree typically cover the independent mental disorders that may account for the symptom (Step 4). The final decision points in most of the decision trees provide the differential diagnosis for those presentations that do not conform to or that fall below the threshold for a specific DSM-5-TR diagnosis. These decision points thus differentiate among Adjustment Disorder, a residual Other Specified or Unspecified Disorder category, and no mental disorder at all (Steps 5 and 6). The important step of considering whether the presenting symptom has been feigned (as in Malingering or Factitious Disorder) has been explicitly included in the following decision trees: Somatic Complaints or Illness/Appearance Anxiety (2.19), Memory Loss or Memory Impairment (2.29), and Cognitive Impairment (2.30), as these are the types of symptoms that are most commonly feigned. However, as discussed in Step 1 in Chapter 1, being on the lookout for the possibility that symptoms might have been feigned potentially applies to the evaluation of all presenting symptoms, especially in certain contexts and settings (e.g., forensic).

As noted above, the order of the 30 decision trees in this handbook corresponds roughly to the organization of the DSM-5-TR disorders. The following lists show the decision trees organized by 1) DSM-5-TR diagnostic grouping and 2) mental status examination domain.

Decision trees organized by DSM-5-TR diagnostic grouping

Neurodevelopmental presentations
2.1   Poor school performance
2.2   Behavioral problems in a child or adolescent
2.3   Speech disturbance
2.4   Distractibility

Schizophrenia and other psychotic presentations
2.5   Delusions
2.6   Hallucinations
2.7   Catatonic symptoms

Decision trees organized by DSM-5-TR diagnostic grouping (continued)

Bipolar presentations
2.8   Elevated or expansive mood
2.9   Irritable mood

Depressive presentations
2.10   Depressed mood
2.11   Suicidal ideation or behavior
2.12   Psychomotor retardation

Anxiety presentations
2.13   Anxiety
2.14   Panic attacks
2.15   Avoidance behavior

Obsessive-compulsive and related symptom presentations
2.16   Repetitive pathological behaviors

Trauma- and stressor-related presentations
2.17   Trauma or psychosocial stressors involved in the etiology

Dissociative symptom presentations
2.18   Depersonalization/derealization

Somatic symptom presentations
2.19   Somatic complaints or illness/appearance anxiety

Feeding and eating presentations
2.20   Appetite or weight change or abnormal eating behavior

Sleep-wake presentations
2.21   Insomnia
2.22   Hypersomnolence

Sexual dysfunction presentations
2.23   Sexual dysfunction in a female
2.24   Sexual dysfunction in a male

Disruptive, impulse-control, and conduct presentations
2.25   Aggressive behavior
2.26   Impulsivity or impulse-control problems
2.27   Self-injurious behavior

Substance-related presentations
2.28   Excessive or problematic substance use

Neurocognitive presentations
2.29   Memory loss or memory impairment
2.30   Cognitive impairment

Decision trees organized by mental status examination domain

Mood/affect
2.8   Elevated or expansive mood
2.9   Irritable mood
2.10 Depressed mood
2.13 Anxiety
2.14 Panic attacks

Behavior
2.2   Behavioral problems in a child or adolescent
2.7   Catatonic symptoms
2.11 Suicidal ideation or behavior
2.15 Avoidance behavior
2.16 Repetitive pathological behaviors
2.25 Aggressive behavior
2.26 Impulsivity or impulse-control problems
2.27 Self-injurious behavior
2.28 Excessive or problematic substance use

Motor
2.12 Psychomotor retardation

Cognition
2.4   Distractibility
2.29 Memory loss or memory impairment
2.30 Cognitive impairment

Thought form/speech
2.3   Speech disturbance

Thought content
2.5   Delusions
2.11 Suicidal ideation or behavior

Perceptual disturbance
2.6   Hallucinations
2.18 Depersonalization/derealization

Somatic symptoms
2.14 Panic attacks
2.19 Somatic complaints or illness/appearance anxiety

Personality features
2.26 Impulsivity or impulse-control problems
2.27 Self-injurious behavior

Sleep/eating/sex
2.20 Appetite or weight change or abnormal eating behavior
2.21 Insomnia
2.22 Hypersomnolence
2.23 Sexual dysfunction in a female
2.24 Sexual dysfunction in a male

Decision trees organized by mental status examination domain *(continued)*

Functioning
2.1   Poor school performance

Etiological factors
2.17   Trauma or psychosocial stressors involved in the etiology
2.28   Excessive or problematic substance use

2.1 Decision Tree for Poor School Performance

Poor school performance is an all-too-common and very nonspecific aspect of childhood and adolescence. On the one hand, clinicians should certainly not assume that every poor student has a mental disorder underlying their poor academic performance. On the other hand, most (if not all) mental disorders occurring in children are likely to have a negative impact on school performance, and, not infrequently, difficulty in school is the chief complaint.

The evaluation for the causes of poor school performance will usually include testing for overall IQ and for deficits in specific academic skills (e.g., reading, mathematics, writing, expressive and receptive language). A definitive diagnosis of a DSM-5-TR neurodevelopmental disorder requires that the learning or communication difficulties be substantially and quantifiably below what would be expected given the individual's age and that the difficulties substantially interfere with school, work, or social functioning. The next step is a careful assessment for the presence of the various psychiatric disorders that have impaired school performance as a consequence. This entails a careful history (supplemented by reports from parents, teachers, and pediatricians), clinical observation, and an evaluation of the role of substance use. For example, is the poor performance in school associated with deficits in intellectual function and adaptive functioning (as in Intellectual Developmental Disorder)? Are there significant deficits in the social use of verbal and nonverbal communication (as in Autism Spectrum Disorder and Social [Pragmatic] Communication Disorder)? Are there clinically significant symptoms of inattention and/or hyperactive-impulsive behavior occurring in two or more different settings (as in Attention-Deficit/Hyperactivity Disorder)? Are there frequent uncontrollable temper tantrums on top of a baseline of persistent anger and irritability (as in Disruptive Mood Dysregulation Disorder)? Is there a pattern of antisocial behaviors such as truancy (as in Conduct Disorder)? Is there school refusal based on an inability to separate from attachment figures (as in Separation Anxiety Disorder)? Is there clinically significant depressed mood (as in Major Depressive Disorder)? Because neurodevelopmental disorders and other mental disorders frequently co-occur, it is important to evaluate for all possibilities in the tree (which may require going through the tree several times) and to make whichever diagnoses are appropriate.

The presence of a psychiatric disorder does not guarantee that it is the cause of problematic school performance. Other factors (e.g., poor work habits, excessive TV watching or video game playing, lack of motivation, poor schooling, disruptive home or community environment) may also play a significant role. Occasionally, the psychiatric disorder (e.g., Adjustment Disorder, Oppositional Defiant Disorder, Major Depressive Disorder) may be more the result of poor school performance than its cause.

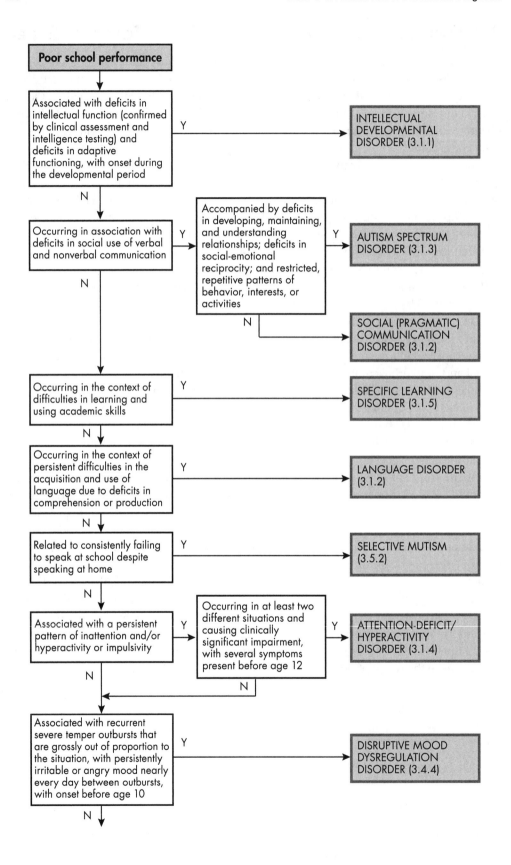

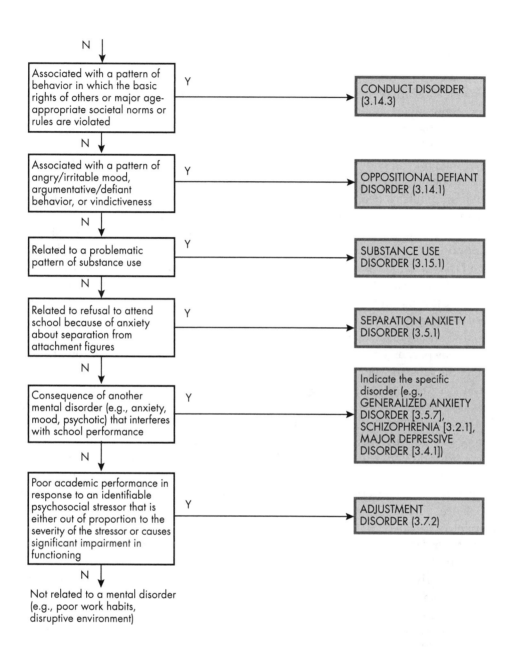

2.2 Decision Tree for Behavioral Problems in a Child or Adolescent

A common reason for referring a child or adolescent to a mental health professional is to request an evaluation and possible treatment for a reported behavioral problem. It goes without saying, however, that many behavioral problems occurring in children or adolescents are not due to a mental disorder. In some instances, the behavioral problems are not of sufficient severity or duration to warrant a diagnosis of a mental disorder. In others, the problem is more a consequence of a disturbance in the family relationship than a problem emanating primarily from the child. Finally, there are some very serious behavioral problems (e.g., shooting, mugging, rape) that occur for reasons outside the domain of the mental disorders covered in DSM-5-TR (e.g., revenge).

Behavioral problems with an onset in early childhood are most often associated with Attention-Deficit/Hyperactivity Disorder, Oppositional Defiant Disorder, Disruptive Mood Dysregulation Disorder, Autism Spectrum Disorder, Stereotypic Movement Disorder, and Intellectual Developmental Disorder (Intellectual Disability). The differential among these is usually straightforward and is determined by a consideration of the accompanying symptoms.

A first onset of behavioral problems during adolescence strongly suggests that substances may play an important role. The behavioral problems may result from the direct effect of the substance on the brain (as in Substance Intoxication), may be a by-product of a Substance Use Disorder (e.g., illegal activities associated with procurement), or may be motivated by gain (e.g., a plan to get rich quick as a drug dealer). Other disorders that often have an onset in later childhood or early adolescence include the Adolescent-Onset Type of Conduct Disorder (which has a better prognosis than the Childhood-Onset Type, occurring before age 10), Major Depressive Disorder, Bipolar Disorder, Schizophrenia, Kleptomania, and Pyromania. Conduct Disorder that has an onset in childhood (i.e., before age 10) is particularly worrisome and is associated with a higher incidence of violence, poorer peer relationships, and an increased likelihood for the child to develop into an adult with Antisocial Personality Disorder.

Behavioral problems occurring in response to a psychosocial stressor suggest either 1) a diagnosis of Posttraumatic Stress Disorder or Acute Stress Disorder, if the stressor is of a particularly traumatic nature and the behavioral problems are accompanied by intrusion symptoms associated with the traumatic event, avoidance of reminders of the event, and a change in cognition, mood, and arousal; or 2) a diagnosis of Adjustment Disorder.

If the behavioral problems are not covered by any of the decision points so far and the problems are clinically significant and represent a psychological or biological dysfunction in the individual, the residual categories—Other Specified/Unspecified Disruptive, Impulse-Control, and Conduct Disorder—would apply, with the choice depending on whether the clinician wishes to record the symptomatic presentation on the chart (in which case Other Specified Disruptive, Impulse-Control, and Conduct Disorder would be used, followed by the specific reason) or not (in which case Unspecified Disruptive, Impulse-Control, and Conduct Disorder would be used). Otherwise, the behavioral problems would be considered problematic but not indicative of a mental disorder, possibly justifying the assignment of Z72.810 Child or Adolescent Antisocial Behavior, which is included in the DSM-5-TR chapter "Other Conditions That May Be a Focus of Clinical Attention."

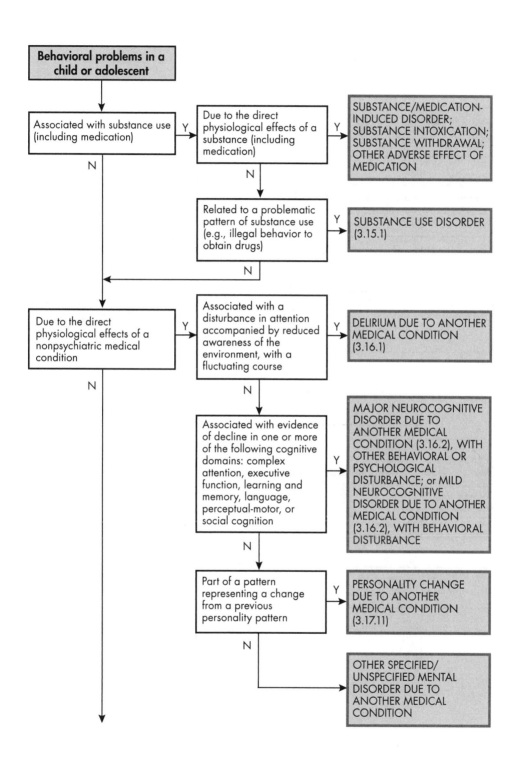

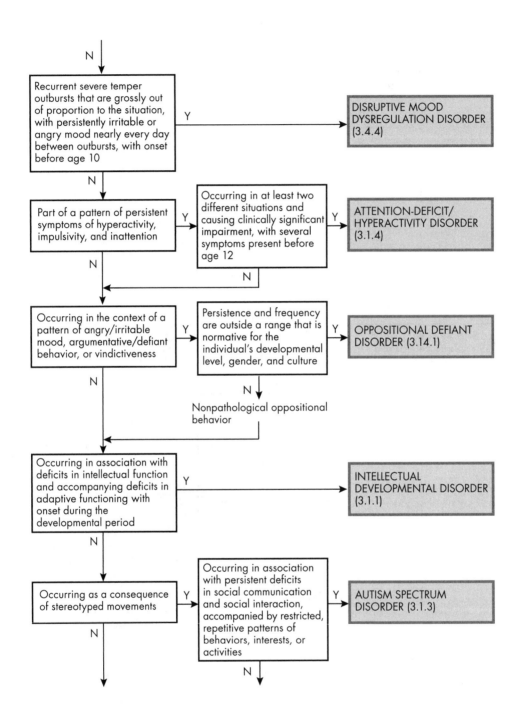

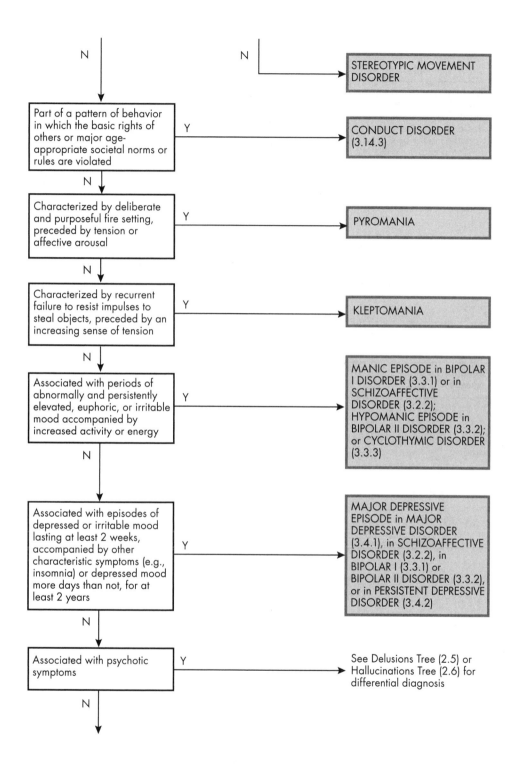

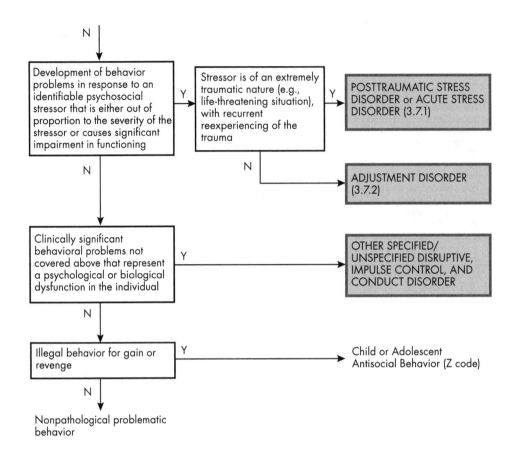

2.3 Decision Tree for Speech Disturbance

The decision tree for speech disturbance covers various types of psychopathology that may manifest in the person's ability to speak or in the quality of the person's speech. *Impaired speech production* may be related to problems with the acquisition and use of language, with the ability to articulate words intelligibly, or with speech fluency. *Disorganized speech* is characterized by the individual's switching from one topic to another without a discernible connection or providing answers to questions that are only obliquely related or unrelated to the question. Other speech disturbances include deficits in understanding and following the social rules of verbal communication, slowed or pressured speech, or repetitive or stereotyped speech.

Disorganized speech is one of the most challenging symptoms to diagnose because there is no standard by which to judge when speech is "disorganized." This judgment depends in part on the clinician's ability to comprehend and on the patient's pattern of speech production. Furthermore, no one speaks in logically coherent and syntactically correct sentences all the time. Many clinicians and trainees have a tendency to overcall mildly illogical speech as clinically significant "loosening of associations." The kinds of "disorganized speech" covered in this decision tree should be obvious even to the most casual observer. If the clinician has difficulty deciding whether or not a patient's speech is disorganized, then it should probably not be considered pathological.

Once it is established that the individual has a disturbance in speech, the next task is to determine which of the many possible mental disorders best accounts for it. This usually requires an evaluation of the context and the accompanying symptoms. Speech disturbance in Delirium is accompanied by a disturbance of attention and awareness, whereas speech disturbance in Major or Mild Neurocognitive Disorder is accompanied by other cognitive deficits. Aphasia (impairment in the understanding or transmission of ideas by language due to injury or disease of the brain centers involved in language) that occurs in the absence of other cognitive symptoms can be diagnosed using the ICD-10-CM symptom code R47.01.

Disorganized speech is a common manifestation of substance use. Usually a diagnosis of Substance Intoxication or Substance Withdrawal will suffice, but severely disorganized speech suggests a diagnosis of Substance Intoxication Delirium or Substance Withdrawal Delirium or an underlying Substance/Medication-Induced Major Neurocognitive Disorder. The differential diagnosis of disorganized speech in a Manic Episode versus Schizophrenia has been the subject of considerable discussion. The disorganized speech in an episode of Schizophrenia (e.g., so-called loosening of associations) presumably is distinguished from the "flight of ideas" in mania based on the observer's ability to follow the train of thought. Theoretically at least, the clinician can discern how the patient got from one topic to the next in a flight of ideas, whereas the derailments in the speech of patients with Schizophrenia are much less understandable. Although this distinction may be helpful in the most classic cases, at the boundary there are many instances in which it is difficult or impossible to distinguish between loosening of associations and flight of ideas. Similarly, whereas rapid or pressured speech is often characteristic of mania, the speech of an excited or agitated patient with Schizophrenia may also be overwhelming. Therefore, it is best to base the differential diagnosis between

Schizophrenia and Manic Episodes on the accompanying symptoms and overall course rather than on an isolated evaluation of the speech pattern.

The decision tree also includes the differential diagnosis for several disorders that are characterized by impaired speech first presenting during development. A diagnosis of a Language Disorder may be warranted if an individual has symptoms such as difficulty understanding words, sentences, or specific types of words; a markedly limited vocabulary; and/or difficulty producing sentences. Difficulties with speech sound production that interfere with intelligibility may warrant a diagnosis of Speech Sound Disorder. Problems in the fluency and time patterning of speech that are inappropriate for age and language skills suggest a diagnosis of Childhood-Onset Fluency Disorder (Stuttering). In Autism Spectrum Disorder and Social (Pragmatic) Communication Disorder, there are deficits in the social use of verbal and nonverbal communication. These problems may be manifested by the person having difficulties with understanding and following social rules of verbal and nonverbal communication in naturalistic contexts, struggles with changing language according to the needs of the listener or situation, and problems following rules for conversations and storytelling. Inappropriate vocal outbursts that occur in the context of otherwise normal speech suggest a Tic Disorder.

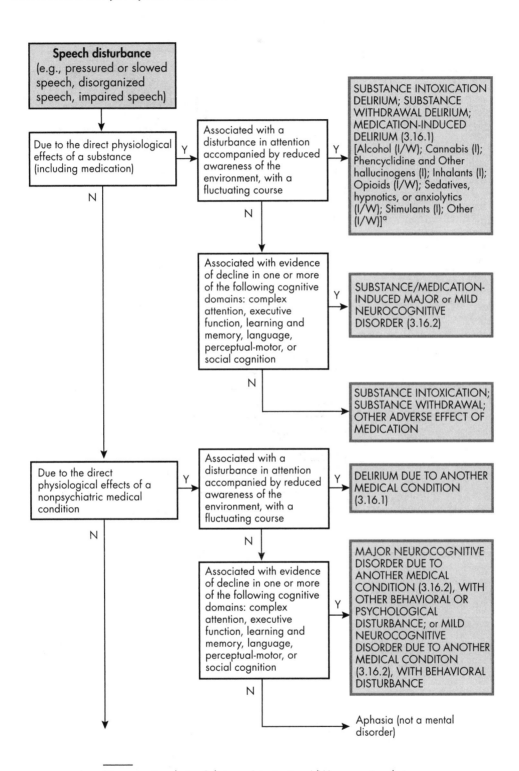

Speech disturbance (e.g., pressured or slowed speech, disorganized speech, impaired speech)

Due to the direct physiological effects of a substance (including medication) — Y → Associated with a disturbance in attention accompanied by reduced awareness of the environment, with a fluctuating course — Y → SUBSTANCE INTOXICATION DELIRIUM; SUBSTANCE WITHDRAWAL DELIRIUM; MEDICATION-INDUCED DELIRIUM (3.16.1) [Alcohol (I/W); Cannabis (I); Phencyclidine and Other hallucinogens (I); Inhalants (I); Opioids (I/W); Sedatives, hypnotics, or anxiolytics (I/W); Stimulants (I); Other (I/W)]ᵃ

↓ N

Associated with evidence of decline in one or more of the following cognitive domains: complex attention, executive function, learning and memory, language, perceptual-motor, or social cognition — Y → SUBSTANCE/MEDICATION-INDUCED MAJOR or MILD NEUROCOGNITIVE DISORDER (3.16.2)

↓ N

SUBSTANCE INTOXICATION; SUBSTANCE WITHDRAWAL; OTHER ADVERSE EFFECT OF MEDICATION

Due to the direct physiological effects of a nonpsychiatric medical condition — Y → Associated with a disturbance in attention accompanied by reduced awareness of the environment, with a fluctuating course — Y → DELIRIUM DUE TO ANOTHER MEDICAL CONDITION (3.16.1)

↓ N

Associated with evidence of decline in one or more of the following cognitive domains: complex attention, executive function, learning and memory, language, perceptual-motor, or social cognition — Y → MAJOR NEUROCOGNITIVE DISORDER DUE TO ANOTHER MEDICAL CONDITION (3.16.2), WITH OTHER BEHAVIORAL OR PSYCHOLOGICAL DISTURBANCE; or MILD NEUROCOGNITIVE DISORDER DUE TO ANOTHER MEDICAL CONDITON (3.16.2), WITH BEHAVIORAL DISTURBANCE

↓ N

Aphasia (not a mental disorder)

ᵃI = occurring during Substance Intoxication; I/W = occurring during Substance Intoxication or Substance Withdrawal, as indicated in DSM-5-TR, Table 1: "Diagnoses associated with substance class," p. 545.

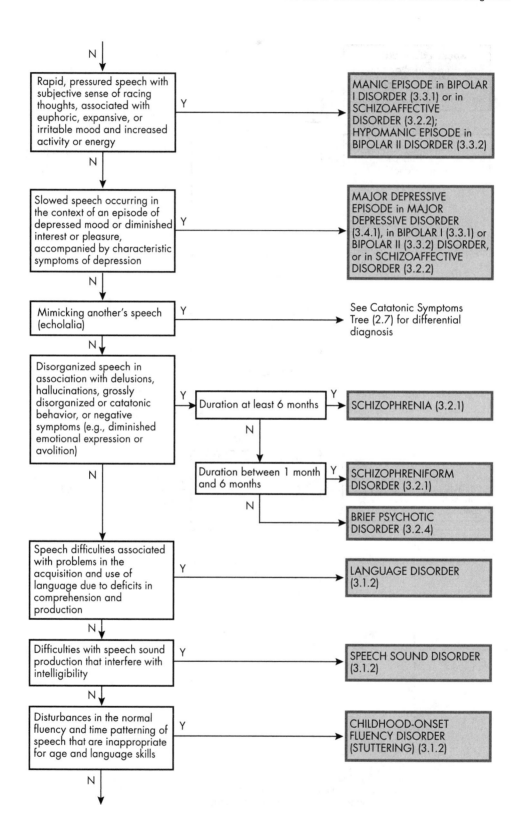

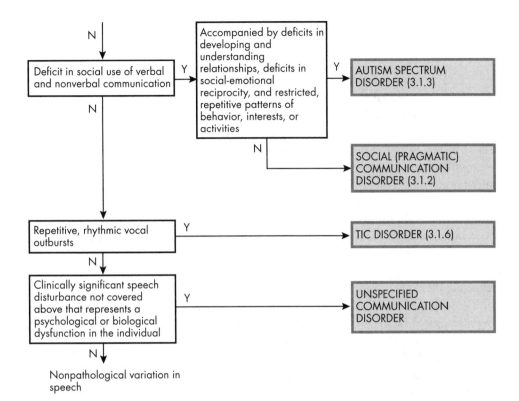

2.4 Decision Tree for Distractibility

Distractibility refers to an inability to filter out extraneous stimuli when attempting to concentrate on a particular task or activity. This is a very nonspecific symptom that occurs in a wide variety of mental disorders, as well as in individuals without any mental disorder. The differential diagnosis rests on the age at onset, severity, the symptoms with which the distractibility is associated, and whether it results from a reaction to an external stressor. Clinically significant inattention with an onset in early childhood suggests a diagnosis of Attention-Deficit/Hyperactivity Disorder. Inattention with onset in adolescence suggests a variety of possible disorders, including recurrent Substance Intoxication or Substance Withdrawal, Major Depressive or Bipolar Disorder, and Schizophrenia. When inattention has a first onset later in life, it is especially important to consider the possible etiological role of a medication, drug of abuse, or nonpsychiatric medical condition.

The clinician should consider a diagnosis of Delirium when inattention is severe and is associated with other cognitive or perceptual symptoms (e.g., disorientation, hallucinations). The hallmark of Delirium is a disturbance of attention and awareness—the patient is unable to appreciate or respond appropriately to the external environment, to filter out irrelevant stimuli, and to follow instructions or reply to questions. Because Delirium is often a medical emergency, it is crucial to identify (and then correct) the underlying etiological factors that may be related to a nonpsychiatric medical condition, substance use (including medication side effects), or some combination of these.

Distractibility is rarely the presenting symptom in disorders other than Attention-Deficit/Hyperactivity Disorder and Delirium. The evaluation of the differential diagnosis depends on what the accompanying features are (e.g., elevated mood in Manic Episode, excessive worry and anxiety in Generalized Anxiety Disorder, persistent psychotic symptoms in Schizophrenia). It is also always useful to determine whether the patient has experienced psychosocial stressors that may be causing or increasing distractibility.

Finally, everyone has differing abilities to filter out extraneous stimuli from the environment. Moreover, the nature and level of stimulation characteristic of the environment can increase or reduce any individual's ability to maintain attention. Whether a particular manifestation of distractibility constitutes an aspect of a mental disorder or should be considered within the normal range depends on its severity and persistence, and on whether it causes clinically significant distress or impairment.

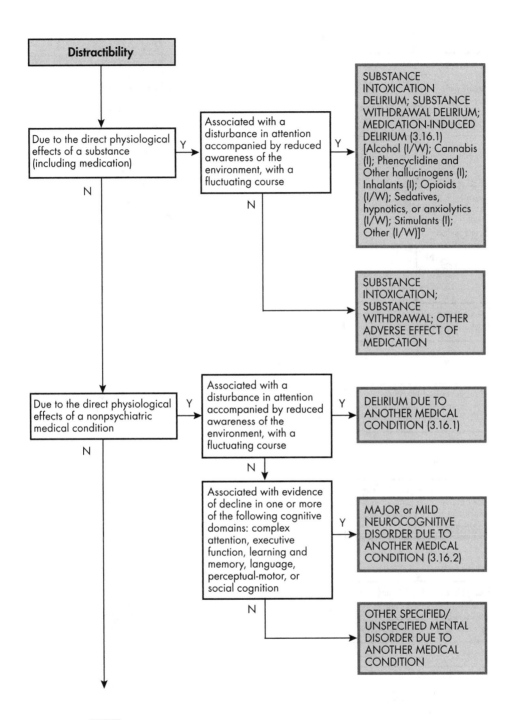

ᵃ I = occurring during Substance Intoxication; I/W = occurring during
Substance Intoxication or Substance Withdrawal, as indicated in DSM-5-TR,
Table 1: "Diagnoses associated with substance class," p. 545.

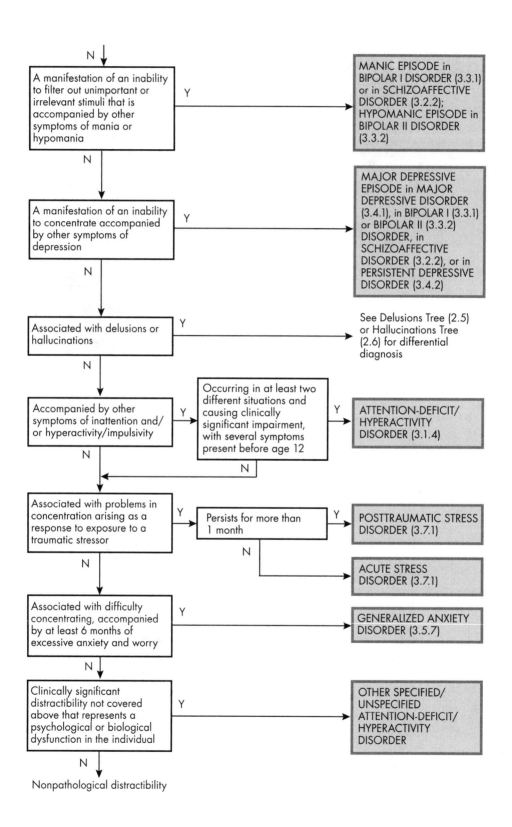

2.5 Decision Tree for Delusions

An all-too-common error regarding the differential diagnosis for delusions is to assume that any firmly held belief that is unusual, strange, or seemingly bizarre (at least from the clinician's perspective) is a delusion. Such misattributions can be avoided through a consideration of the degree to which the person's belief comports with the definition of *delusion* in the DSM-5 glossary (the glossary was omitted from DSM-5-TR because of overlap with revised text):

> A false belief based on incorrect inference about external reality that is firmly held despite what almost everyone else believes and despite what constitutes incontrovertible and obvious proof or evidence to the contrary. The belief is not ordinarily accepted by other members of the person's culture or subculture ([e.g.,] it is not an article of religious faith). When a false belief involves a value judgment, it is regarded as a delusion only when the judgment is so extreme as to defy credibility. (DSM-5, p. 819)

Several aspects of this DSM-5 glossary definition are helpful to keep in mind when attempting to determine whether a patient's beliefs should be considered delusional. Delusional convictions are impervious to compelling evidence of their implausibility, and the person remains completely convinced of their veracity, rejecting alternative explanations out of hand. In deciding whether a belief is fixed and false enough to be considered a delusion, the clinician should first determine that a serious error in inference and reality testing has occurred and then determine the strength of the conviction. It may be helpful to ask the patient to talk at length about their conviction, because it is often only in the specific details of the belief and how the person arrived at that belief that the errors of inference become apparent. In evaluating the strength of the delusional conviction, the clinician should present alternative explanations (e.g., the possibility that suspicious phone hang-ups are due to people dialing a wrong number). The patient who cannot acknowledge even the possibility of these explanations is most likely to have a delusion.

It should be noted that the determination of whether a religious belief is a delusion can be especially challenging because religious beliefs cannot be subjected to a determination of whether the belief is "true" or "false" and thus cannot be challenged with incontrovertible evidence or proof to the contrary. In such situations, the clinician must consider the parameters of the belief system that is characteristic of the religion to which the person ascribes and determine whether the person's beliefs deviate markedly from what others within the same religious persuasion believe. If the clinician is unfamiliar with the belief system of the individual's cultural or religious background, consultation with other individuals who are familiar with the patient's culture or religion is often necessary to avoid misdiagnosing a religious belief as a delusion. As noted in the first step of this decision tree, fixed beliefs that are sanctioned by that person's culture or religion should not be considered to be delusions.

Once the clinician determines that a delusion is present, the next task is to consider which DSM-5-TR disorder best accounts for it. The particular content and form of a delusion are much less important in making the diagnosis than is the context in which the delusion occurs. The most common diagnostic error here is to overlook the critically important role of substances (including medications) and nonpsychiatric medical conditions in the etiology of delusions. In younger individuals presenting with delusions, a careful history and drug screening are especially important to rule out the role of drugs of abuse. First onset of delusional thinking at a late age should always raise a red flag for a possible underlying nonpsychiatric medical condition or a medication side effect.

Once substance and nonpsychiatric medical etiologies have been ruled out, the first decision involves determining whether the delusions occur only in the context of a Manic Episode or Major Depressive Episode, in which case the diagnosis is Bipolar I Disorder With Psychotic Features, Bipolar II Disorder With Psychotic Features, or Major Depressive Disorder With Psychotic Features, depending on whether there has been a Manic Episode (Bipolar I Disorder), a Hypomanic Episode and a Major Depressive Episode (Bipolar II Disorder), or a Major Depressive Episode in the absence of any Manic or Hypomanic Episodes (Major Depressive Disorder).

The next step involves considering the duration of the delusions. If the delusions are present for less than 1 month (but for at least 1 day), the diagnosis is Brief Psychotic Disorder. For delusions lasting for 1 month or longer, the differential diagnosis depends on whether or not the delusions are accompanied by hallucinations, disorganized speech, grossly disorganized or catatonic behavior, or negative symptoms, thus meeting Criterion A of Schizophrenia and Schizophreniform Disorder (i.e., two or more Criterion A symptoms, each present for a significant portion of time during a 1-month period). If so, the differential is between Schizophrenia or Schizophreniform Disorder and Schizoaffective Disorder, and depends first on whether or not there has been a history of Major Depressive or Manic Episodes. If there has been no history of mood episodes, the diagnosis depends on the duration of the psychotic disturbance: Schizophreniform Disorder if the duration is less than 6 months, and Schizophrenia if the duration is 6 months or longer.

If there has been a history of mood episodes, the tree goes through each of the Schizoaffective criteria in turn: whether the psychotic symptoms are concurrent with mood episodes during an uninterrupted period of illness (Criterion A); whether delusions or hallucinations have been present for at least 2 weeks in the absence of a major mood episode (Criterion B), and whether mood episodes have been present for a majority of the total duration of the active and residual periods of the illness (Criterion C). If any of these criteria are not met, the diagnosis is Schizophrenia or Schizophreniform Disorder (depending on the duration), plus a comorbid diagnosis of Other Specified Bipolar and Related Disorder or Other Specified Depressive Disorder to indicate the presence of the relevant type of mood episodes. If all of the mood episodes are superimposed on the psychotic disturbance, a comorbid diagnosis of Other Specified/Unspecified Bipolar and Related Disorder or Other Specified/Unspecified Depressive Disorder can be given if the mood episodes are clinically significant. However, if any of the mood episodes occurred at times other than during the psychotic dis-turbance, an additional comorbid diagnosis of Bipolar I Disorder, Bipolar II Disorder, or Major Depressive Disorder is given instead.

If delusions lasting at least 1 month occur in the absence of symptoms meeting Criterion A of Schizophrenia (i.e., at least 1 month of hallucinations, disorganized speech, grossly disorganized or catatonic behavior, or negative symptoms), the diagnosis depends on whether or not there has also been a history of Major Depressive or Manic Episodes. If there is no such history, the diagnosis is Delusional Disorder. If there is a history of Manic or Major Depressive Episodes, the diagnosis can still be Delusional Disorder if the total duration of the mood episodes is brief compared to the total duration of the delusional periods (e.g., less than 25% of the total duration of the delusions). In such cases, the presence of the mood episodes can be indicated by giving a comorbid diagnosis of Other Specified/Unspecified Bipolar and Related Disorder or Other Specified/Unspecified Depressive Disorder if all of the mood episodes are superimposed on the delusional periods. However, if any of the mood episodes occurred at times other than during the delusional periods, a comorbid diagnosis of Bipolar I Disorder (if any Manic Episodes), Bipolar II Disorder (if Hypomanic and Major Depressive Episodes), or Major Depressive Disorder (if only Major Depressive Episodes) is given instead.

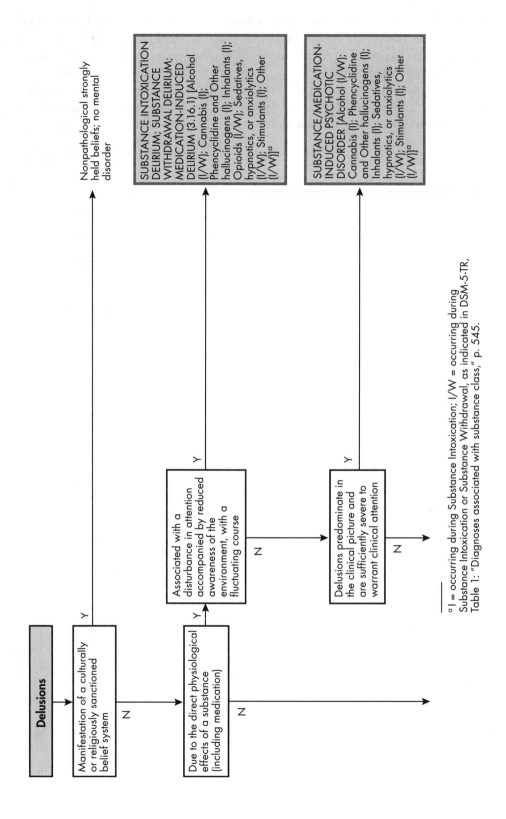

Delusions

Manifestation of a culturally or religiously sanctioned belief system

— N →

Due to the direct physiological effects of a substance (including medication)

— N →

Y ↑ Nonpathological strongly held beliefs; no mental disorder

Y ↑

Associated with a disturbance in attention accompanied by reduced awareness of the environment, with a fluctuating course

— N →

Delusions predominate in the clinical picture and are sufficiently severe to warrant clinical attention

— N →

Y ↑

SUBSTANCE INTOXICATION DELIRIUM; SUBSTANCE WITHDRAWAL DELIRIUM; MEDICATION-INDUCED DELIRIUM (3.16.1) [Alcohol (I/W); Cannabis (I); Phencyclidine and Other hallucinogens (I); Inhalants (I); Opioids (I/W); Sedatives, hypnotics, or anxiolytics (I/W); Stimulants (I); Other (I/W)]ᵃ

Y ↑

SUBSTANCE/MEDICATION-INDUCED PSYCHOTIC DISORDER [Alcohol (I/W); Cannabis (I); Phencyclidine and Other hallucinogens (I); Inhalants (I); Sedatives, hypnotics, or anxiolytics (I/W); Stimulants (I); Other (I/W)]ᵃ

ᵃ I = occurring during Substance Intoxication; I/W = occurring during Substance Intoxication or Substance Withdrawal, as indicated in DSM-5-TR, Table 1: "Diagnoses associated with substance class," p. 545.

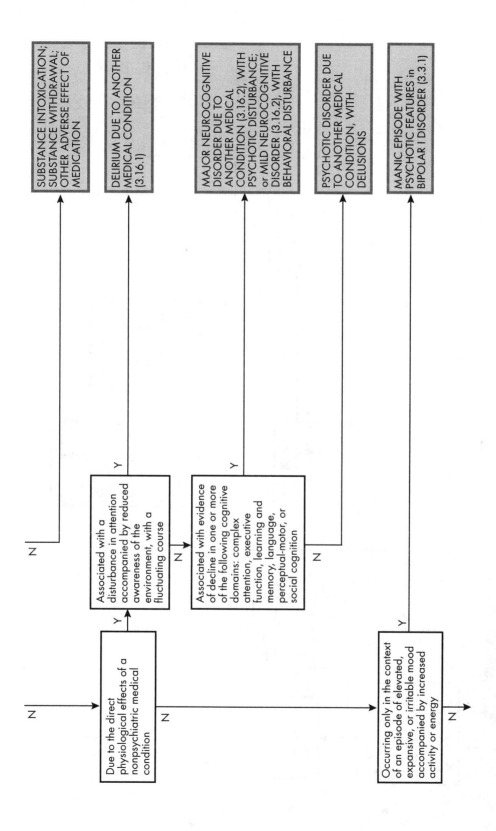

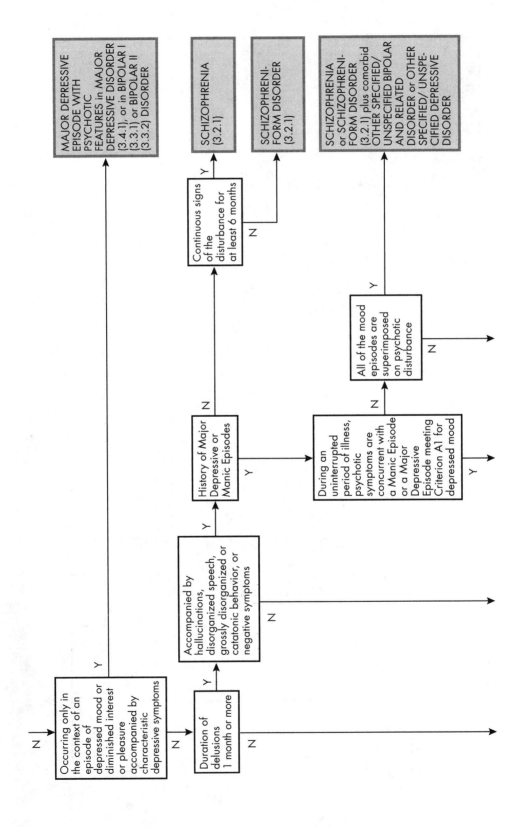

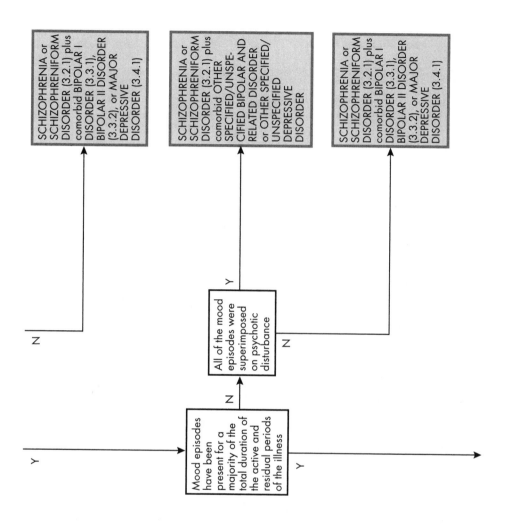

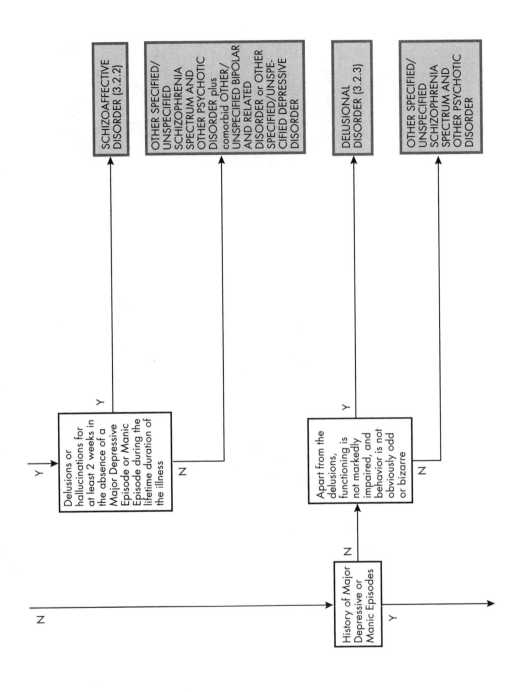

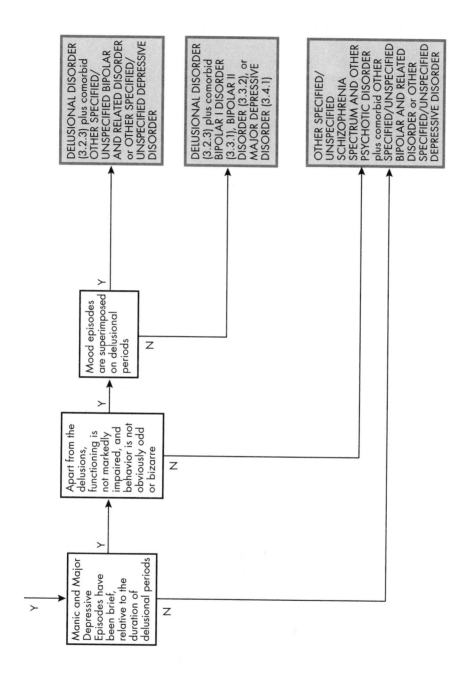

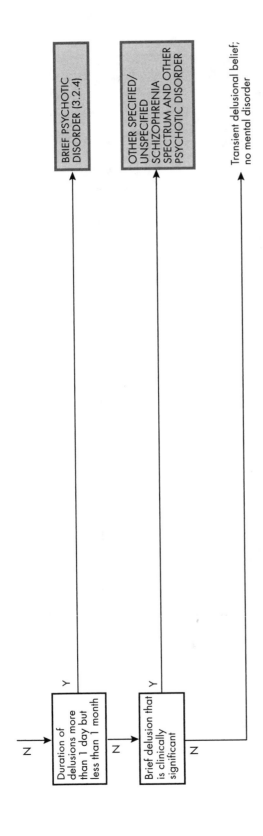

2.6 Decision Tree for Hallucinations

Hallucinations are sensory perceptions without external stimulation. *Illusions,* on the other hand, involve a misperception of an actual stimulus. When illusions occur in the absence of hallucinations, they do not count toward a diagnosis of a psychotic disorder and instead suggest Delirium, Substance Intoxication or Substance Withdrawal, Schizotypal Personality Disorder, or no mental disorder.

When trying to determine the etiology of a hallucination, the clinician needs to consider the sensory modality involved (i.e., whether the hallucination is auditory, visual, gustatory, olfactory, or tactile). As a general rule, visual, gustatory, and olfactory hallucinations are especially suggestive of an etiological substance or nonpsychiatric medical condition and demand a careful medical workup. Similarly, a late age at first onset of hallucinations in any modality suggests the need for an especially careful medical workup. Hallucinations can occur in the context of a Delirium (either substance- or medication-induced or due to a nonpsychiatric medical condition); in the context of a Major or Mild Neurocognitive Disorder Due to Another Medical Condition (in which case the diagnosis would be Major Neurocognitive Disorder, With Psychotic Disturbance, or Mild Neurocognitive Disorder, With Behavioral Disturbance); in the absence of accompanying cognitive impairment as a direct physiological consequence of a substance/medication or nonpsychiatric medical condition (diagnosed respectively as a Substance/Medication-Induced Psychotic Disorder or a Psychotic Disorder Due to Another Medical Condition); or as a typical feature of a Substance Intoxication or Substance Withdrawal.

After ruling out a nonpsychiatric medical condition or substance as an etiological factor, the clinician must then consider whether the hallucination is indicative of an independent psychotic disorder. There are four circumstances in which "hallucinations" should not count toward the diagnosis of a psychotic disorder: 1) hallucinatory experiences that are part of a religious ritual or are a culturally sanctioned experience (e.g., hearing the voice of a dead relative giving advice); 2) hypnopompic or hypnagogic hallucinations that occur at the beginning or end of sleep episodes; 3) substance-induced hallucinations that occur with intact reality testing (e.g., an individual who is cognizant that the perceptual disturbances are due to recent hallucinogen use); and 4) hallucinations that occur in the context of Functional Neurological Symptom Disorder (i.e., conversion hallucinations), which tend to affect multiple sensory modalities at the same time and to have psychologically meaningful content presented to the clinician in the form of an interesting story.

The next task is to determine whether clinically significant mood symptoms are present and, if so, the relationship between the hallucinations and the mood symptoms. The presence of a Manic or Major Depressive Episode raises the possibility that the hallucinations are part of a Bipolar I Disorder With Psychotic Features, Bipolar II Disorder With Psychotic Features, Major Depressive Disorder With Psychotic Features, or Schizoaffective Disorder. The differential diagnosis here depends on the temporal relationship between the hallucinations and the mood episodes. If the hallucinations are confined entirely to the mood episodes, then the diagnosis is Bipolar I Disorder With Psychotic Features, Bipolar II Disorder With Psychotic Features, or Major Depressive Disorder With Psychotic Features. Such hallucinations can be mood congruent (e.g., castigating accusatory voices in an individual with depression) or mood incongruent (i.e., hallucinations that have nothing to do with the prevailing mood).

The next step in the process involves considering the duration of the hallucinations: if the hallucinations have been present for less than 1 month (but for at least 1 day, the diagnosis is Brief Psychotic Disorder. For hallucinations lasting for 1 month or longer, the differential diagnosis depends on whether or not the hallucinations are accompanied by delusions, disorganized speech, grossly disorganized or catatonic behavior, or negative symptoms, thus meeting Criterion A of Schizophrenia or Schizophreniform Disorder (i.e., two or more Criterion A symptoms, each present for a significant portion of time during a 1-month period). If so, the differential is between Schizophrenia or Schizophreniform Disorder and Schizoaffective Disorder, and the diagnosis depends first on whether or not there is a history of Major Depressive or Manic Episodes. If there is no history of mood episodes, the diagnosis depends on the duration of the psychotic disturbance: Schizophreniform Disorder if the duration is less than 6 months, and Schizophrenia if the duration is 6 months or longer.

If there has been a history of mood episodes, the tree goes through each of the Schizoaffective criteria in turn: whether the psychotic symptoms are concurrent with mood episodes during an uninterrupted period of illness (Criterion A); whether delusions or hallucinations have been present for at least 2 weeks in the absence of a major mood episode (Criterion B); and whether mood episodes have been present for a majority of the total duration of the active and residual periods of the illness (Criterion C) (e.g., a 2-year psychotic disturbance with 1½ years of mood symptoms). If any of these criteria are not met, Schizoaffective Disorder is ruled out, and the diagnosis is either Schizophrenia or Schizophreniform Disorder (depending on the duration), plus a comorbid bipolar or depressive disorder diagnosis to indicate the presence of the relevant type of mood episodes. If all of the mood episodes are superimposed on the psychotic disturbance, a comorbid diagnosis of Other Specified/Unspecified Bipolar and Related Disorder or Other Specified/Unspecified Depressive Disorder can be given if the mood episodes are clinically significant. However, if any of the mood episodes occurred at times other than during the psychotic disturbance, an additional comorbid diagnosis of Bipolar I Disorder, Bipolar II Disorder, or Major Depressive Disorder is given instead.

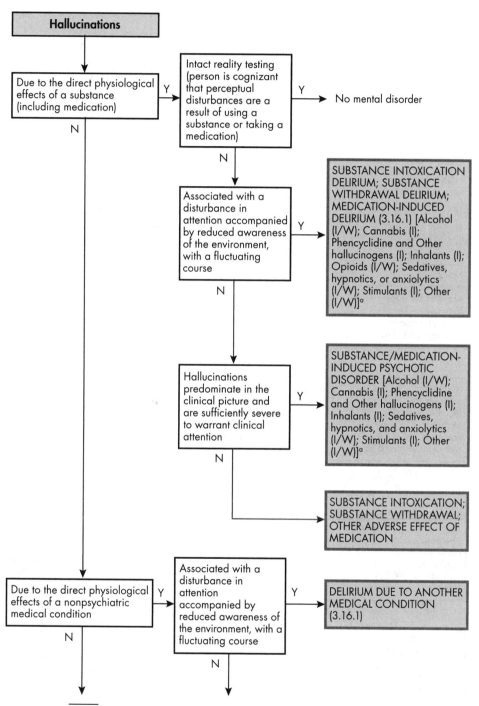

ᵃ I = occurring during Substance Intoxication; I/W = occurring during Substance Intoxication or Substance Withdrawal, as indicated in DSM-5-TR, Table 1: "Diagnoses associated with substance class," p. 545.

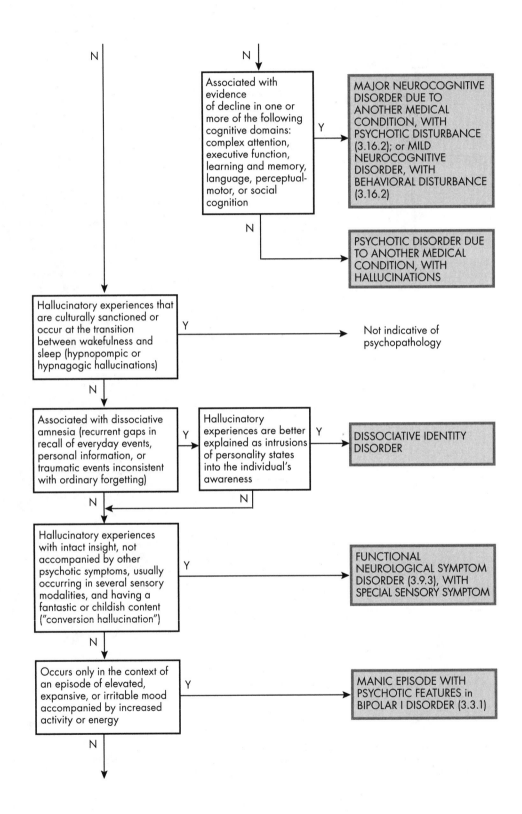

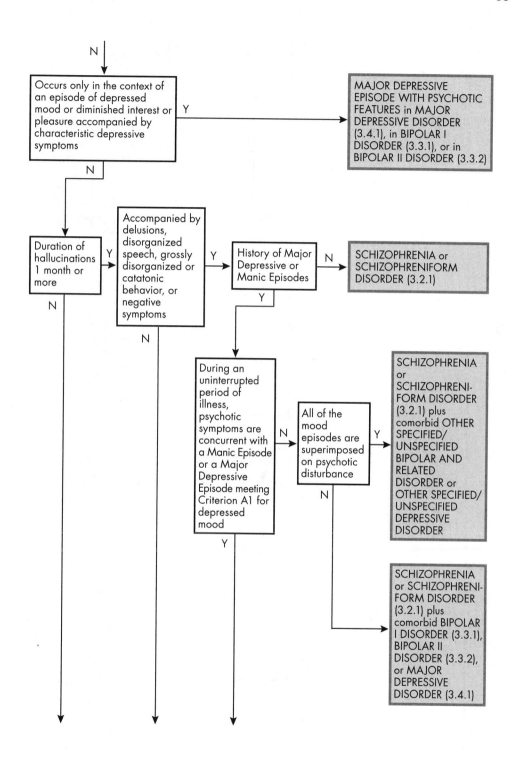

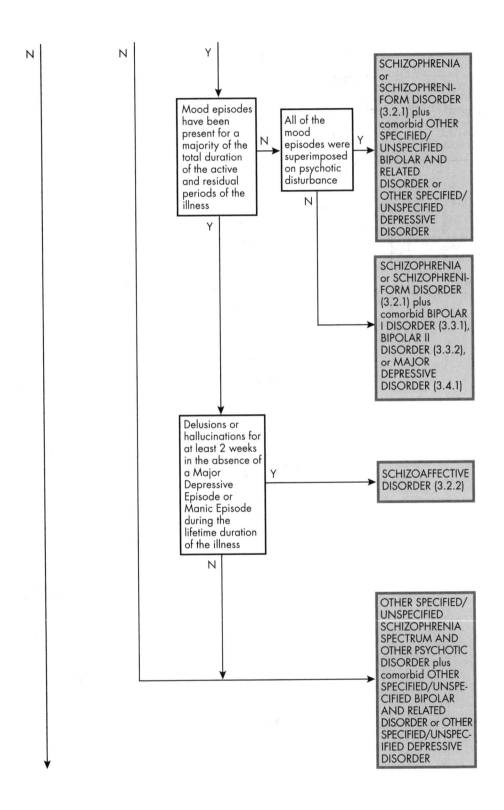

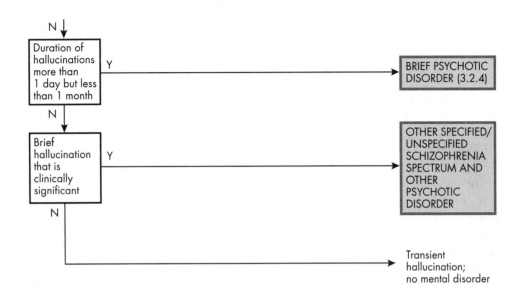

2.7 Decision Tree for Catatonic Symptoms

The catatonic symptoms covered here include stupor (i.e., no psychomotor activity, no active relating to environment), catalepsy (i.e., passive induction of a posture held against gravity), waxy flexibility (i.e., slight, even resistance to positioning by the examiner), mutism (i.e., no, or very little, verbal response), negativism (i.e., opposing or not responding to instructions or external stimuli), posturing (i.e., spontaneous and active maintenance of a posture against gravity), mannerisms (i.e., odd, circumstantial caricatures of normal actions), stereotypy (i.e., repetitive, abnormally frequent, non-goal-directed movements), agitation (not influenced by external stimuli), grimacing, echolalia (i.e., mimicking another's speech), and echopraxia (i.e., mimicking another's movements).

The initial task is to determine whether the "syndrome" of catatonia is present (i.e., three or more catatonic symptoms). This can be difficult because a number of the individual items resemble other types of symptoms characteristic of DSM-5-TR disorders (e.g., catatonic excitement may resemble psychomotor agitation in a Manic or Major Depressive Episode, catatonic stupor may resemble extreme psychomotor retardation in a Major Depressive Episode or Delirium, catatonic mutism may resemble alogia and avolition in Schizophrenia). The judgment about these distinctions is based in part on the context in which the symptom occurs (i.e., the presence of multiple catatonic symptoms vs. the presence of symptoms characteristic of the other disorder) and on its presentation (i.e., individuals with catatonic symptoms appear to be oblivious to external environmental stimuli, although they may later report accurately what was happening around them).

If catatonic symptoms are present but do not constitute the syndrome of catatonia, a substance- or medication-induced etiology for the symptoms should first be considered. If the symptoms are due to the direct physiological effects of substance use, such as from Phencyclidine Intoxication, a diagnosis of Substance Intoxication or Substance Withdrawal would apply. If the catatonic-like symptoms are judged to be due to the use of an antipsychotic medication or other dopamine receptor blocking agent, then one of the medication-induced movement disorders (i.e., Neuroleptic Malignant Syndrome, Medication-Induced Acute Dystonia, or Medication-Induced Parkinsonism) would apply. Otherwise, for catatonic symptoms below the threshold for the catatonia syndrome (i.e., fewer than three catatonic symptoms) that are judged to be clinically significant and to represent a psychological or behavioral dysfunction, thus meeting the definitional requirements of a mental disorder, the residual category Unspecified Catatonia would apply. Note that because the DSM-5-TR diagnoses of Catatonic Disorder Due to Another Medical Condition and Catatonia Associated With Another Mental Disorder require the presence of the syndrome of catatonia, presentations of one or two catatonic symptoms that are due to a nonpsychiatric medical condition or associated with another mental disorder are therefore diagnosed as Unspecified Catatonia.

Once the syndrome of catatonia has been established, the next step is to determine the etiology. A catatonic syndrome can be due to the direct physiological effects of a neurological or other nonpsychiatric medical condition (in which case Catatonic Disorder Due to Another Medical Condition is diagnosed). The syndrome of catatonia can be a manifestation of a Manic Episode, a Major Depressive Episode, or Autism Spectrum Disorder, in which case Catatonia Associated With Bipolar I Disorder, Bipolar II Disorder, Major Depressive Disorder, or Autism Spectrum Disorder, respectively, is diagnosed). A catatonic syndrome can also occur in the context of other psychotic symptoms such as delusions, hallucinations, or disorganized speech, in which case Catatonia Associated With [appropriate psychotic disorder (e.g., Schizophrenia)] would be diagnosed).

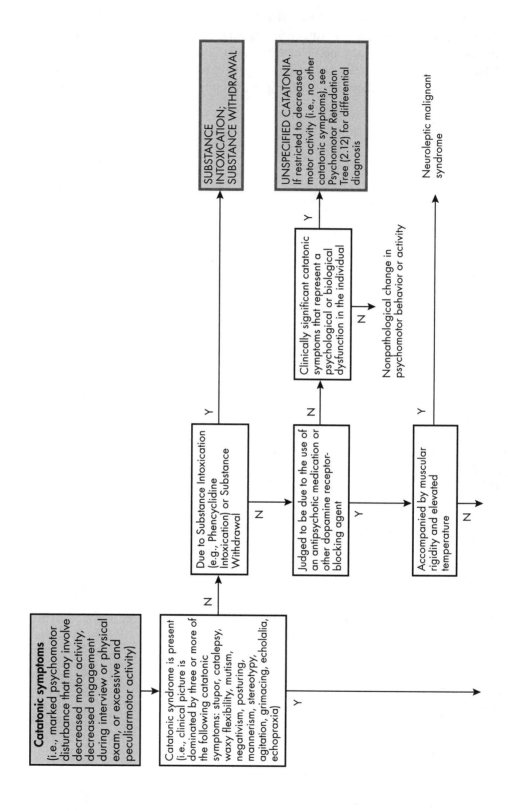

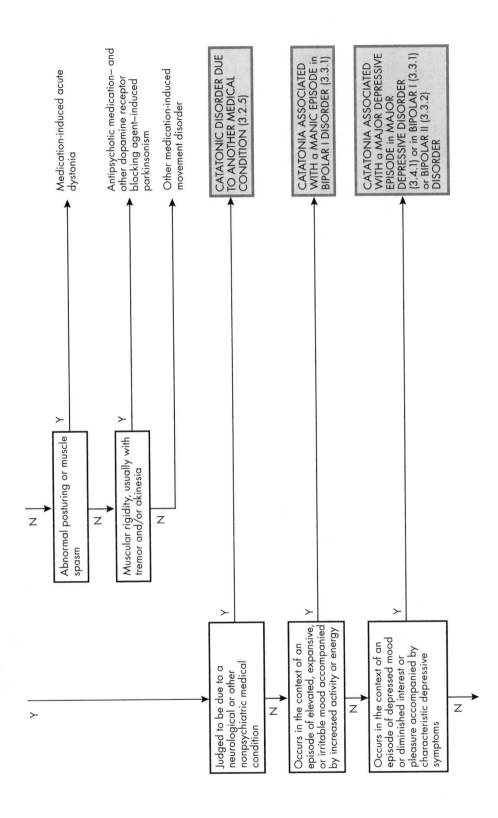

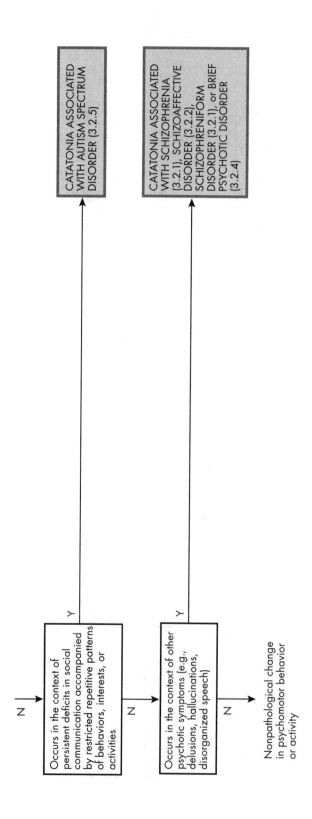

2.8 Decision Tree for Elevated or Expansive Mood

Most people have experienced at least some periods of elevated or expansive mood in their lives, usually in response to a particularly wonderful event or experience, such as falling in love, having a child, graduating from school, landing a coveted job, being victorious at a sporting event, or winning money at a game of chance. These mood states become a concern only when they are *abnormally* elevated or expansive and are disconnected from contextual factors.

The first step in the differential diagnosis is to ensure that the mood disturbance is not caused by substance/medication use or a nonpsychiatric medical condition. The clinician's first reflex, particularly for any late onset of these symptoms, should be to conduct a thorough medical workup and to evaluate whether the individual is using any medications (or drugs of abuse) that may produce mood changes as a side effect. In younger individuals, there is always a strong possibility that the changes in mood are caused by the effects of Substance Intoxication or Substance Withdrawal. Nonpsychiatric medical conditions that can cause elevated or expansive mood include Cushing's disease, multiple sclerosis, stroke, traumatic brain injuries, and anti-*N*-methyl-D-aspartate receptor encephalitis.

The next step is to determine whether the elevated mood is part of a Manic or Hypomanic Episode. As described in the DSM-5-TR criteria, such episodes form the building blocks for the bipolar disorders. It should be noted that the symptomatic definitions of Manic and Hypomanic Episodes are essentially the same. The boundary between them depends on clinical judgment as to the severity of and the impairment caused by the mood disturbance. By definition, a Hypomanic Episode does not cause marked impairment or distress and may even be compatible with improved social and job performance. The bipolar disorders are made up of combinations of Manic, Hypomanic, and Major Depressive Episodes. Bipolar I Disorder consists of one or more Manic Episodes and (optionally) one or more Major Depressive Episodes. The term *bipolar* is used even for individuals who have had only unipolar Manic Episodes (with no depressive episodes), because the vast majority of such individuals will eventually go on to have Major Depressive Episodes, and the course, family loading, and treatment issues are equivalent to individuals who have had both Manic and Major Depressive Episodes. Bipolar II Disorder consists of one or more Major Depressive Episodes with intercurrent Hypomanic Episodes.

If there have been one or more Manic Episodes, the diagnosis will depend on whether there is a history of delusions or hallucinations. If there is no such history, the diagnosis is Bipolar I Disorder. If there is such a history and the delusions and hallucinations have been confined to Manic or Major Depressive Episodes, then the diagnosis is Bipolar I Disorder, With Psychotic Features. If delusions or hallucinations occur outside of the confines of Manic or Major Depressive Episodes, then a Schizophrenia Spectrum or Other Psychotic Disorder will need to be diagnosed to account for the psychotic symptoms (refer to the Delusions Tree [2.5] or Hallucinations Tree [2.6] for the psychotic disorder diagnosis).

If there have been Hypomanic Episodes (and no Manic Episodes), and there has been at least one Major Depressive Episode, the diagnosis would similarly depend on whether there is a history of delusions or hallucinations. If there is no such history, the diagnosis is

Bipolar II Disorder. If there is such a history and the delusions and hallucinations have been confined to Major Depressive Episodes, then the diagnosis is Bipolar II Disorder, With Psychotic Features. If delusions and or hallucinations occur outside of the confines of Major Depressive Episodes, then a Schizophrenia Spectrum or Other Psychotic Disorder will need to be diagnosed to account for the psychotic symptoms (refer to the Delusions Tree [2.5] or Hallucinations Tree [2.6] for the psychotic disorder diagnosis).

Cyclothymic Disorder is a relatively uncommon Bipolar and Related Disorder, characterized by numerous alternating periods of hypomania and depression that are less severe than a Manic, Hypomanic, or Major Depressive Episode.

Finally, because for most people, periods of elevated and expansive mood are intermittently common during gambling (i.e., at least when a person is winning), it is important *not* to diagnose such symptoms as evidence of mania if they are confined to sessions of gambling. However, given that some individuals might engage in (often reckless) gambling behavior during Manic Episodes, the combination of gambling and expansive mood does not necessarily rule out a diagnosis of Bipolar I Disorder.

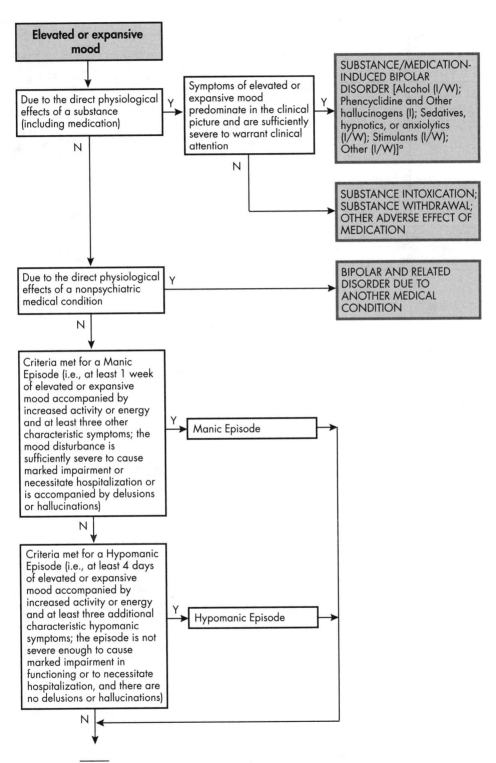

ᵃ I = occurring during Substance Intoxication; I/W = occurring during Substance Intoxication or Substance Withdrawal, as indicated in DSM-5-TR, Table 1: "Diagnoses associated with substance class," p. 545.

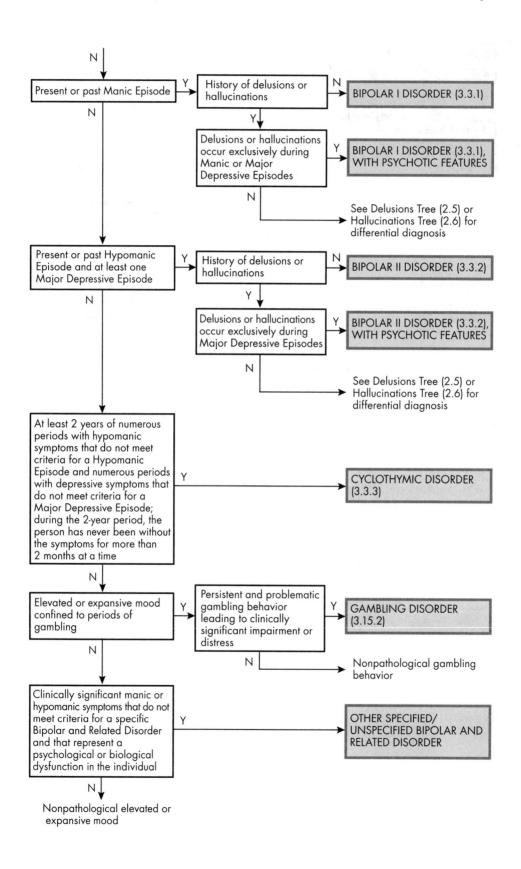

2.9 Decision Tree for Irritable Mood

All people can become more or less irritable under the right set of circumstances (e.g., not enough sleep, caught in traffic, under deadline pressure). The decision tree for irritable mood is not meant to apply to everyday experiences of irritable mood but instead to periods of irritability that are either so persistent or so severe that they cause clinically significant distress or impairment.

The first step in the differential diagnosis is to ensure that the irritability is not caused by substance/medication use or a nonpsychiatric medical condition. The clinician's first reflex, particularly for any late onset of these symptoms, should be to conduct a thorough medical workup and to evaluate whether the individual is using any medication (or drugs of abuse) that may produce irritability as a side effect. In younger individuals, there is always a strong possibility that the irritability is caused by the effects of Substance Intoxication or Substance Withdrawal. Nonpsychiatric medical conditions that can cause irritable mood include chronic pain, hyperthyroidism, hypoglycemia, traumatic brain injury, Wilson's disease, and polycystic ovary syndrome.

The next step is to determine whether the irritable mood is part of a Manic or Hypomanic Episode. Distinct episodes of abnormally and persistently irritable mood accompanied by increased activity or energy and at least four other characteristic symptoms define a Manic Episode or Hypomanic Episode. Note that four associated manic or hypomanic symptoms (rather than the typical three) are required to make a diagnosis of a Manic or Hypomanic Episode in the absence of elevated or expansive mood so that the episode can more easily be differentiated from a Major Depressive Episode with associated irritability. As described in the DSM-5-TR criteria, these mood episodes form the building blocks for the bipolar disorders. Bipolar I Disorder consists of one or more Manic Episodes and (optionally) one or more Major Depressive Episodes. Bipolar II Disorder consists of one or more Major Depressive Episodes with intercurrent Hypomanic Episodes.

If there have been one or more Manic Episodes, the diagnosis will depend on whether there is a history of delusions or hallucinations. If there is no such history, the diagnosis is Bipolar I Disorder. If there is such a history and the delusions and hallucinations have been confined to Manic or Major Depressive Episodes, then the diagnosis is Bipolar I Disorder, With Psychotic Features. If delusions and or hallucinations occur outside of the confines of Manic and Major Depressive Episodes, then a Schizophrenia Spectrum or Other Psychotic Disorder will need to be diagnosed to account for the psychotic symptoms (refer to the Delusions Tree [2.5] or Hallucinations Tree [2.6] for the psychotic disorder diagnosis).

If there have been Hypomanic Episodes (and no Manic Episodes), and there has been at least one Major Depressive Episode, the diagnosis would similarly depend on whether there is a history of delusions or hallucinations. If there is no such history, the diagnosis is Bipolar II Disorder. If there is such a history and the delusions and hallucinations have been confined to Major Depressive Episodes, then the diagnosis is Bipolar II Disorder, With Psychotic Features. If delusions and or hallucinations occur outside of the confines of Major Depressive Episodes, then a Schizophrenia Spectrum or Other Psychotic Disorder will need to be diagnosed to account for the psychotic symptoms (refer to the Delusions Tree [2.5] or Hallucinations Tree [2.6] for the psychotic disorder diagnosis).

In Cyclothymic Disorder, which is characterized by a persistent pattern of alternation between periods of hypomania and depression symptoms that do not meet criteria for a Hypomanic or Major Depressive Episode, irritable mood may occur during the periods of hypomania symptoms.

Up to this point, the Irritable Mood Tree closely resembles the Elevated or Expansive Mood Tree, but because irritability is also commonly associated with depressive disorders, this tree must also inquire about the possibility that the irritable mood is indicative of a depressive disorder rather than a bipolar disorder. According to the original DSM-III definition, Major Depressive Episode was defined in terms of a "dysphoric mood," which was characterized by symptoms such as feeling depressed, sad, blue, hopeless, low, down in the dumps, *or irritable.* One remnant of that DSM-III definition that appears in subsequent editions of DSM is that irritable mood is still included as an alternative Criterion A1 mood symptom in children and adolescents. Therefore, the next steps in the decision tree involve considering whether the irritable mood occurs in the context of a Major Depressive Episode, Persistent Depressive Disorder, or Premenstrual Dysphoric Disorder. In those cases in which criteria have been met for a Major Depressive Episode, the final diagnosis depends on whether there has been a history of delusions or hallucinations and whether the depressive disorder is "persistent" (i.e., duration of 2 years or longer). If there is no history of delusions or hallucinations, and the depressive disorder is not persistent, the diagnosis is simply Major Depressive Disorder. However, if there is a period of depressed mood for most of the day, more days than not, for at least 2 years, an additional diagnosis of Persistent Depressive Disorder, With Persistent Major Depressive Episode, is made if the criteria have been met for a Major Depressive Episode for the entire 2-year period; alternatively, a diagnosis of Persistent Depressive Disorder, With Intermittent Major Depressive Episodes, would be made to indicate the chronicity of the depression. If there is a history of delusions or hallucinations occurring exclusively during the Major Depressive Episodes, Major Depressive Disorder With Psychotic Features is diagnosed in place of Major Depressive Disorder (i.e., Major Depressive Disorder With Psychotic Features plus Persistent Depressive Disorder, With Persistent Major Depressive Episode; Major Depressive Disorder plus Persistent Depressive Disorder, With Intermittent Major Depressive Episodes; or Major Depressive Disorder With Psychotic Features). If the delusions or hallucinations occur outside of Major Depressive Episodes, refer to the Delusions Tree (2.5) or the Hallucinations Tree (2.6) to determine the differential diagnosis of which Schizophrenia Spectrum or Other Psychotic Disorder is most applicable.

A diagnosis of Persistent Depressive Disorder, With Pure Dysthymic Disorder, by itself is warranted for presentations characterized by chronic depression persisting for at least 2 years that is consistently below the symptom threshold for a Major Depressive Episode. Periods of depressed mood that are regularly present in the final week before the onset of menses and that become absent in the week postmenses are diagnosed as Premenstrual Dysphoric Disorder.

Next in the differential are two disorders with prominent irritability that have their onset in childhood: Disruptive Mood Dysregulation Disorder, which is characterized by frequent severe temper outbursts that are grossly out of proportion to the situation, with persistently angry or irritable mood between the outbursts; and Oppositional Defiant Disorder, which is also characterized by a pattern of persistent angry and irritable mood that is accompanied by argumentativeness, defiance, and vindictiveness. If the irritability is a fundamental part of the person's characteristic repertoire of mood states, then a diagnosis of a Personality Disorder may be most appropriate. Also, two of the DSM-5-

TR personality disorders, Borderline Personality Disorder and Antisocial Personality Disorder, include chronic irritability among their characteristic features.

Finally, clinically significant irritability that is not covered so far could qualify for a diagnosis of Adjustment Disorder if the irritability occurs as a maladaptive response to a psychosocial stressor. Otherwise, clinically significant irritability that does not meet the criteria for any other mental disorder and is judged to represent a psychological or biological dysfunction in the individual could qualify for one of the residual unspecified categories. Given that irritable mood can be characteristic of either a Bipolar and Related Disorder or a Depressive Disorder, the specific choice is a matter of clinical judgment. If the presentation is judged to be more consistent with a Bipolar and Related Disorder, Unspecified Bipolar and Related Disorder should be diagnosed. If it is more consistent with a Depressive Disorder, Unspecified Depressive Disorder should be diagnosed. If the presentation is not clearly best considered bipolar or depressive, Unspecified Mood Disorder can be diagnosed pending additional clarifying information.

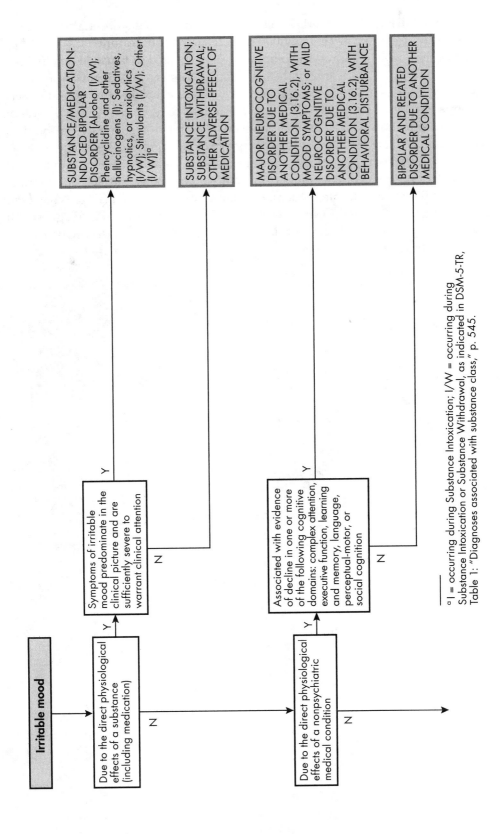

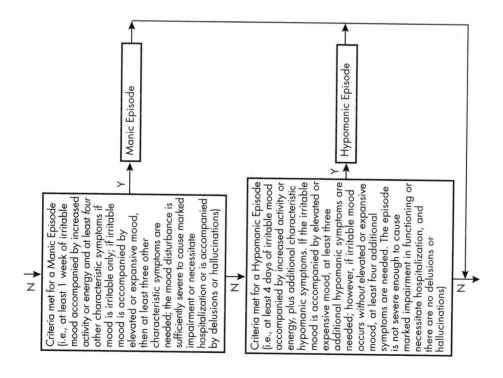

Criteria met for a Manic Episode (i.e., at least 1 week of irritable mood accompanied by increased activity or energy and at least *four* other characteristic symptoms if mood is irritable only; if irritable mood is accompanied by elevated or expansive mood, then at least three other characteristic symptoms are needed; the mood disturbance is sufficiently severe to cause marked impairment or necessitate hospitalization or is accompanied by delusions or hallucinations)

Manic Episode

Criteria met for a Hypomanic Episode (i.e., at least 4 days of irritable mood accompanied by increased activity or energy, plus additional characteristic hypomanic symptoms. If the irritable mood is accompanied by elevated or expansive mood, at least three additional hypomanic symptoms are needed; however, if irritable mood occurs *without* elevated or expansive mood, at least four additional symptoms are needed. The episode is not severe enough to cause marked impairment in functioning or necessitate hospitalization, and there are no delusions or hallucinations)

Hypomanic Episode

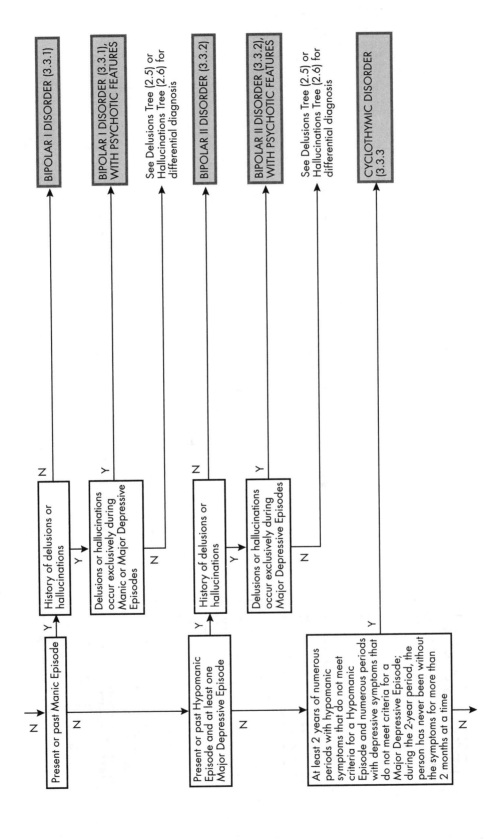

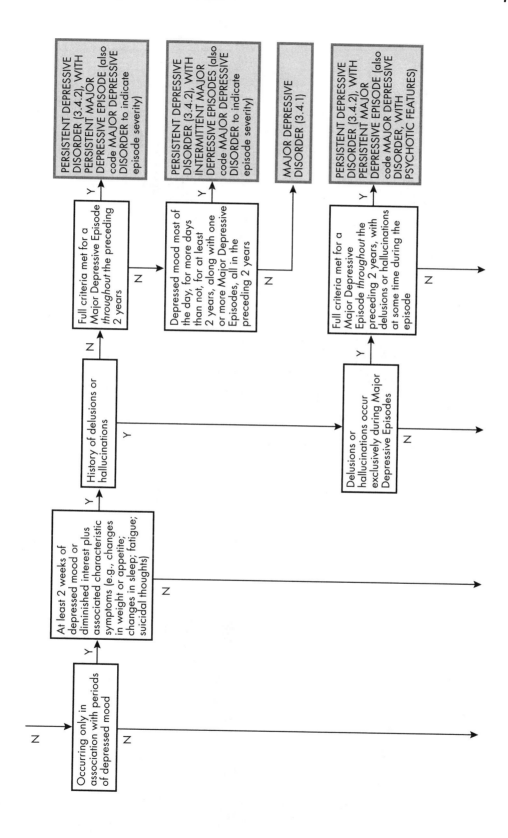

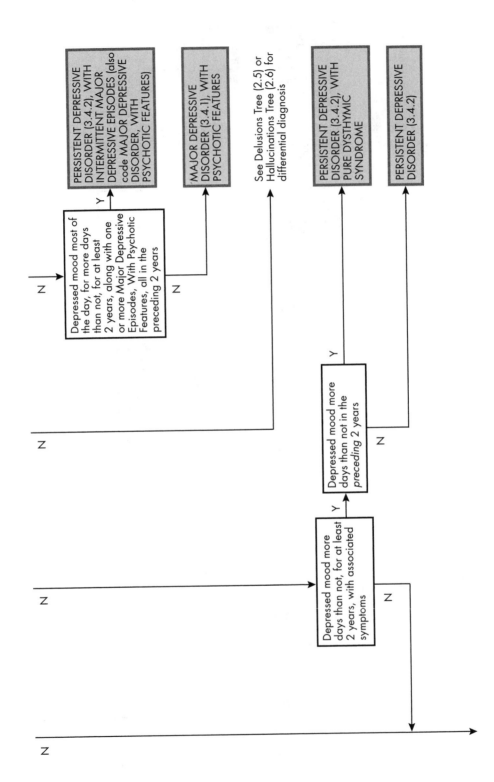

PERSISTENT DEPRESSIVE DISORDER (3.4.2), WITH INTERMITTENT MAJOR DEPRESSIVE EPISODES (also code MAJOR DEPRESSIVE DISORDER, WITH PSYCHOTIC FEATURES)

MAJOR DEPRESSIVE DISORDER (3.4.1), WITH PSYCHOTIC FEATURES

See Delusions Tree (2.5) or Hallucinations Tree (2.6) for differential diagnosis

PERSISTENT DEPRESSIVE DISORDER (3.4.2), WITH PURE DYSTHYMIC SYNDROME

PERSISTENT DEPRESSIVE DISORDER (3.4.2)

Depressed mood most of the day, for more days than not, for at least 2 years, along with one or more Major Depressive Episodes, With Psychotic Features, all in the preceding 2 years

Depressed mood more days than not in the preceding 2 years

Depressed mood more days than not, for at least 2 years, with associated symptoms

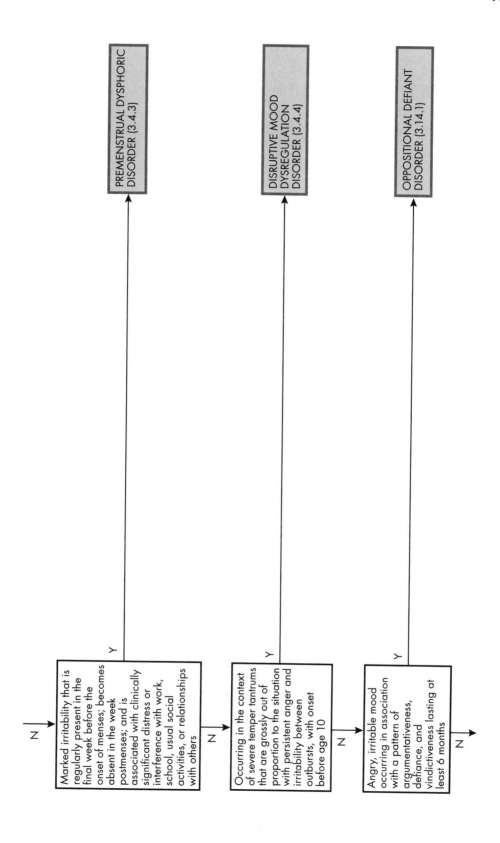

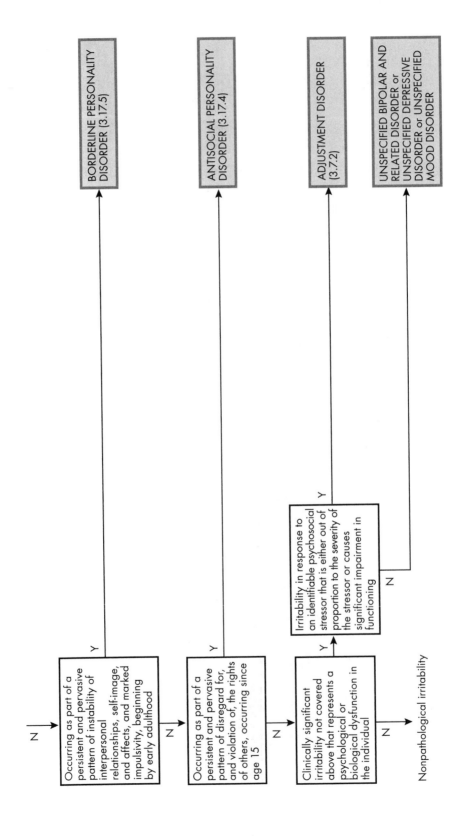

2.10 Decision Tree for Depressed Mood

Depressed mood is one of the most common presenting symptoms in mental health settings and is a component of many psychiatric conditions. The differential diagnosis of
depressed mood requires consideration of both the context in which the depression occurs and the clustering and duration of symptoms.

Substances (including both drugs of abuse and medication side effects) must first be
ruled out as the cause of the depressed mood. Depression can arise in the context of Substance Intoxication (e.g., with cannabis use), result from taking or withdrawing from a
medication, or be part of Substance Withdrawal (e.g., from cocaine). Because depressed
mood is a frequent concomitant of Substance Intoxication and Substance Withdrawal, it
usually does not require a separate diagnosis. However, if the depressive symptoms predominate in the clinical presentation and are sufficiently severe to warrant clinical attention, then a diagnosis of Substance/Medication-Induced Depressive Disorder may be
more appropriate than simply giving the diagnosis of Substance Intoxication or Substance
Withdrawal. The differential between Substance/Medication-Induced Depressive Disorder and a non-substance-induced depressive disorder can be made historically by docu-
menting that the depressed mood occurs only in relation to substance/medication use.
When such a history is not forthcoming, a period of abstinence is usually required to determine whether the depressed mood resolves once the effects of the substance wear off.
DSM-5-TR suggests waiting for "about 1 month" after cessation of substance use to see
whether the mood symptoms spontaneously resolve, although the actual required period of time to wait varies depending on the drug and the clinical situation. Other factors
that should be considered include previous history of Major Depressive Episodes, family history, and the likelihood that this type of substance in the amount used could have
caused the depressive symptoms. See Step 2, "Rule Out Substance Etiology (Including
Drugs of Abuse, Medications")" in Chapter 1, "Differential Diagnosis, Step by Step." If
the mood symptoms continue to persist after a reasonable waiting period, then a Sub-
stance/Medication-Induced Depressive Disorder is unlikely and the diagnosis should
be a non-substance-induced depressive disorder.

One of the most difficult differential diagnostic determinations in psychiatry is to distinguish between independent depressive disorders and those that are the direct physiological consequence of a nonpsychiatric medical condition. A number of nonpsychiatric
medical conditions are known to cause depression through their direct effect on the brain.
If severe cognitive impairment is also present, Major Neurocognitive Disorder Due to Another Medical Condition must be considered. However, it is important not to assume that
severe cognitive impairment necessarily indicates a diagnosis of Neurocognitive Disorder
Due to Another Medical Condition. The cognitive impairment that can occur as part of a
Major Depressive Episode can be severe enough to mimic a Major Neurocognitive Disorder. Often, only time, serial evaluations, and sequential antidepressant treatment trials
will confirm whether a particular presentation is better explained by a Major Neurocognitive Disorder or a Major Depressive Episode with severe cognitive symptoms.

The next step is to determine whether there have been any Major Depressive, Manic,
or Hypomanic Episodes, because the diagnosis of an episodic mood disorder in DSM-5-
TR depends on the combination of these episodes: Major Depressive Disorder requires

at least one Major Depressive Episode and never any Manic or Hypomanic Episodes; Bipolar I Disorder requires at least one Manic Episode (with or without Major Depressive Episodes); and Bipolar II Disorder requires at least one Hypomanic Episode and at least one Major Depressive Episode but never any Manic Episodes. Tree 2.10 first checks for the presence (or history) of a Major Depressive Episode (i.e., a period of depressed mood, present for most of the day, nearly every day, for at least 2 weeks, accompanied by at least four characteristic symptoms such as diminished interest, changes in appetite and sleep, feeling worthless or guilty, and suicidal thoughts or behavior). However, if criteria are also met at the same time for a Manic Episode, the episode is instead a Manic Episode With Mixed Features rather than a Major Depressive Episode.

The next question about manic or hypomanic symptoms is intended to determine whether the final diagnosis will be a Bipolar and Related Disorder (Bipolar I Disorder, Bipolar II Disorder, or Other Specified/Unspecified Bipolar and Related Disorder) or a Depressive Disorder. If criteria have ever been met for a Manic Episode, the final diagnosis depends on whether there has been a history of delusions or hallucinations. If there is no such history, the diagnosis is Bipolar I Disorder. If delusions and/or hallucinations occur exclusively during Manic Episodes, the diagnosis is Bipolar I Disorder, Manic, With Psychotic Features; however, if delusions and/or hallucinations occur at other times than during Manic Episodes, the diagnosis is one of the Schizophrenia Spectrum and Other Psychotic Disorders. If criteria have been met for a Hypomanic Episode in addition to the Major Depressive Episode, the final diagnosis also depends on whether there has been a history of delusions or hallucinations during the Major Depressive Episodes. If there is no such history, the diagnosis is Bipolar II Disorder. If delusions and/or hallucinations occur exclusively during Major Depressive Episodes, the diagnosis is Bipolar II Disorder, Depressed, With Psychotic Features; however, if delusions and/or hallucinations occur at other times than during Major Depressive Episodes, the diagnosis is one of the Schizophrenia Spectrum and Other Psychotic Disorders. In cases in which there is a Major Depressive Episode with clinically significant manic or hypomanic symptoms that do not meet criteria for a Manic or Hypomanic Episode, the final diagnosis also depends on whether there has been a history of delusions or hallucinations. If there is no such history, the diagnosis is Other Specified/Unspecified Bipolar and Related Disorder plus Major Depressive Disorder. If delusions and/or hallucinations occur exclusively during Major Depressive Episodes, the diagnosis is Other Specified/Unspecified Bipolar and Related Disorder plus Major Depressive Disorder With Psychotic Features; and if not, the diagnosis is one of the Schizophrenia Spectrum and Other Psychotic Disorders. Finally, if there have been 2 or more years of numerous periods with hypomanic symptoms and numerous periods with depressive symptoms (and no history of Major Depressive, Manic, or Hypomanic Episodes), the diagnosis is Cyclothymic Disorder.

Once the presence of lifetime manic or hypomanic symptoms has been ruled out, the remaining decision points in the tree determine which depressive disorder best accounts for the symptomatic presentation. In those cases in which criteria have been met for a Major Depressive Episode, the final diagnosis depends on whether there has been a history of delusions or hallucinations and whether the depressive disorder is "persistent" (i.e., duration of 2 years or longer). If there is no history of delusions or hallucinations, and the depressive disorder is not persistent, the diagnosis is simply Major Depressive Disorder. However, if there is a period of depressed mood for most of the day, more days than not, for at least 2 years, an additional diagnosis of Persistent Depressive Disorder, With Persistent Major Depressive Episode, is made if the criteria have been met for a Major Depressive Episode for an entire 2-year period; alternatively, a diagnosis of Persistent Depressive Disorder, With Intermittent Major Depressive Episodes, would be made to indicate the chronicity of the depression. If there is a history of delusions or hallucinations occurring exclusively during the Major Depressive Episodes, Major Depressive Disorder With Psychotic Features is diagnosed in place of Major Depressive Disorder (i.e., Major Depressive Disorder With Psychotic Features plus Persistent Depressive Disorder, With Persistent Major Depressive Episode; Major Depressive Disorder plus Persistent Depressive Disorder, With Intermittent Major Depressive Episodes; or Major Depressive Disorder With Psychotic Features). If the delusions or hallucinations occur outside of Major Depressive Episodes, refer to the Delusions Tree [2.5] or Hallucinations Tree [2.6] to determine the differential diagnosis of which Schizophrenia Spectrum and Other Psychotic Disorder is most applicable.

A diagnosis of Persistent Depressive Disorder, With Pure Dysthymic Syndrome, by itself is warranted for presentations characterized by chronic depression persisting for at least 2 years that is consistently below the symptom threshold for a Major Depressive Episode (referred to in prior editions of the DSM as "dysthymia"). Periods of depressed mood that are regularly present in the final week before the onset of menses and that become absent in the week postmenses are diagnosed as Premenstrual Dysphoric Disorder.

Finally, if the depression is not adequately explained by any of the decision points so far in the tree, it may still justify a DSM-5-TR diagnosis. If the depression is a symptomatic manifestation of a maladaptive response to an identifiable psychosocial stressor, a diagnosis of Adjustment Disorder With Depressed Mood might apply. If not, and the depression is clinically significant and represents a psychological or biological dysfunction in the individual (thus qualifying as a mental disorder), the residual category Other Specified/ Unspecified Depressive Disorder would apply. Otherwise, the depression would be considered part of "normal" everyday blues and not indicative of a mental disorder.

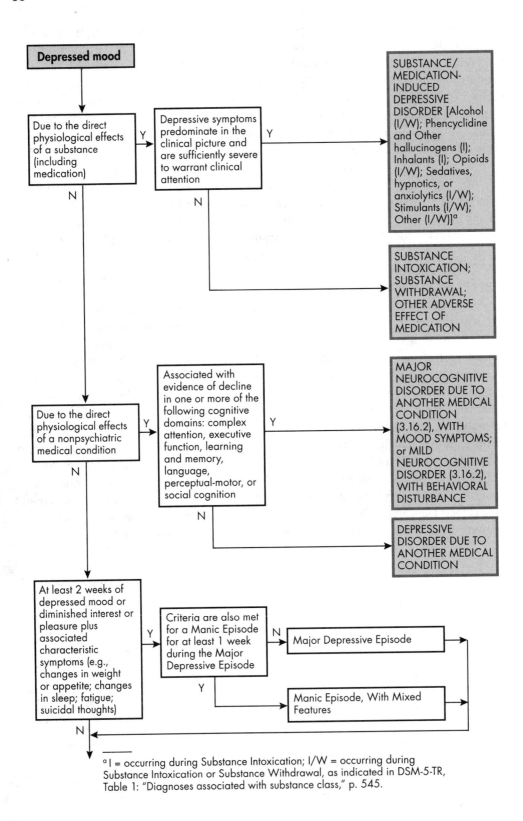

a I = occurring during Substance Intoxication; I/W = occurring during Substance Intoxication or Substance Withdrawal, as indicated in DSM-5-TR, Table 1: "Diagnoses associated with substance class," p. 545.

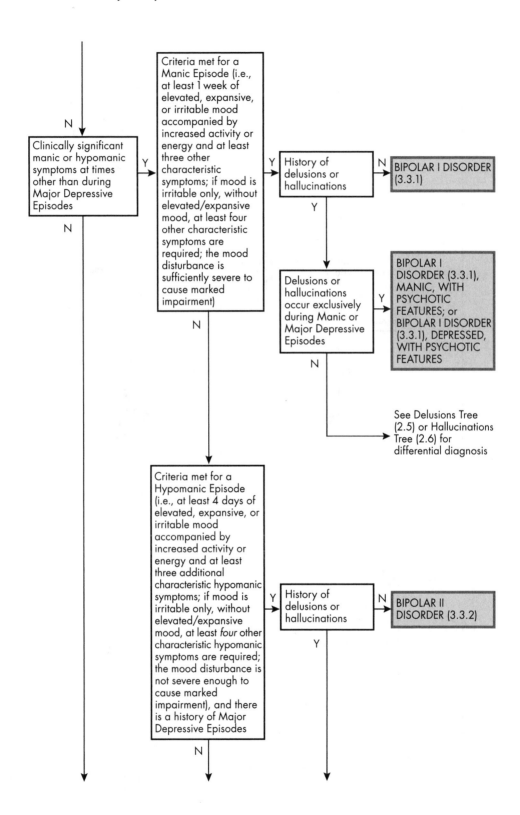

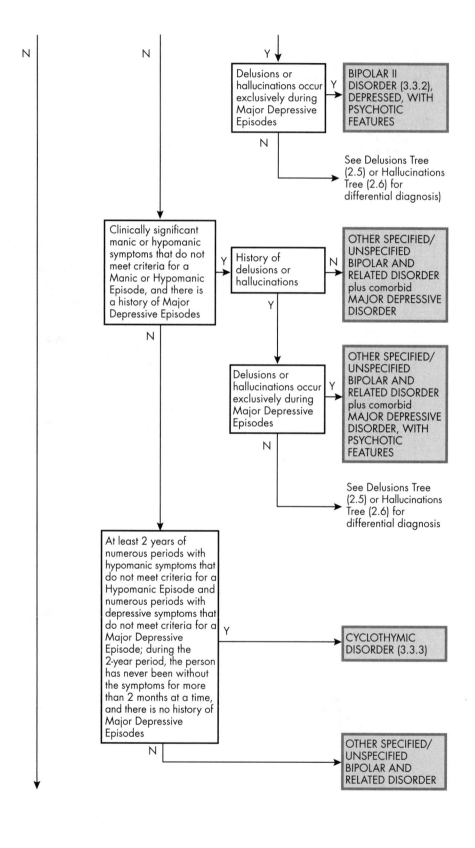

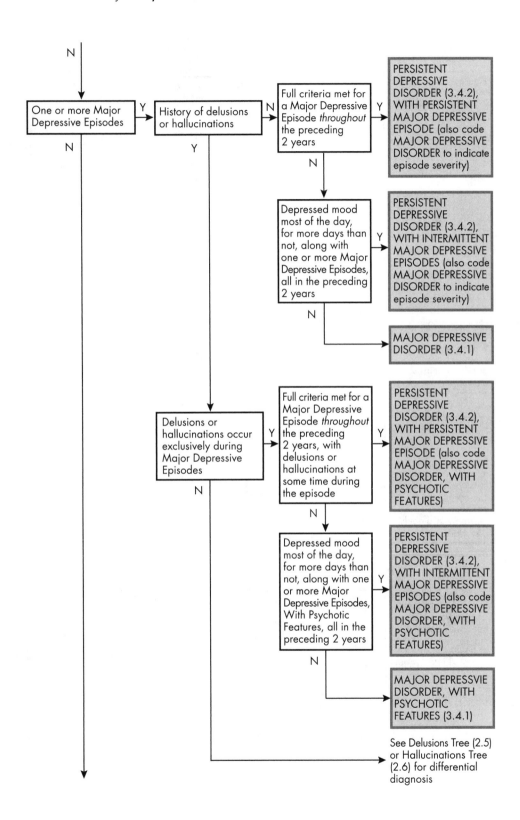

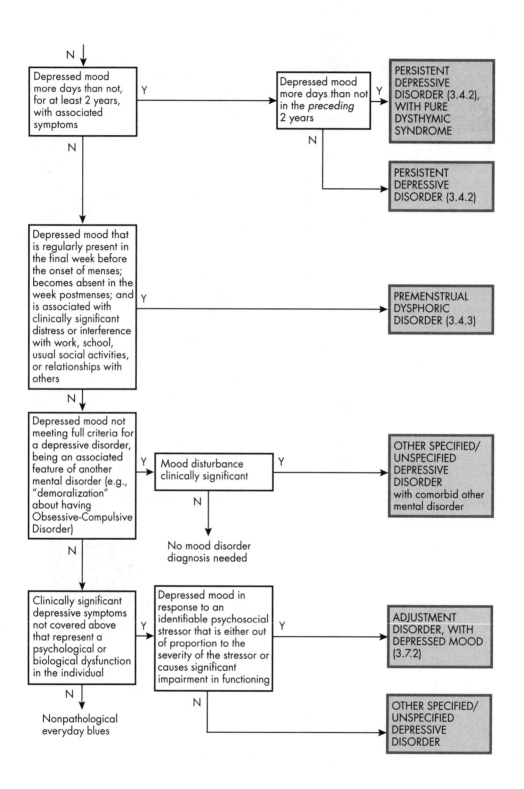

2.11 Decision Tree for Suicidal Ideation or Behavior

When the clinician is evaluating suicidality, it is important to determine the urgency of current suicidal thoughts, the degree to which definite plans have been formulated and acted on, the availability of a means of suicide, the lethality of the method, the urgency of the impulse, the presence of psychotic symptoms, the history of previous suicidal thoughts and attempts, family history of suicidal behavior, and current and past substance use. The degree of suicidality is on a continuum ranging from recurrent wishes to be dead, to feelings that others would be better off if the person were dead ("passive suicidal thoughts"), to formulating suicidal plans, to overt suicidal behaviors.

Suicidal behavior is explicitly mentioned in the diagnostic criteria for only four conditions—Bipolar I Disorder, Bipolar II Disorder, and Major Depressive Disorder (in Criterion A9 of the Major Depressive Episode component), and Criterion 5 in Borderline Personality Disorder—potentially giving the misleading impression that suicidal behavior is not a central concern in other conditions such as Schizophrenia, Substance Use Disorder, and Posttraumatic Stress Disorder, each of which is associated with elevated rates of suicidal behavior. Taking advantage of the fact that the ICD-10-CM classification includes codes for recording the presence of psychiatric symptoms, the DSM-5-TR chapter "Other Conditions That May Be a Focus of Clinical Attention" provides ICD-10-CM codes to indicate current suicidal behavior, as well as a history of suicidal behavior. These symptom codes can be used in addition to the codes for the particular mental disorder judged to be associated with the suicidal behavior, or they can be used as a stand-alone code if there is no associated mental disorder. Consequently, this decision tree begins by assigning the code for current suicidal behavior if there is potentially self-injurious behavior with at least some intent to die (i.e., the definition of suicidal behavior) and then continues with the differential diagnosis of disorders most associated with suicidal behavior.

Because suicidal behavior is part of the diagnostic criteria for Major Depressive Episode, most people associate suicide most closely with mood disorders. For this reason, the fourth and fifth branches of the tree offer "mini-differential diagnoses" of those DSM-5-TR conditions associated with depressed mood and suicidal ideation/behavior, and those with a concurrent mixture of depressive and manic symptoms (so-called mixed states). As this decision tree illustrates, although suicidal ideation is a characteristic feature of mood disorders, it must be considered in the management of a wide array of DSM-5-TR disorders. Moreover, the risk of suicide increases dramatically when the individual has more than one disorder, because each disorder may independently contribute to the risk (e.g., a particularly common and dangerous combination is that of Major Depressive Disorder, Alcohol Use Disorder, and Borderline Personality Disorder).

Suicidal behavior may be associated with symptoms other than depressed mood. For example, suicidal behavior may occur under the direction of delusions or command hallucinations (e.g., in Schizophrenia, Bipolar Disorder With Psychotic Features, or Major Depressive Disorder With Psychotic Features), may be related to confusion or other cognitive impairment (e.g., in Delirium, Major Neurocognitive Disorder, Substance Intoxication, or Substance Withdrawal), or may result from disinhibition (e.g., in a Manic Episode or Substance Intoxication). Individuals with Borderline Personality Disorder or Antisocial Personality Disorder have a 5%–10% risk of successful suicide, perhaps resulting from the impulsivity, labile moods, low frustration tolerance, and high rates of substance use characteristic of these disorders. Similarly, Conduct Disorder is an important predictor of suicide in adolescents, particularly when it is accompanied by substance use and mood symptoms.

The evaluation of suicidal ideation or behavior must take into account the fact that such symptoms are sometimes feigned as a way of gaining admission to the hospital or of "solving" other life problems. Patients quickly learn the power of saying the phrase, "I want to kill myself," as a way of influencing clinicians, family members, and other important individuals in their lives. In Malingering, the patient's motivation is some obvious external reward (e.g., getting transferred from prison to hospital, getting a place to spend the night). In contrast, although the presumed motivation is a psychological need to assume the sick role in Factitious Disorder, it is not necessary to determine the individual's motivation in order to make the diagnosis, so long as their behavior is evident even in the absence of external rewards. Adjustment Disorder applies to those individuals who develop suicidal ideation or behavior in response to an identifiable psychosocial stressor and in the absence of other symptoms that meet the criteria for a specific DSM-5-TR disorder that would explain the suicidal ideation or behavior. This diagnosis is most commonly used to describe suicidal behavior in adolescents.

Another possibility is that in certain extreme circumstances (e.g., an intractable terminal illness), the desire to kill oneself may not necessarily represent a mental disorder at all. However, before a clinician can arrive at this conclusion, a thorough evaluation is necessary to rule out all other more treatable causes of suicidal ideation (e.g., depression, pain, insomnia, psychosis, Delirium).

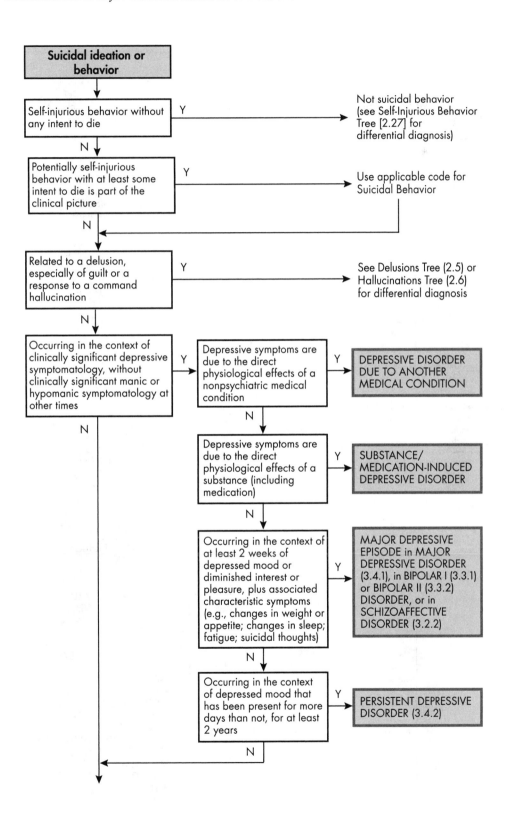

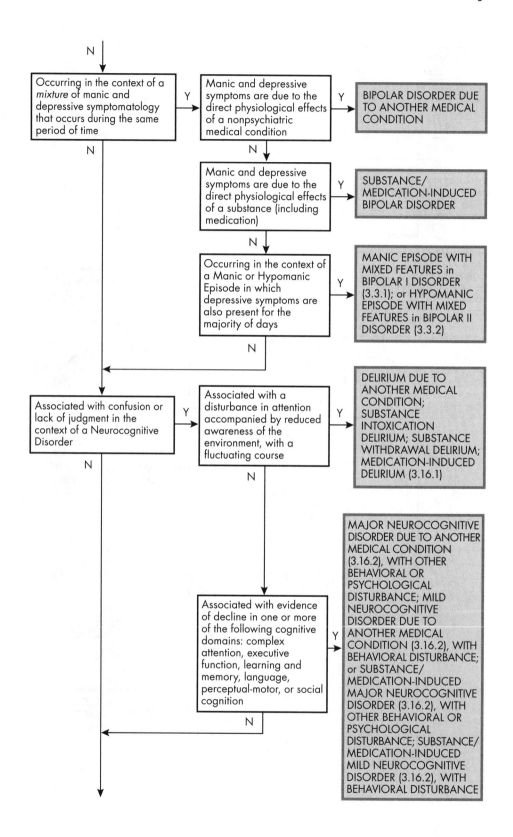

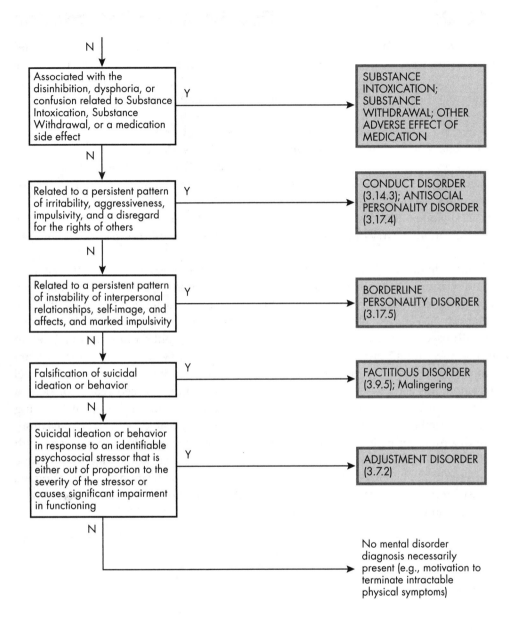

2.12 Decision Tree for Psychomotor Retardation

Psychomotor retardation is defined as visible generalized slowing of movements and speech. In its extreme form, psychomotor retardation may be characterized by unresponsiveness and mutism that is indistinguishable from catatonic stupor. The symptom of psychomotor retardation should be distinguished from other similar symptoms:

- *Fatigue* is a subjective sense of having decreased energy or being tired all the time but is not characterized by visible evidence of slowed movements.
- *Leaden paralysis* is the individual's subjective sense that their arms and legs are as "heavy as lead" and is a part of the "atypical" pattern of symptoms in a Major Depressive Episode With Atypical Features.
- *Avolition* (one of the negative symptoms of Schizophrenia) is characterized by a lack of motivation to carry out behaviors rather than being physically slowed down.

Nonpsychiatric medical conditions may cause psychomotor retardation that usually does not warrant a separate mental disorder diagnosis. It is important to remember that psychomotor changes associated with Delirium can be characterized by either agitation or retardation. Very few clinicians miss the dramatic presentations of Delirium associated with psychomotor agitation (e.g., the patient pulling out an intravenous line). In contrast, the "quiet" cases of Delirium associated with psychomotor retardation are much more likely to go unrecognized; these scenarios are noted by specifying the level of psychomotor activity as "hypoactive." Another common "missed" cause of slowed movements is Antipsychotic Medication– and Other Dopamine Receptor Blocking Agent–Induced Parkinsonism. This differentiation is complicated by the fact that a number of disorders for which antipsychotic medications are given also can manifest with psychomotor retardation (e.g., Schizophrenia, Bipolar Disorder or Major Depressive Disorder With Psychotic Features, Delirium). A change in medication (e.g., reducing the dosage of antipsychotic medication or administering anticholinergic medication) can often be helpful in making the distinction.

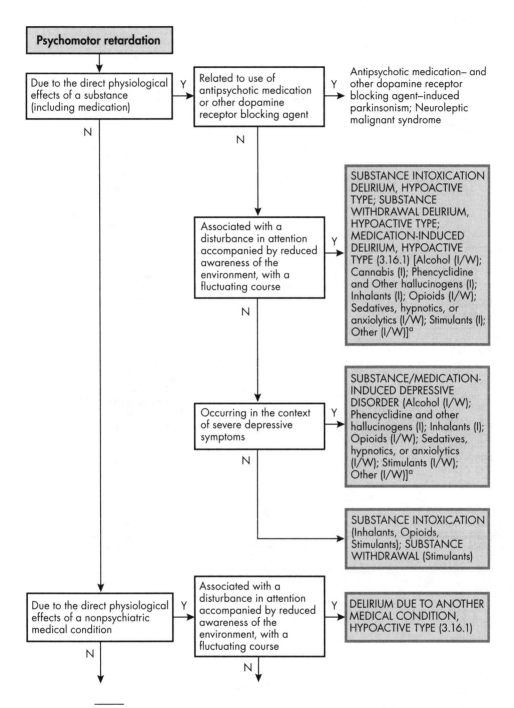

ᵃ I = occurring during Substance Intoxication; I/W = occurring during
Substance Intoxication or Substance Withdrawal, as indicated in DSM-5-TR,
Table 1: "Diagnoses associated with substance class," p. 545.

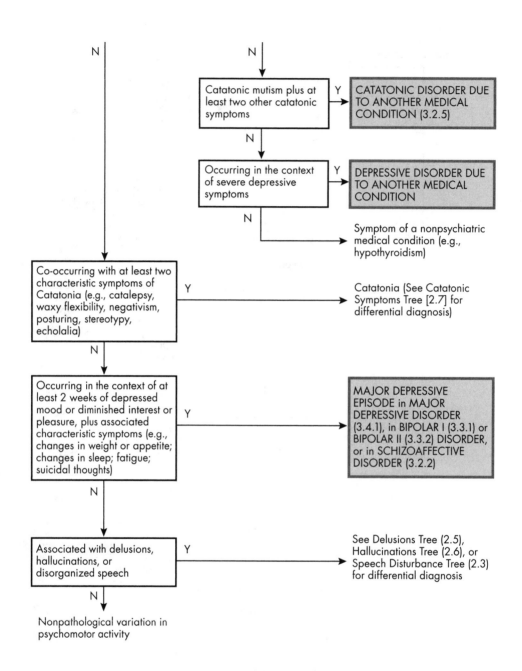

2.13 Decision Tree for Anxiety

As is always the case, the first step in the differential diagnosis is to rule out substance/medication use or a nonpsychiatric medical condition as the direct physiological cause of a patient's anxiety. Because anxiety can be an associated feature of Delirium and Major or Mild Neurocognitive Disorder, these more specific conditions are also considered within this section of the decision tree.

When the anxiety occurs in discrete episodes with a sudden onset and is accompanied by a number of somatic symptoms (e.g., palpitations, shortness of breath, dizziness) and cognitive symptoms (e.g., fear of going crazy or having a heart attack), it is considered to be a Panic Attack (or, if the number of characteristic symptoms falls short of the minimum threshold of four, a "limited-symptom attack"). Because of the specific treatment implications of panic attacks, a separate decision tree (2.14) is provided for them.

The remaining decision points in the anxiety tree differentiate among the Anxiety Disorders by determining what the individual is fearful of, what situations are avoided, and whether the anxiety is in response to an identifiable psychosocial stressor. In Panic Disorder, the anxiety is related to the fear of having additional panic attacks and the possible consequences of these attacks. Agoraphobia is similar in that the person is afraid of places or situations from which escape would be difficult or embarrassing in the event of a Panic Attack or panic-like symptoms, but the focus is on the fear and avoidance of the places and situations that might trigger a Panic Attack rather than on the Panic Attack itself. Reflecting the more generalized nature of the avoidance in Agoraphobia (compared with the more limited nature of avoided situations in conditions such as Specific Phobia), a diagnosis of Agoraphobia requires that the individual must be fearful of situations from at least two "agoraphobic clusters": public transportation, open spaces, enclosed spaces, standing in a line or being in a crowd, and being outside the home alone. Separation Anxiety Disorder, Social Anxiety Disorder, and Specific Phobia each have a specific focus of fear and avoidance (i.e., separation from major attachment figures, situations in which the person may be exposed to the scrutiny of others, exposure to a feared object [e.g., spider] or situation [e.g., flying in an airplane], respectively). Individuals whose anxiety is about health or having or acquiring a serious illness can be diagnosed as having Somatic Symptom Disorder or Illness Anxiety Disorder, depending on whether their anxiety is accompanied by distressing somatic symptoms (Somatic Symptom Disorder) or focused on having or acquiring a serious illness (Illness Anxiety Disorder). Both Hoarding Disorder and Body Dysmorphic Disorder may be associated with clinically significant anxiety (e.g., anxiety associated with the person being forced to discard personal items; anxiety and embarrassment about others observing the imagined defects or flaws in physical appearance).

Anxiety that develops in response to exposure to a traumatic stressor may be indicative of Posttraumatic Stress Disorder or Acute Stress Disorder if the other characteristic features of these disorders are also present (i.e., intrusion and avoidance symptoms related to the traumatic stressor or its circumstances, negative alterations in cognitions and mood, and alterations in arousal and activity); the differentiation is based on duration (i.e., 1 month or less for Acute Stress Disorder, greater than 1 month for Posttraumatic Stress Disorder). Marked anxiety is also common in Obsessive-Compulsive Disorder, especially when the individual is confronted with situations that trigger their obsessions or compulsions (e.g., an individual with a contamination obsession and handwashing compulsion who accidently touches a soiled object).

Anxiety occurs so commonly with Major Depressive Episodes, Manic Episodes, and Hypomanic Episodes that its co-occurrence is more the rule than the exception. The clinician can indicate the presence of anxiety with the specifier With Anxious Distress, including the severity of the anxiety (ranging from mild to severe), when the following occurs: if symptoms of anxiety are present for the majority of days of the current or most recent Major Depressive Episode in Major Depressive Disorder, Bipolar I Disorder, or Bipolar II Disorder; the current or most recent Manic Episode in Bipolar I Disorder; or the current or most recent Hypomanic Episode in Bipolar I Disorder or Bipolar II Disorder.

Finally, if the anxiety is not adequately explained by any of the decision points so far in the tree, a DSM-5-TR diagnosis may still be justified. If the anxiety is a symptomatic manifestation of a maladaptive response to an identifiable psychosocial stressor, the diagnosis is Adjustment Disorder With Anxiety. If the anxiety does not occur in this context yet is clinically significant and represents a psychological or biological dysfunction in the individual (thus qualifying as a mental disorder), a residual category would apply. The choice of the diagnosis depends on whether the clinician wishes to record the symptomatic presentation on the chart (in which case Other Specified Anxiety Disorder would be used, followed by the specific reason) or not (in which case Unspecified Anxiety Disorder would be used). Otherwise, the anxiety would be considered part of the normal repertoire of emotional expression and not indicative of a mental disorder.

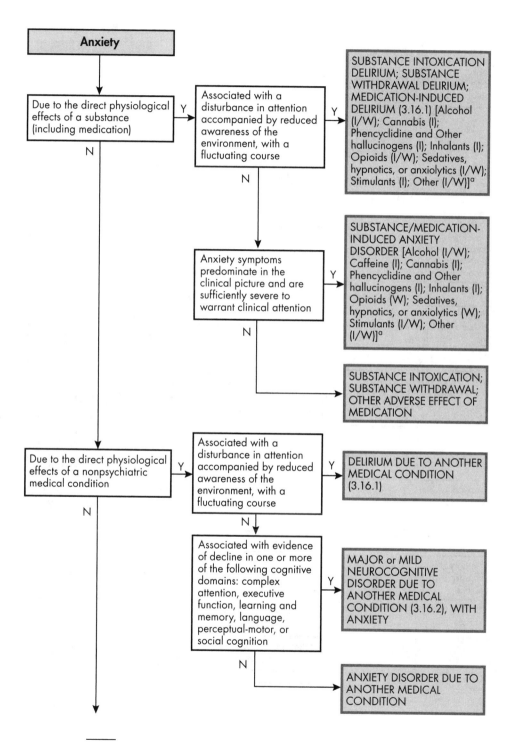

ᵃ I = occurring during Substance Intoxication; I/W = occurring during
Substance Intoxication or Substance Withdrawal; W = occurring during
Substance Withdrawal, as indicated in DSM-5-TR, Table 1: "Diagnoses
associated with substance class," p. 545.

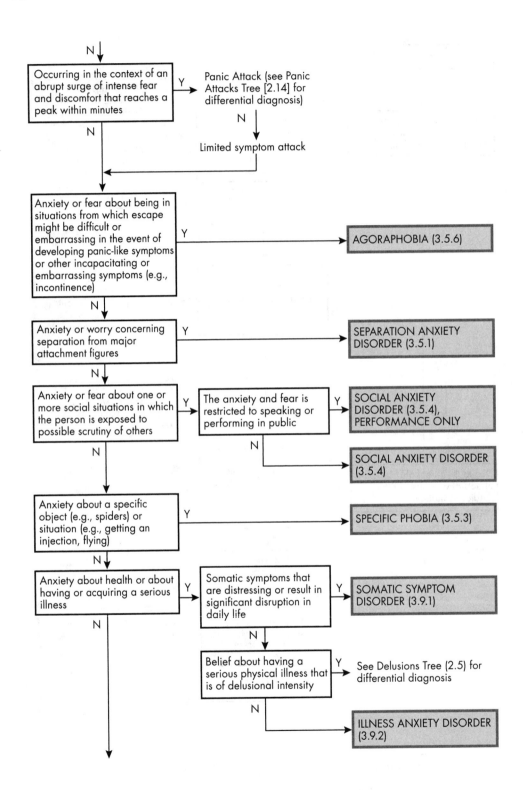

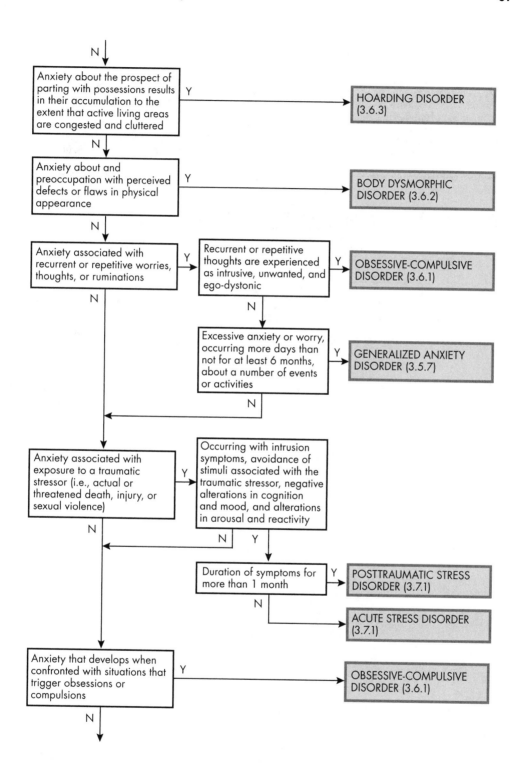

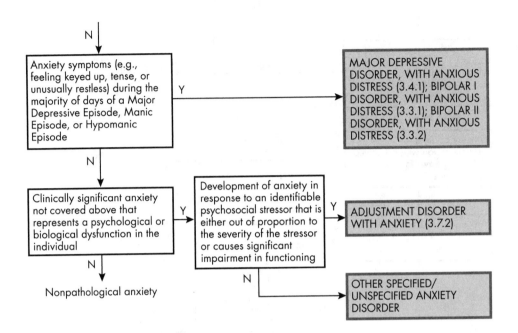

2.14 Decision Tree for Panic Attacks

Panic attacks are discrete episodes of intense fear or discomfort accompanied by symptoms such as palpitations, shortness of breath, sweating, trembling, derealization, and a fear of losing control or dying. Although panic attacks are required for a diagnosis of Panic Disorder, they also occur in association with a number of other DSM-5-TR disorders listed in the tree. For example, if a patient with a snake phobia goes on a hike and steps on a snake, that experience could easily result in a Panic Attack that would be indicative of a Specific Phobia rather than Panic Disorder.

The first step in the differential diagnosis for a Panic Attack is to rule out the presence of etiological substance/medication use. When taken in high enough doses or during Substance Withdrawal, a number of substances and medications can lead to a Panic Attack. Because caffeine is a common but covert culprit in this regard, taking a careful history of the consumption of caffeine-containing substances is important. If substance/medication-related Panic Attacks warrant clinical attention, Substance/Medication-Induced Anxiety Disorder should be diagnosed; otherwise, a diagnosis of Substance Intoxication or Substance Withdrawal will suffice. Sometimes, individuals have their first Panic Attack while taking a substance or a medication and then go on to have additional attacks even when they are not taking any substances or medications. Such subsequent attacks should not be considered substance/medication-induced Panic Attacks but instead might warrant a diagnosis of Panic Disorder.

Next, possible etiological nonpsychiatric medical conditions, such as hyperthyroidism or a pheochromocytoma, should be considered. If evidence indicates that such a medical condition is the direct cause of the Panic Attack (e.g., the onset of the Panic Attacks was parallel to the onset of the nonpsychiatric medical condition, and the Panic Attacks remitted after initiation of successful treatment for the nonpsychiatric medical condition), that would suggest the diagnosis of Anxiety Disorder Due to Another Medical Condition.

Once it is clear that the Panic Attacks are not the direct physiological consequence of a substance or nonpsychiatric medical condition, the next step is to determine the relationship between the Panic Attacks and a possible situational trigger. By definition, at least two of the panic attacks in Panic Disorder must be unexpected—that is, there is no relationship between the attacks and a situational cue (i.e., they arise "out of the blue"). In contrast, the panic attacks that occur in patients with Social Anxiety Disorder, Specific Phobia, Separation Anxiety Disorder, Posttraumatic Stress Disorder or Acute Stress Disorder, Illness Anxiety Disorder, Obsessive-Compulsive Disorder, and Generalized Anxiety Disorder are closely related to the pertinent situational trigger (e.g., social situations such as public speaking, a specific situation such as closed places, being separated from major attachment figures, being exposed to reminders of the trauma, the possibility of having a serious illness, obsessive concerns such as contamination fears, and worry about a number of events or situations, respectively). If the Panic Attacks are not an associated feature of a specific DSM-5-TR disorder but nonetheless are judged to be clinically significant, either a diagnosis of Adjustment Disorder (if the Panic Attacks are a response to an identifiable psychosocial stressor) or a diagnosis of a residual category (Other Specified/Unspecified Anxiety Disorder) may be appropriate. Finally, Panic Attacks triggered by a realistic threat (e.g., being held up at gunpoint) or the experience of a single isolated Panic Attack (or rare Panic Attacks) does not warrant a diagnosis of a mental disorder.

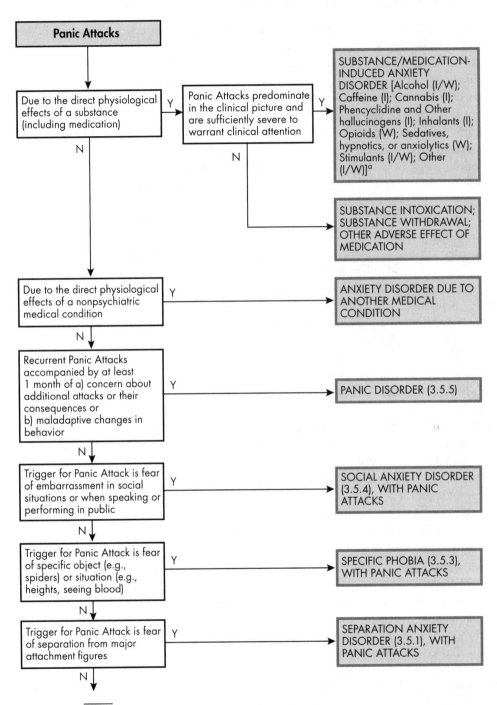

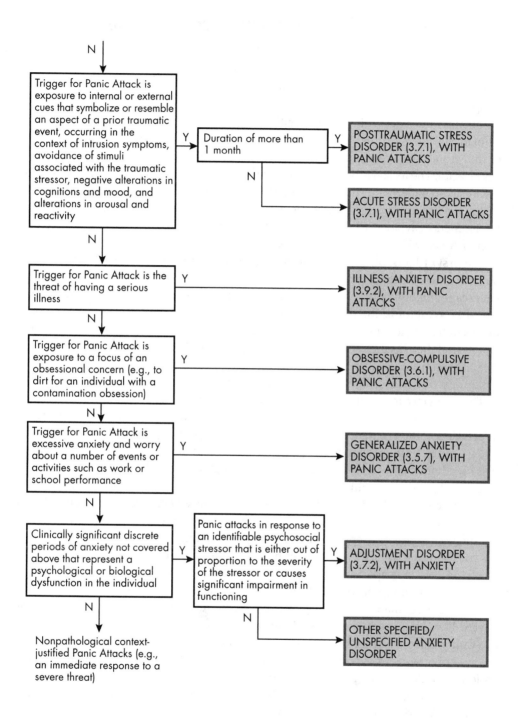

2.15 Decision Tree for Avoidance Behavior

Avoidance behavior (particularly of realistically harmful situations) is often adaptive. This decision tree applies only when the avoidance is based on unrealistic or excessive fears and leads to clinically significant distress or impairment. Avoidance is a fairly ubiquitous and nonspecific symptom and is an associated feature of many disorders. The evaluation of this symptom requires determining the specific circumstances triggering the avoidance. This is one of the few decision trees included in this handbook that does not include a decision point for ruling out substance/medication use or a nonpsychiatric medical condition as an etiological factor. The reason is because avoidance behavior is almost invariably a psychological reaction to an underlying anxiety or fear. Although substance/medication use or a nonpsychiatric medical condition can cause anxiety, the lack of contextual associations makes the development of avoidance behavior related to Substance/Medication-Induced Anxiety Disorder or Anxiety Disorder Due to Another Medical Condition unlikely.

The first order of business is determining whether the avoidance behavior involves multiple situations and places. If so, and if the situations are avoided due to thoughts that escape might be difficult or help might not be available in the event of developing panic-like symptoms, the diagnosis of Agoraphobia might apply. Individuals associate the risk of having a Panic Attack or panic-like symptoms with particular locations or situations that then become conditioned stimuli particularly likely to trigger additional attacks. The individuals then avoid what appear to be "triggering" situations in an effort to minimize the chance of having panic attacks or panic-like symptoms.

The avoidance in Social Anxiety Disorder is related to the fear of social embarrassment. This avoidance comes in two forms: the performance anxiety form of Social Anxiety Disorder concerns the avoidance of public activities (e.g., speaking, playing music, acting, eating, urinating, writing) that can easily be performed by the individual in the privacy of their own home, and can be indicated by the "Performance Only" specifier; the generalized form includes virtually any situation that involves social interaction and in many cases may be virtually identical to Avoidant Personality Disorder. The Specific Phobias probably involve some interaction between evolutionarily predetermined inborn fears and the occurrence of aversive early-life experiences that reinforce them. In Separation Anxiety Disorder, which can occur in both childhood and in adulthood, situations in which the person is apart from major attachment figures are avoided. In Posttraumatic Stress Disorder and Acute Stress Disorder, the individual avoids situations that are reminiscent of the traumatic stressor (e.g., someone who resembles the assailant, loud sounds that recall wartime, tremors that recall a major earthquake). Some individuals with Obsessive-Compulsive Disorder learn that avoiding certain triggering situations will prevent the onset of obsessions (e.g., avoidance of handshakes will help reduce contamination obsessions). Similarly, some individuals with Illness Anxiety Disorder will avoid situations that they feel might jeopardize their health (e.g., visiting sick family members) lest they trigger ruminations about having contracted a serious illness.

Many other psychiatric disorders can have avoidance as an associated feature. For example, in Psychotic Disorders, avoidance behavior can occur in the context of a particular delusion, such as when a patient with a delusion avoids going outside for fear that the FBI is after them. Low motivation, which may be due to the anhedonia in a Major Depressive Episode or as part of the negative symptoms in Schizophrenia, may lead to a generalized avoidance of going out of the house. Because of a sexual dysfunction, sexual situations may be avoided because of anxiety about poor sexual performance. Individuals with Anorexia Nervosa and Avoidant/Restrictive Food Intake Disorder avoid certain foods (e.g., high-calorie foods in Anorexia Nervosa, aversive foods in Avoidant/Restrictive Food Intake Disorder), leading to clinically significant weight loss and potential malnutrition. A generalized pattern of avoidance characterizes Avoidant Personality Disorder, which by definition has its onset by early adulthood and tends to be relatively persistent and stable over the course of the person's lifetime.

Finally, if the avoidance behavior is not adequately explained by any of the decision points so far in the tree, a DSM-5-TR diagnosis might still be justified. If the avoidance behavior develops in response to an identifiable psychosocial stressor that is either out of proportion to the severity of the stressor or causes significant impairment in functioning, a diagnosis of Adjustment Disorder might apply. If the avoidance behavior did not develop in response to a stressor, yet it represents a psychological or biological dysfunction in the individual that is judged to be clinically significant (thus qualifying as a mental disorder), a residual category would apply. DSM-5-TR does not include a residual category for avoidance behavior per se. The closest residual category would be Other Specified/Unspecified Anxiety Disorder, because most likely the avoidance is serving to prevent some sort of anxiety. The choice of category depends on whether the clinician wishes to record the symptomatic presentation on the chart (in which case Other Specified Anxiety Disorder would be used, followed by the specific reason) or not (in which case Unspecified Anxiety Disorder would be used). Otherwise, the avoidance would be considered part of the normal repertoire of human behavior and not indicative of a mental disorder.

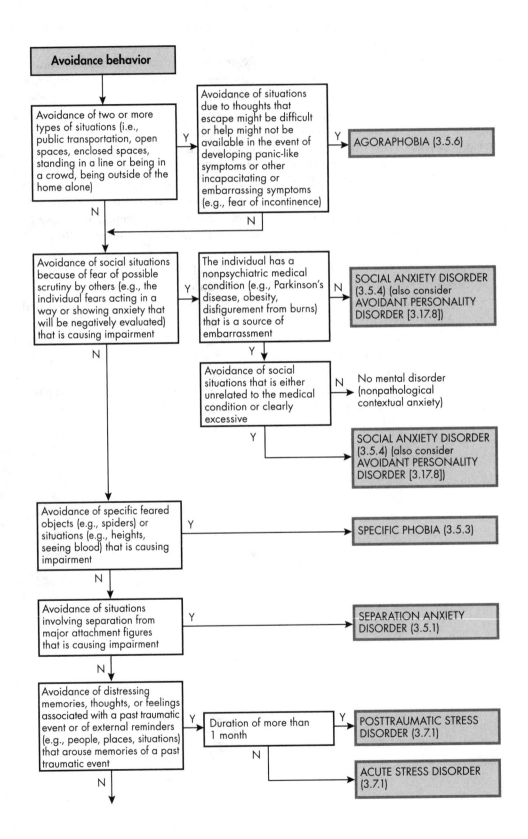

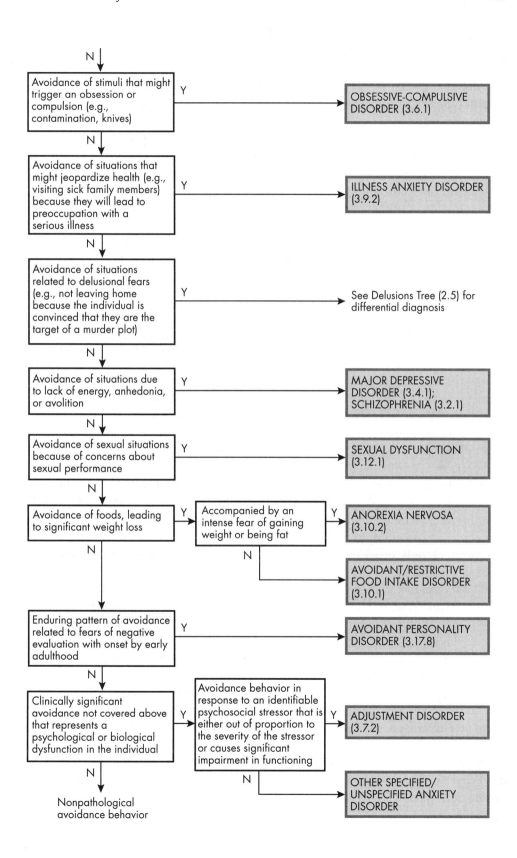

2.16 Decision Tree for Repetitive Pathological Behaviors

This decision tree covers a range of repetitive behaviors that may be indicative of psychopathology by virtue of their distressing nature or their negative impact on functioning. For the purposes of this decision tree, *repetitive behaviors* refer to behaviors that are repeated over and over again in short succession (e.g., stereotyped motor movements, tics, compulsions, hair pulling) that the individual usually finds difficult to control.

The first step involves determining whether the repetitive behaviors are due to the direct physiological effects of a nonpsychiatric medical condition (e.g., liver failure causing repetitive skin picking). Certain sleep disorders, such as Restless Legs Syndrome and Periodic Limb Movement Disorder, also cause repetitive movements, particularly of the lower extremities at night. Both of these conditions should be considered examples of an etiological nonpsychiatric medical condition and thus warrant the selection of the "Yes" branch for this decision point. While periodic leg movements are not part of the diagnostic criteria for Restless Legs Syndrome, if periodic limb movements occur only in the context of Restless Legs Syndrome, a separate diagnosis of Periodic Limb Movement Disorder is not given.

The next step involves a consideration of whether the repetitive movements are due to substance use (e.g., cocaine use causing repeated checking behavior) or a medication. Of note, the DSM-5-TR chapter "Medication-Induced Movement Disorders and Other Adverse Effects of Medication" includes two medication-induced movement disorders characterized by repetitive movements: Tardive Dyskinesia (repetitive, involuntary movements of the tongue, jaw, trunk, or extremities) and Medication-Induced Acute Akathisia (e.g., intense sense of restlessness accompanied by repetitive movements of the lower extremities, such as rocking back and forth from foot to foot).

The decision tree proceeds with the differential diagnosis of disorders characterized by repetitive behaviors with onset during the neurodevelopmental period (i.e., Autism Spectrum Disorder, Stereotypic Movement Disorder, and Tic Disorders). Autism Spectrum Disorder has two main requirements: persistent deficits in social communication and social interaction across multiple contexts (Criterion A); and restricted repetitive patterns of behaviors, interests, or activities (Criterion B), one of which (Criterion B1) involves stereotyped or repetitive motor movements. Therefore, if repetitive behaviors are accompanied by at least one other Criterion B item (i.e., insistence on sameness; inflexible adherence to routines or ritualized behaviors; restricted fixated interests; or hyper- or hyporeactivity to sensory input) plus all three Criterion A items (deficits in social-emotional reciprocity; deficits in nonverbal communication behaviors used for social interaction; and deficits in developing, maintaining, and understanding relationships), then a diagnosis of Autism Spectrum Disorder would apply. Repetitive stereotyped behavior (such as hand waving, body rocking, or head banging) with onset during the neurodevelopmental period in the absence of other symptoms sufficient to meet criteria for Autism Spectrum Disorder would justify a diagnosis of Stereotyped Movement Disorder. Finally, if the repetitive behaviors are characterized by motor movements or vocalizations that are sudden, rapid, and nonrhythmic, a diagnosis of one of the DSM-5-TR Tic Disorders (i.e., Tourette's Disorder, Persistent Motor or Vocal Tic Disorder, or Provisional Tic Disorder) would apply, depending on whether the tics are motor, vocal, or both, and their overall duration.

Next, the decision tree continues with the Obsessive-Compulsive and Related Disorders (excluding Hoarding Disorder), which are characterized by, among other symptoms, repetitive behaviors. In Obsessive-Compulsive Disorder (OCD), the repetitive behaviors (compulsions) are typically performed in response to an obsession and are intended to reduce the anxiety and distress brought on by that obsession (e.g. repetitive hand-washing in response to a contamination obsession). In cases of OCD without obsessions (less than 10%), the repetitive behaviors must be performed according to certain rules that must be applied rigidly. In Body Dysmorphic Disorder, the repetitive behaviors take the form of mirror checking, excessive grooming, skin picking, and seeking reassurance from others, each of which helps, even if temporarily, to reduce the distress associated with the perceived defects or flaws in physical appearance. Trichotillomania (Hair-Pulling Disorder) and Excoriation (Skin-Picking) Disorder, collectively known as body-focused repetitive behavior disorders, are characterized by repetitive behaviors targeting the body (hair pulling and skin picking) that the individual makes repeated attempts to stop.

Repetitive behaviors (such as repeatedly checking the body for evidence of illness, spending inordinate amounts of time searching for information about a feared illness, and repeatedly seeking reassurance from doctors) can occur in both Somatic Symptom Disorder and Illness Anxiety Disorder. The main difference between these two disorders is whether the repetitive behaviors occur in the context of the distressing somatic symptoms that the person fears might be evidence of a life-threatening illness (Somatic Symptom Disorder), or if the presentation is confined to the preoccupation with having a serious illness (Illness Anxiety Disorder).

Stereotypies (repetitive, abnormally frequent, non-goal-directed movements) can occur in Schizophrenia, Catatonia, and other psychotic disorders. If stereotypies occur in the context of other psychotic symptoms, the differential diagnosis of psychotic symptoms needs to be considered. If the stereotypies are accompanied by delusions, hallucinations, or catatonic symptoms, refer to the Delusions Tree (2.5), the Hallucinations Tree (2.6), or the Catatonic Symptoms Tree (2.7), respectively, for the differential diagnosis.

Sudden, rapid, recurrent nonrhythmic motor movements or vocalizations (i.e., tics) with onset after age 18 are diagnosed as Other Specified/Unspecified Tic Disorder, which appears at the end of this tree, because the earlier branch in which Tic Disorders are diagnosed starts with the requirement that the repetitive behaviors have their onset during the neurodevelopmental period (i.e., before age 18).

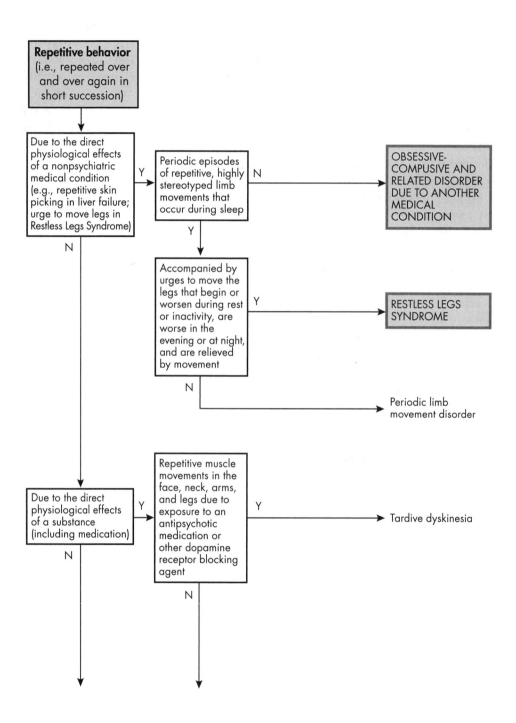

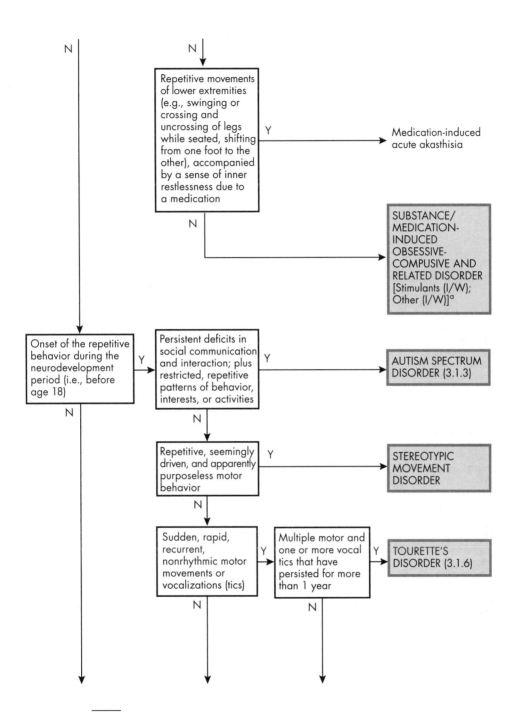

ᵃ I/W = occurring during Substance Intoxication or Substance Withdrawal, as indicated in DSM-5-TR, Table 1: "Diagnoses associated with substance class," p. 545.

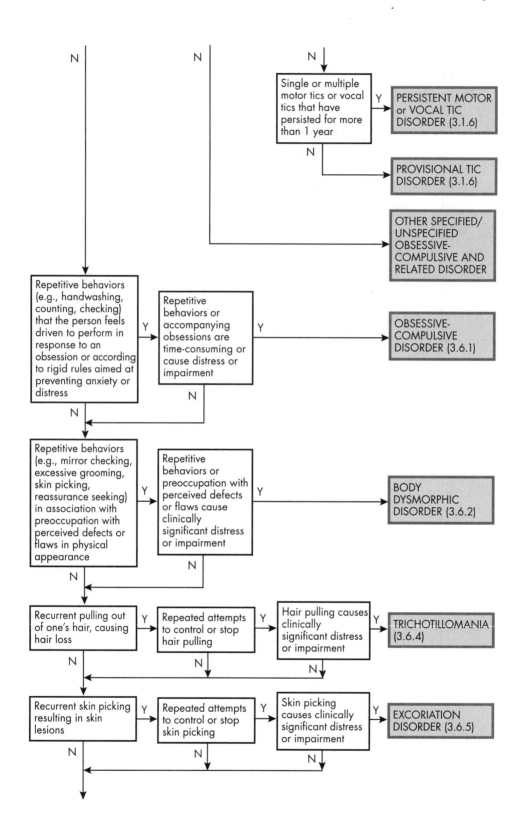

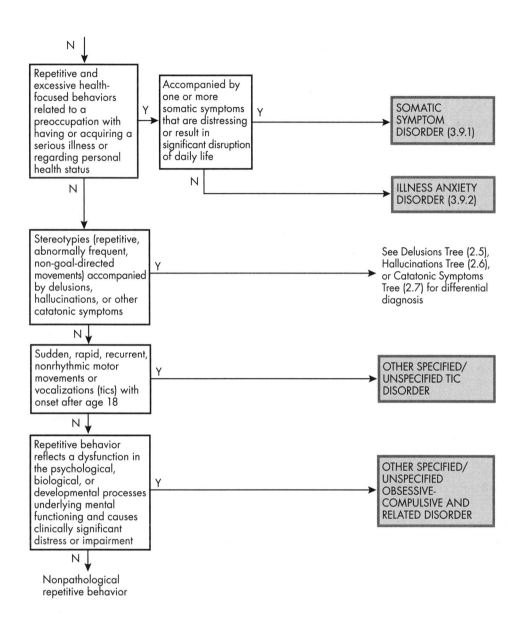

2.17 Decision Tree for Trauma or Psychosocial Stressors Involved in the Etiology

Psychosocial stressors are important in the pathogenesis of all of the DSM-5-TR disorders, but their specific etiological role serves as a defining feature for only a few. Four disorders in DSM-5-TR can be diagnosed only if the individual has been exposed to an extreme stressor: Posttraumatic Stress Disorder, Acute Stress Disorder, Reactive Attachment Disorder, and Disinhibited Social Engagement Disorder. Posttraumatic Stress Disorder requires exposure to an event that involved actual or threatened death, serious injury, or sexual violation, and is characterized by persistent intrusion symptoms associated with the traumatic event (e.g., intrusive memories of the event, distressing dreams, flashbacks, distress upon exposure to cues reminiscent of the event), avoidance of stimuli associated with the event, negative alterations in cognitions and moods associated with the event (e.g., the individual's negative beliefs about themselves and the world, distorted blame of self or others, feelings of detachment, persistent negative state, inability to experience positive emotions), and marked alterations in reactivity and arousal. The symptom profile of Acute Stress Disorder closely resembles that of Posttraumatic Stress Disorder, except that the symptoms have lasted for less than 1 month. Reactive Attachment Disorder and Disinhibited Social Engagement Disorder both require extended exposure to extremes of insufficient care as a young child, such as frequent changes in primary caregivers or being raised in poorly staffed institutional settings.

Although not required as part of the disorder definition, Brief Psychotic Disorder, Dissociative Amnesia, and Functional Neurological Symptom Disorder (Conversion Disorder) often develop in response to a severe psychosocial stressor. A diagnosis of Brief Psychotic Disorder applies if the reaction to an extreme stressor involves the development of psychotic symptoms lasting for less than 1 month. If the individual is unable to recall important autobiographical information related to a traumatic experience, then the diagnosis of Dissociative Amnesia might apply. If the person develops symptoms of altered voluntary motor or sensory function that are incompatible with any recognized neurological condition in response to a psychosocial stressor, then a diagnosis of Functional Neurological Symptom Disorder would apply. Although the development of each of these disorders is often related to exposure to a traumatic stressor, any of these three conditions can develop without exposure to a stressor.

In cases where the psychosocial stressor involves the death of a loved one, multiple psychiatric diagnoses, including Prolonged Grief Disorder, Major Depressive Disorder, and Posttraumatic Stress Disorder may be applicable. A diagnosis of Prolonged Grief Disorder should be considered if, after at least 12 months have elapsed since the death of a person to whom the bereaved individual was close (or after 6 months, if the bereaved individual is a child or adolescent), severe impairing grief symptoms continue to persist. It should be noted that from a symptomatic perspective, the characteristic symptoms of Prolonged Grief Disorder, such as intense yearning/longing for the deceased and preoccupation with thoughts and memories of the deceased, are also characteristic of a normal grief reaction. What makes it a disorder is the persistence of impairing grief symptoms nearly every day beyond the first year following the loss. In cases where the circumstances of the loved one's death qualify as a Criterion A Posttraumatic Stress Disorder traumatic event to the individual (e.g., the individual observes the loved one being shot to death during a robbery; the individual survives an automobile accident that resulted in the death of the loved one), an additional diagnosis of Posttraumatic Stress Disorder might also apply. In some cases, a grief reaction might evolve into a full-blown Major Depressive Episode, in which case a diagnosis of Major Depressive Disorder, Bipolar I Disorder, or Bipolar II Disorder might be applicable. Finally, if clinically significant symptoms that do not meet criteria for a Major Depressive Episode or any other specific disorder have developed in response to the loss of a loved one, then the most appropriate diagnosis would be Adjustment Disorder.

Many clinicians are confused about the relationship between the Adjustment Disorders and the other conditions in DSM-5-TR that are often precipitated by the presence of a psychosocial stressor. Adjustment Disorder is diagnosed for those presentations in which the maladaptive response to the stressor causes clinically significant distress or impairment but does not meet the threshold requirements for any specific DSM-5-TR disorder. In contrast, when the criteria are met for a specific DSM-5-TR disorder, that disorder is diagnosed regardless of the presence or absence of associated stressors. For example, if a depressive reaction occurs in response to a job loss or the individual learning that they have a serious illness, the diagnosis is Major Depressive Disorder if the reaction meets the full criteria for a Major Depressive Episode. A less severe, but nonetheless clinically significant, depressive reaction might instead be diagnosed as Adjustment Disorder With Depressed Mood.

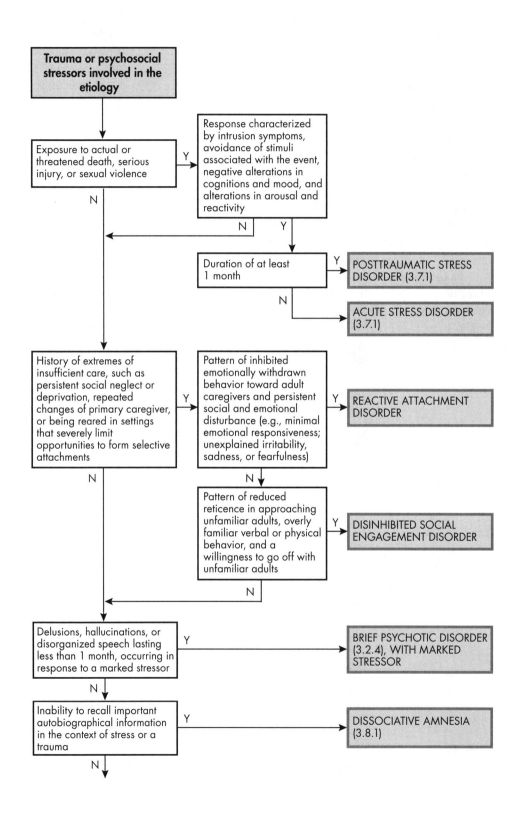

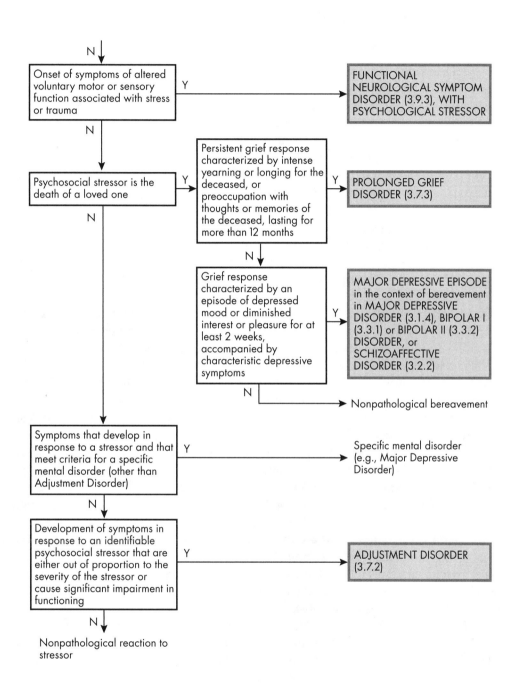

2.18 Decision Tree for Depersonalization/ Derealization

Dissociation is a mental process of the individual disconnecting from their thoughts, feelings, memories, or sense of identity. Dissociation is a commonly experienced normal phenomenon and not necessarily evidence of psychopathology. Everyday examples include daydreaming, blanking out while driving until missing an exit, "getting lost" in a book or movie, and zoning out during a lecture and then realizing 10–15 minutes have passed. Each of these examples involve the individual briefly losing touch with awareness of their immediate surroundings before reconnecting to their present place, time, and established identity. In contrast, pathological dissociation can range in severity along a continuum from distressing episodes of the individual feeling detached from their body, mind, feelings, or sensation (depersonalization); feeling detached from other people, objects, or surroundings (derealization); having significant gaps in memory about everyday events, personal information, or past traumatic events; to the co-existence of two or more distinct identities or personality states accompanied by changes in behavior, memory, perception, and thinking.

Transient symptoms of depersonalization and/or derealization are common in the general population, with a prevalence reported to range from 26% to 74% and between 31% to 66% at the time of a traumatic event (e.g., a motor vehicle accident). This is in contrast to the relatively low prevalence of Dissociative Disorders, each with a reported 12-month prevalence of between 1% and 2%. Even though dissociation is a hallmark of the DSM-5-TR Dissociative Disorders, depersonalization and derealization in particular can occur as a symptom of any number of other DSM-5-TR disorders, such as Panic Disorder and Posttraumatic Stress Disorder.

Like most psychiatric symptoms, depersonalization and derealization can be caused by the direct effects of a substance or medication on the central nervous system (e.g., Cannabis Intoxication, Alcohol Withdrawal), as well as be part of the symptomatic presentation of a nonpsychiatric medical condition such as a seizure disorder or migraines. In contrast to the other DSM-5-TR diagnostic classes that include specific diagnoses for symptomatic presentations that are induced by a substance/medication or due to a medical condition (e.g., Caffeine-Induced Anxiety Disorder, Anxiety Disorder Due to Hyperthyroidism, respectively), there is no substance/medication-induced dissociative disorder or dissociative disorder due to a medical condition in DSM-5-TR. Instead, dissociative symptoms induced by substance or medication use must be diagnosed as Substance Intoxication (if the dissociative symptoms occur during intoxication), Substance Withdrawal (if symptoms occur during withdrawal), or an Adverse Effect of Medication (if the dissociative symptoms are a side effect of a medication; e.g., some antihistamines). Clinically significant dissociative symptoms caused by a medical condition can be diagnosed by using the residual category Other Specified Mental Disorder Due to Another Medical Condition (e.g., Other Specified Mental Disorder Due to Seizure Disorder).

After the clinician rules out substances and medical conditions as the cause of the symptoms of depersonalization or derealization, the next step is to consider whether the symptoms are associated with delusions or hallucinations that may be indicative of a diagnosis of Schizophrenia (given that depersonalization and derealization are included among its associated features; DSM-5-TR, p. 116). If depersonalization or derealization is associated with hallucinations, the clinician must consider whether these hallucinatory experiences are better explained by intrusions of personality states into the individual's awareness, which are indicative of Dissociative Identity Disorder. If that is the case (i.e., hallucinatory experiences are not indicative of psychosis), the clinician continues with the remainder of the Depersonalization/Derealization Tree to make the diagnosis of Dissociative Identity Disorder. Otherwise, the clinician needs to continue with either the Delusions Tree (2.5) or the Hallucinations Tree (2.6) to determine whether a diagnosis of a Schizophrenia Spectrum and Other Psychotic Disorder may be appropriate.

Next, the clinician considers whether depersonalization and/or derealization are part of the clinical presentation of Acute Stress Disorder or Posttraumatic Stress Disorder, consistent with the association between dissociative symptoms and exposure to trauma. Acute Stress Disorder includes dissociative flashbacks as Criterion B3, depersonalization/derealization as Criterion B6, and dissociative amnesia as Criterion B7. Posttraumatic Stress Disorder includes dissociative flashbacks as Criterion B3, dissociative amnesia as Criterion D1, and a specifier "With Dissociative Symptoms" if there is recurrent depersonalization or derealization.

Depersonalization and derealization can be part of the presentation of the DSM-5-TR Dissociative Disorders. Even though neither depersonalization nor derealization is an explicit defining feature of Dissociative Identity Disorder (subjective division and disconnection of personality states) or Dissociative Amnesia (disconnection from memories), depersonalization and derealization are part of presentations of both of these disorders. Because the diagnosis of Dissociative Identity Disorder requires the presence of Dissociative Amnesia, to differentiate between these diagnoses, the tree inquires first about the inability to recall important information and then asks about disruption in identity. Next in the decision tree, the decision point about apparently purposeful travel or bewildered wandering reflects whether the Dissociative Fugue subtype applies to the diagnosis of Dissociative Amnesia.

Depersonalization, derealization, and other dissociative symptoms such as dissociative amnesia are often associated with episodes of Functional Neurological Symptom Disorder (Conversion Disorder), especially at times of symptom onset. In fact, some individuals with Dissociative Identity Disorder present to clinical attention with functional neurological symptoms (e.g., nonepileptic seizures, sensory deficits, motor disturbances). While Functional Neurological Symptom Disorder is classified in DSM-5-TR as a Somatic Symptom Disorder (with the focus on its presenting symptoms), the World Health Organization classifies such presentations in the Dissociative Disorders chapter of ICD-10 and ICD-11 (i.e., Dissociative Neurological Symptom Disorder) because of its presumed mechanism (an involuntary discontinuity in the normal integration of motor, sensory, or cognitive functions).

Depersonalization/derealization is one of the 13 symptoms that can accompany the abrupt surge of intense fear and discomfort that characterizes a Panic Attack. Along with paranoid ideation, depersonalization/derealization also characterizes the transient stress-related episodes that can occur in Borderline Personality Disorder (Criterion 9) and Schizotypal Personality Disorder (Criterion 3). Finally, after all other explanations for the symptoms of depersonalization/derealization have been considered and ruled out, the diagnosis of Depersonalization/Derealization Disorder can be made if the persistent or recurrent experiences of depersonalization/derealization cause clinically significant distress or impairment.

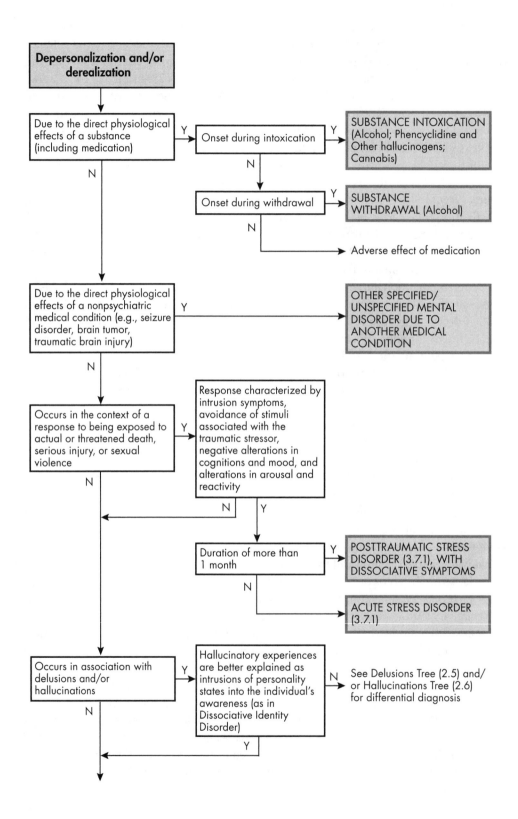

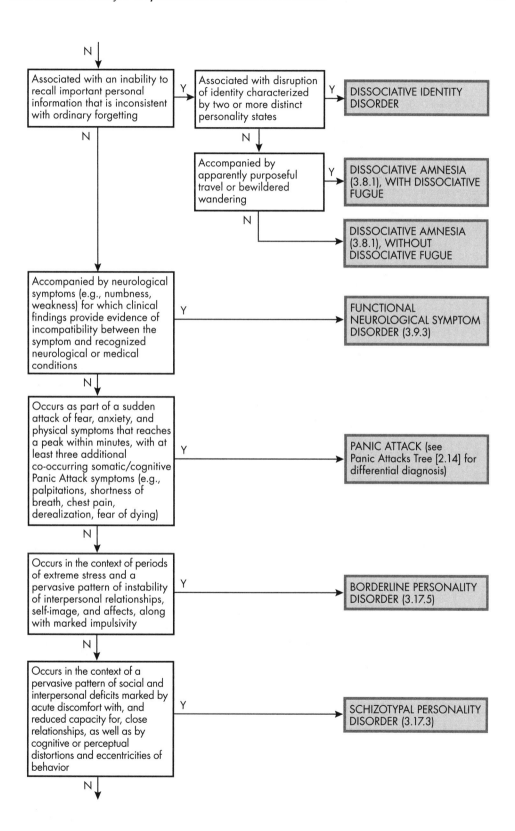

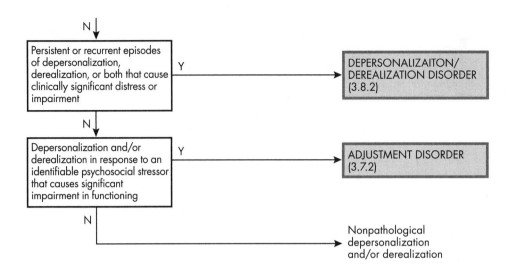

2.19 Decision Tree for Somatic Complaints or Illness/Appearance Anxiety

When a patient presents with distressing somatic complaints, the focus of the differential diagnosis is usually on which nonpsychiatric medical condition best explains the somatic complaints. However, when the somatic complaints are accompanied by abnormal thoughts, feelings, and behaviors related to the somatic symptoms, the presence of a Somatic Symptom Disorder or other mental disorder should be considered.

Physical complaints that are feigned by the individual warrant either the mental disorder diagnosis Factitious Disorder or the nondisordered condition known as Malingering. The differentiation between these two conditions depends on a consideration of the context in which the somatic symptoms developed. If the feigning of the symptoms occurs in the absence of obvious external rewards, the diagnosis is Factitious Disorder, whereas feigning in settings in which the presence of the somatic symptoms provides an obvious financial or other benefit to the patient suggests Malingering.

Somatic complaints can occur as a manifestation of a wide variety of psychiatric conditions. Substance Intoxication or Substance Withdrawal is typically manifested as a characteristic syndrome of somatic and behavioral symptoms. States of high anxiety are typically associated with a variety of somatic complaints. Consequently, somatic symptoms (e.g., muscle tension, chest pain) are included in the diagnostic criteria for Panic Disorder and Generalized Anxiety Disorder and may be the primary reason that patients with these disorders seek treatment. In other cases, the somatic complaints are related to the manifestations of a psychotic disorder (e.g., somatic delusions) or an Obsessive-Compulsive and Related Disorder, such as the preoccupation with an imagined physical defect in Body Dysmorphic Disorder.

When the somatic complaints themselves are the patient's central focus, a diagnosis of one of the DSM-5-TR Somatic Symptom and Related Disorders might be most appropriate. Patients presenting with neurological symptoms such as paralysis or seizures which, upon examination and laboratory investigation, do not conform to a pattern characteristic of a known neurological or other medical condition, can be diagnosed with Functional Neurological Symptom Disorder (Conversion Disorder). Other types of somatic complaints, when accompanied by disproportionate thoughts about the seriousness of the illness, persistently high levels of anxiety about health or about symptoms, or the devotion of excessive time and energy to symptoms or health concerns, may warrant a diagnosis of Somatic Symptom Disorder. In contrast to the DSM-IV Somatoform Disorder diagnoses, in which the somatic complaints were by definition medically unexplained, a diagnosis of Somatic Symptom Disorder in DSM-5-TR can be given to patients with a bona fide medical illness. The DSM-5-TR diagnosis depends on the presence of cognitions, feelings, and behaviors that are, in the clinician's judgment, "excessive" given the nature of the nonpsychiatric medical condition. To avoid pathologizing appropriate reactions to serious or disabling nonpsychiatric medical conditions, this diagnosis should be used very cautiously in medically ill individuals, being reserved only for cases in which the person's reactions to having the medical illness are clearly extreme and maladaptive.

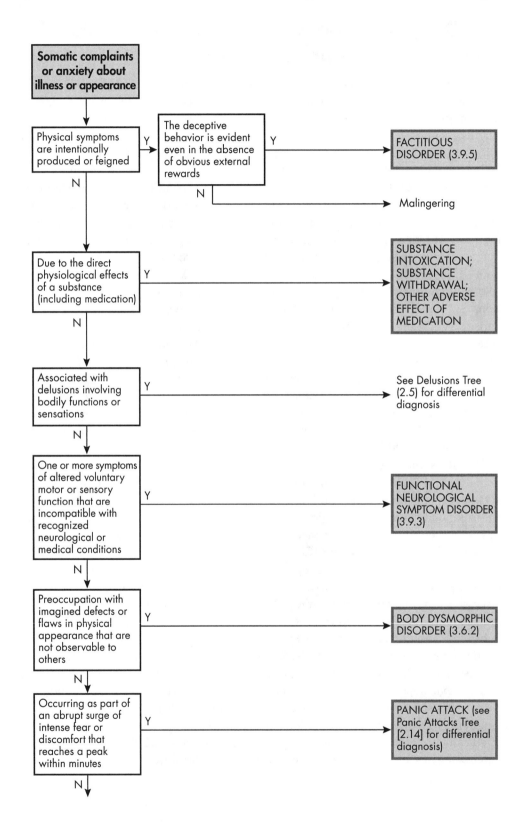

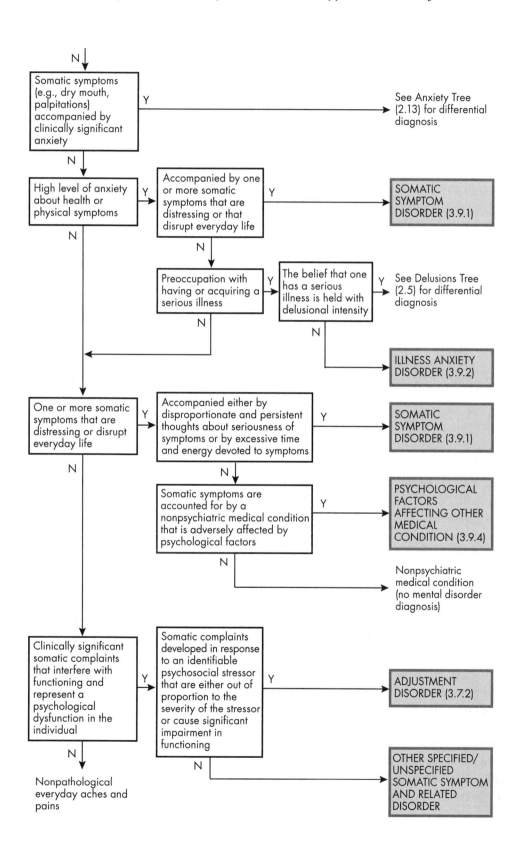

2.20 Decision Tree for Appetite or Weight Change or Abnormal Eating Behavior

This decision tree covers the wide range of disorders in the differential diagnosis of changes in appetite or weight, as well as differential diagnosis of abnormal eating behaviors; this includes consideration of mood disorders, psychotic disorders, and feeding and eating disorders. Because changes in appetite and weight are commonly caused by nonpsychiatric medical conditions, the clinician's first thought should always be to rule out cancer, endocrine disturbances, chronic infections, and other illnesses before assuming that the symptoms are psychiatric. This approach is especially important when weight loss or gain is of major proportions and occurs in conjunction with other physical symptoms. Note that in the assessment of an etiological nonpsychiatric medical condition, in the branch of the decision tree covering the differential diagnosis of weight gain, obesity is listed as one of the possible etiological nonpsychiatric medical conditions. Obesity (defined as a body mass index [BMI] ≥30) by itself is not considered a mental disorder but instead a nonpsychiatric medical condition. A BMI of ≥30 would be considered a feature of a psychiatric disorder only when it is a consequence of a disturbed eating pattern (such as in Binge-Eating Disorder).

Changes in appetite and weight (in both directions) are also frequently caused by the use of certain drugs of abuse (especially stimulants and cannabis) and certain prescribed medications. In fact, one of the major reasons for noncompliance with many of the psychotropic medications (e.g., selective serotonin reuptake inhibitors, serotonin-norepinephrine reuptake inhibitors, tricyclic antidepressants, lithium, divalproex, monoamine oxidase inhibitors, atypical antipsychotics) is the fear of weight gain that not infrequently accompanies their use. Identifying the cause of weight changes can be difficult precisely because many of the conditions treated by these psychotropic medications are themselves associated with changes in weight, independent of the use of medication. For example, if a patient with depression gains weight while being treated with an antidepressant, this could be a side effect of the antidepressant, a characteristic symptom of the depression, or a desirable treatment effect (e.g., improved appetite in someone previously experiencing loss of appetite).

Because changes in appetite and gains or losses in weight are common in many different psychiatric disorders, they are relatively nonspecific on their own in providing clues to the differential diagnosis. Therefore, the clinician must rely on the temporal relationship of the appetite or weight changes with the other presenting symptoms in deciding which is the most appropriate explanation for the change. For example, is the individual not eating because of a delusion that the food is poisoned (as in Schizophrenia, Delusional Disorder, or a Mood Disorder with Psychotic Features); because of a feeling of being unworthy or a loss of pleasure in eating (as in Major Depressive Episode); or because of a diminished appetite or being "too busy" (as in Manic Episode)?

The decision tree is split into three sections: one that provides the differential diagnosis for decreased appetite, weight loss, or failure to make expected weight gains (in a child or adolescent); the second for increased appetite or weight gain not due to binge eating; and the third for increased weight due to binge eating. Decreased appetite or loss of weight is a common feature of disorders with prominent depressive or dysphoric mood: Major Depressive Disorder, Persistent Depressive Disorder, Premenstrual Dysphoric Disorder, and Major Depressive Episodes in Bipolar I and Bipolar II Disorder or Schizoaffective Disorder. Weight loss can also occur as an associated feature of a Manic Episode, related to the accompanying increase in activity or energy and neglect of regular mealtimes. In Anorexia Nervosa, the pathological fear of being (or becoming) fat can result in an often dangerously low weight. Some individuals have a significant weight loss (or a failure to make expected weight gain) in the absence of a fear of gaining weight or being fat. Instead, their weight loss occurs in the context of an eating or feeding disturbance (e.g., lack of interest in eating; avoidance of food based on extreme sensitivity to its sensory characteristics, such as its appearance, color, texture, temperature, taste); or in anticipation of aversive consequences to eating, such as choking. Such individuals may be diagnosed with Avoidant/Restrictive Food Intake Disorder.

Although binge eating can occur in Anorexia Nervosa (Binge-Eating/Purging Type) and in Bulimia Nervosa, these disorders typically do not result in weight gain because in both conditions, the individual engages in compensatory behavior to counteract the consequences of binge eating (e.g., purging, fasting, excessive exercise). In contrast, individuals with Binge-Eating Disorder engage in regular binge eating (i.e., at least once per week for at least 3 months) without employing any inappropriate compensatory mechanisms to keep from gaining weight. Thus, these individuals are typically overweight.

Clinically significant changes in appetite and weight that are the result of a psychological or biological dysfunction in the individual and that are judged to have occurred in response to an identifiable psychosocial stressor can be diagnosed as Adjustment Disorder. Finally, it is important to remember that fad dieting and concerns about gaining and losing weight are fairly ubiquitous aspects of life. A diagnosis of Other Specified or Unspecified Feeding or Eating Disorder should be given only if the eating disturbance represents a psychological or biological dysfunction in the individual.

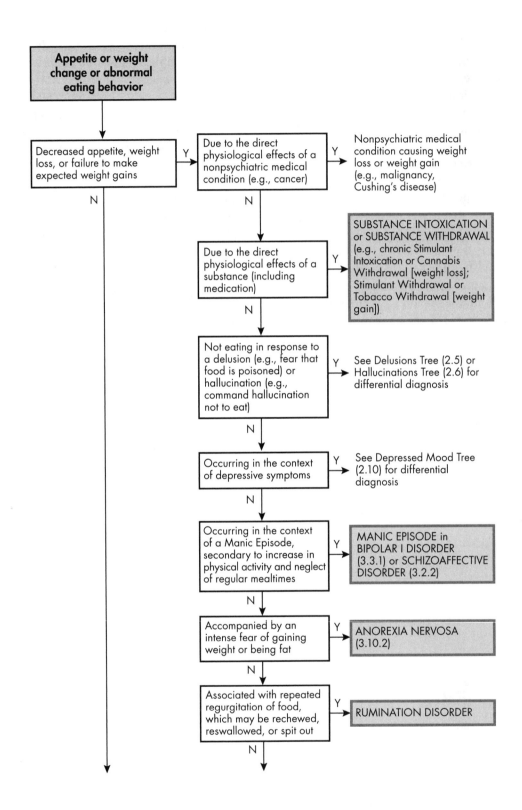

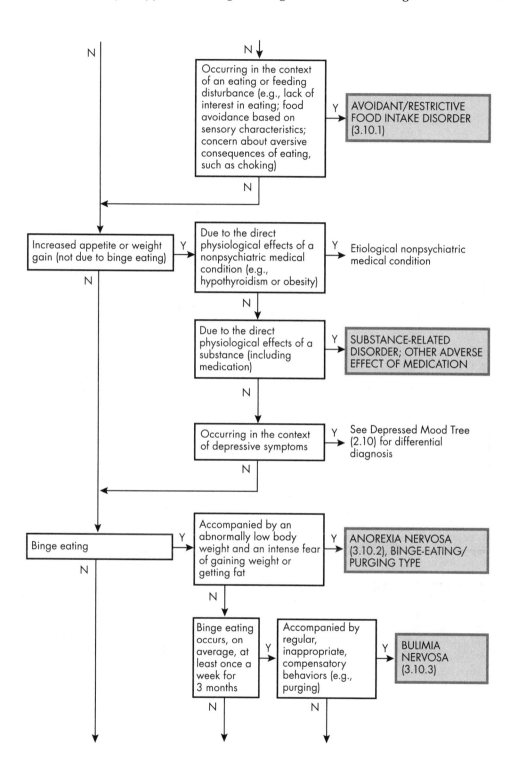

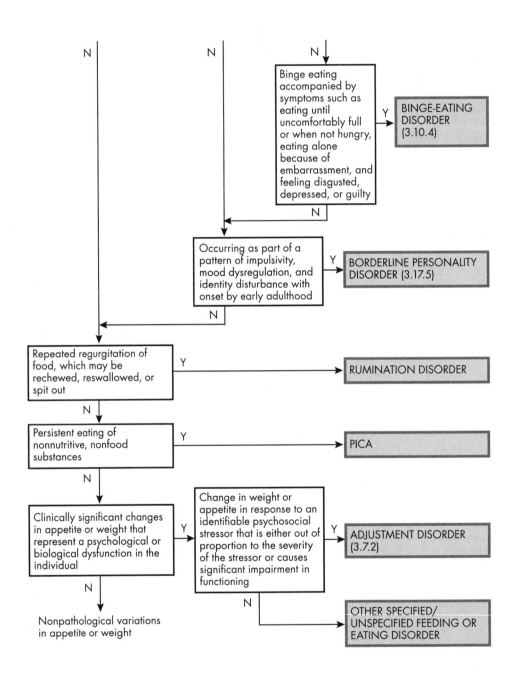

2.21 Decision Tree for Insomnia

Insomnia is defined in DSM-5-TR as dissatisfaction with sleep quantity or quality with complaints of difficulty initiating or maintaining sleep. Drugs of abuse and many prescribed and over-the-counter medications have insomnia as a significant side effect. For drugs of abuse, typically a diagnosis of Substance Intoxication or Substance Withdrawal will suffice to cover the symptoms of insomnia. A diagnosis of Substance/Medication-Induced Sleep Disorder, Insomnia Type, should be considered only if the insomnia predominates in the clinical picture and is sufficiently severe to warrant clinical attention. A diagnosis of Substance/Medication-Induced Sleep Disorder can also be given for clinically notable insomnia related to medications.

The clinician must then rule out other sleep disorders as the cause of the insomnia, because the manifestations of these other sleep disorders can interrupt nighttime sleep:

- DSM-5-TR includes three distinct disorders under the general rubric of Breathing-Related Sleep Disorders, each of which can cause insomnia because of middle-of-the-night awakenings.
  1. Obstructive Sleep Apnea Hypopnea, the most common form of Breathing-Related Sleep Disorder, is characterized by repeated episodes of upper airway obstruction during sleep.
  2. Central Sleep Apnea is characterized by repeated episodes of apneas and hypopneas during sleep caused by variability in respiratory effort.
  3. Sleep-Related Hypoventilation is characterized by episodes of decreased respiration during sleep, which are associated with elevated CO_2 levels.
- Non–Rapid Eye Movement Sleep Arousal Disorder is characterized by recurrent episodes of incomplete awakening from sleep, usually during the first third of the night, which can take the form of Sleep Terrors or Sleepwalking.
- Nightmare Disorder and REM Sleep Behavior Disorder describe problematic phenomena occurring during REM sleep: extended, extremely dysphoric, and well-remembered dreams in the case of Nightmare Disorder; and repeated arousals during REM sleep with vocalizations or complex motor behavior in the case of REM Sleep Behavior Disorder.
- Restless Legs Syndrome is characterized by recurrent or persistent urges to move the legs in response to unpleasant sensations.
- Circadian Rhythm Sleep-Wake Disorder is characterized by a mismatch between the individual's schedule and natural sleep-wake patterns.

Insomnia that occurs exclusively during, and is better explained by, any of these sleep disorders does not warrant a separate diagnosis of Insomnia Disorder. However, if the severity of the insomnia exceeds what would be expected from the other sleep disorder (and thus is not better explained by the other sleep disorder) or occurs at times other than when that sleep disorder is present, a comorbid diagnosis of Insomnia Disorder may be appropriate.

The next step in the assessment is to consider whether the insomnia is actually a symptom of another mental disorder. A number of mental disorders, such as Major Depressive Disorder, may include prominent symptoms of insomnia. If the insomnia is adequately explained by the mental disorder, only the mental disorder is diagnosed and an additional diagnosis of Insomnia Disorder is generally not made. If, however, the insomnia predominates in the clinical picture and warrants clinical attention, then a comorbid diagnosis of Insomnia Disorder may be appropriate. Similarly, a number of nonpsychiatric medical conditions, such as back pain, may significantly disrupt sleep. An additional diagnosis of Insomnia Disorder may also be appropriate in such cases if the insomnia is not adequately explained by the nonpsychiatric medical condition.

Some difficulty falling asleep (or maintaining sleep) is to be expected in everyone's life, especially in association with psychosocial stressors and as part of advancing age. Insomnia should be considered as evidence of a mental disorder only if the insomnia is severe, is prolonged, and results in clinically significant distress or impairment.

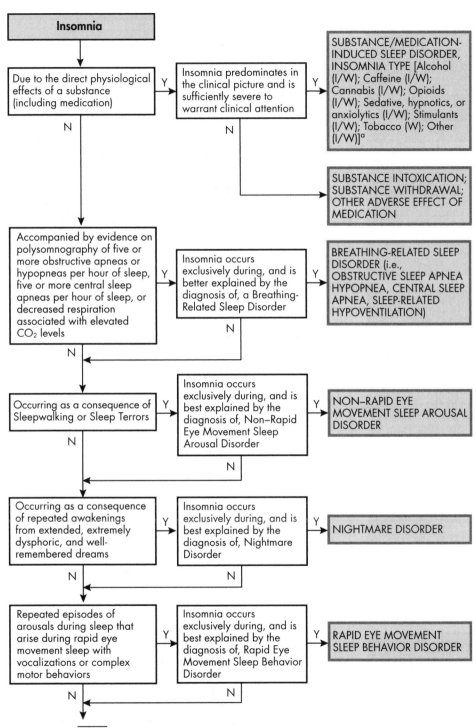

a I = occurring during Substance Intoxication; I/W = occurring during Substance Intoxication or Substance Withdrawal; W = occurring during Substance Withdrawal, as indicated in DSM-5-TR, Table 1: "Diagnoses associated with substance class," p. 545.

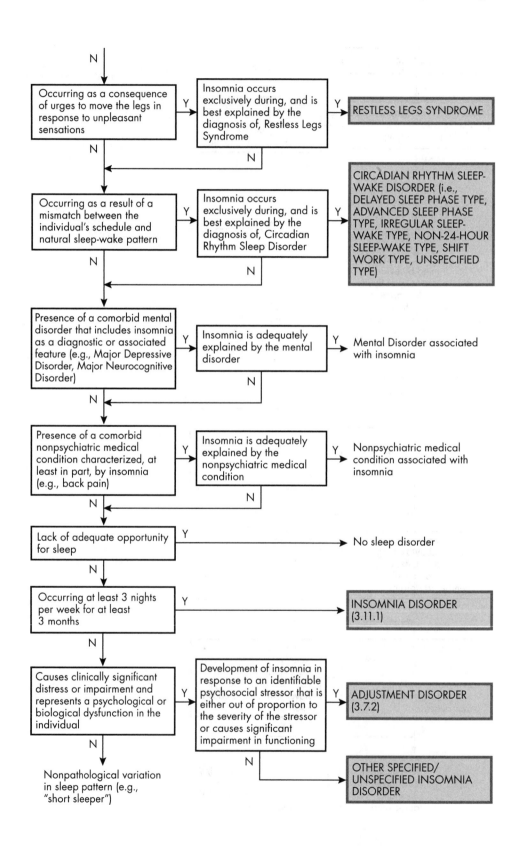

2.22 Decision Tree for Hypersomnolence

Hypersomnolence is a broad diagnostic term and includes symptoms of excessive quantity of sleep (e.g., extended nighttime sleep or involuntary daytime naps), deteriorated quality of wakefulness (e.g., difficulty awakening or inability to remain awake when required), and sleep inertia (i.e., a period of impaired performance and reduced vigilance upon awakening). A diagnosis of Hypersomnolence Disorder should be considered only if the person has been regularly getting adequate amounts of sleep—individuals would not qualify for this diagnosis if they are sleep deprived either because of insomnia or to accommodate their overscheduled lives.

Drugs of abuse and many prescribed and over-the-counter medications have daytime drowsiness as a significant side effect. For drugs of abuse, typically a diagnosis of Substance Intoxication or Substance Withdrawal will suffice to cover the hypersomnolence. A diagnosis of Substance-Induced Sleep Disorder, Daytime Sleepiness Type, should be considered only if the hypersomnolence predominates in the clinical picture and is sufficiently severe to warrant clinical attention. A diagnosis of Medication-Induced Sleep Disorder can also be given for clinically notable hypersomnolence related to medications.

The clinician must then rule out other specific sleep disorders as the cause of the hypersomnolence, given that daytime sleepiness is a characteristic feature of some specific sleep disorders (e.g., Narcolepsy) or might be a consequence of the disturbance in nighttime sleep caused by another sleep disorder (e.g., Nightmare Disorder).

- Narcolepsy is characterized by recurrent periods of an irrepressible need for sleep accompanied by cataplexy (i.e., brief periods of sudden bilateral loss of muscle tone precipitated by laughter), hypocretin deficiency (as measured in cerebrospinal fluid), or characteristic polysomnographic findings (i.e., rapid eye movement [REM] sleep latency of 15 minutes or less, or a multiple sleep latency test with mean sleep latency of 8 minutes or less and two or more sleep-onset REM periods).
- DSM-5-TR includes three distinct disorders under the general rubric of Breathing-Related Sleep Disorders, each of which can cause daytime fatigue.
  1. Obstructive Sleep Apnea Hypopnea, the most common form of Breathing-Related Sleep Disorder, is characterized by repeated episodes of upper airway obstruction during sleep.
  2. Central Sleep Apnea is characterized by repeated episodes of apneas and hypopneas during sleep caused by variability in respiratory effort.
  3. Sleep-Related Hypoventilation is characterized by episodes of decreased respiration during sleep, which are associated with elevated CO_2 levels.
- Non–Rapid Eye Movement Sleep Arousal Disorder is characterized by recurrent episodes of incomplete awakening from sleep, usually during the first third of the night, which can take the form of Sleep Terrors or Sleepwalking.
- Nightmare Disorder and REM Sleep Behavior Disorder describe problematic phenomena occurring during REM sleep: extended, extremely dysphoric, and well-remembered dreams in the case of Nightmare Disorder; and repeated arousals during REM sleep with vocalizations or complex motor behavior in the case of REM Sleep Behavior Disorder.

- Restless Legs Syndrome is characterized by recurrent or persistent urges to move the legs in response to unpleasant sensations.
- Circadian Rhythm Sleep-Wake Disorder is characterized by a mismatch between the individual's schedule and natural sleep-wake patterns.
- Insomnia Disorder is characterized by a predominant complaint of dissatisfaction with sleep quality or quantity, associated with difficulty falling asleep, maintaining sleep, or early-morning awakening.

Hypersomnolence that occurs exclusively during, and is better explained by, any of these sleep disorders does not warrant a separate diagnosis of Hypersomnolence Disorder. However, if the severity of the hypersomnolence exceeds what would be expected from another sleep disorder (and thus is not better explained by the other sleep disorder) or occurs at times other than when that sleep disorder is present, a comorbid diagnosis of Hypersomnolence Disorder may be appropriate.

The next step in the assessment is to consider whether the hypersomnolence is actually a symptom of another mental disorder. A number of mental disorders may include prominent symptoms of hypersomnolence, especially in Major Depressive Episodes With Atypical Features, as seen in Major Depressive Disorder, Bipolar I Disorder, and Bipolar II Disorder. If the daytime fatigue is adequately explained by the mental disorder, only the mental disorder is diagnosed and an additional diagnosis of Hypersomnolence Disorder is not made. If, however, the hypersomnolence predominates in the clinical picture and warrants clinical attention, then a comorbid diagnosis of Hypersomnolence Disorder may be appropriate. Similarly, a number of nonpsychiatric medical conditions, such as mononucleosis, may be characterized by daytime fatigue. An additional diagnosis of Hypersomnolence Disorder may also be appropriate in such cases if the degree of hypersomnolence is not adequately explained by the nonpsychiatric medical condition.

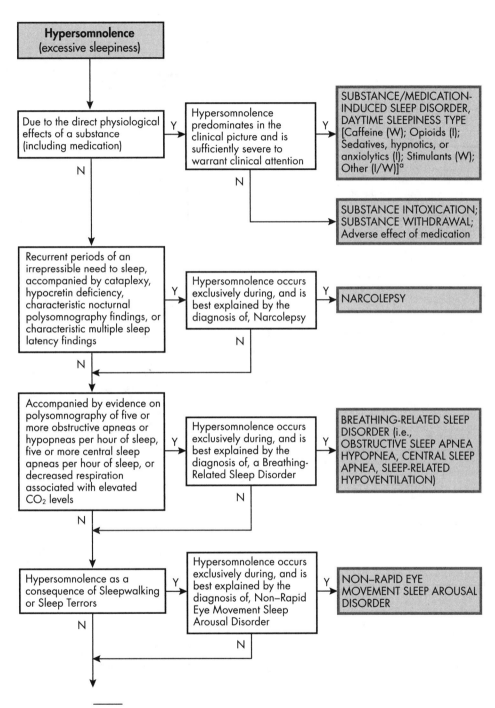

ᵃ I = occurring during Substance Intoxication; I/W = occurring during
Substance Intoxication or Substance Withdrawal; W = occurring during
Substance Withdrawal, as indicated in DSM-5-TR, Table 1: "Diagnoses
associated with substance class," p. 545.

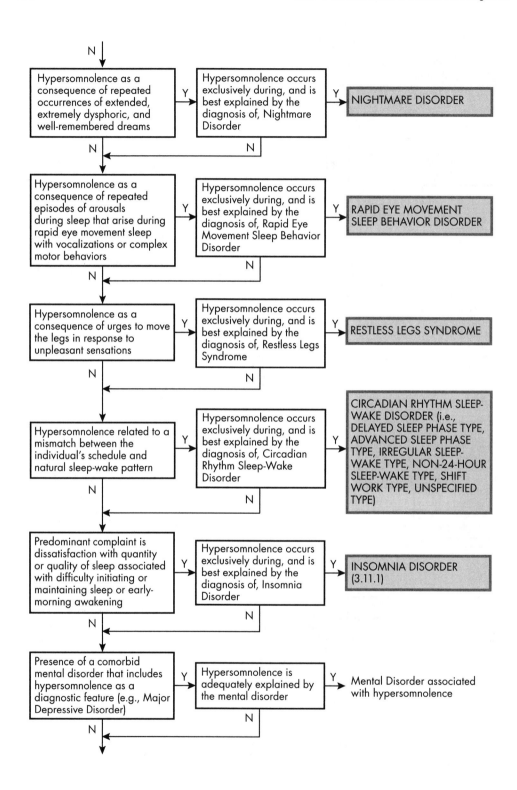

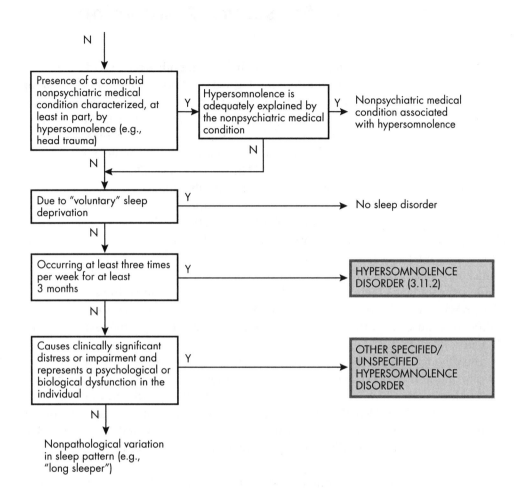

2.23 Decision Tree for Sexual Dysfunction in a Female

The major difficulty in evaluating sexual dysfunctions in both women and men is that there are no accepted guidelines for determining what is "normal" sexual functioning. The threshold for normal sexual functioning varies with the woman's age and prior sexual experience, the availability and novelty of partners, and the expectations and standards characteristic of the woman's cultural, ethnic, or religious group. Successful arousal and orgasm require a level of sexual stimulation that is adequate in focus, intensity, and duration. A diagnosis of Female Sexual Interest/Arousal Disorder or Female Orgasmic Disorder therefore requires a clinical judgment that the woman has experienced adequate stimulation. Moreover, occasional sexual dysfunction is an inherent part of human sexuality and is not indicative of a disorder unless the symptoms have persisted for at least approximately 6 months and result in marked distress or interpersonal difficulty.

Once the clinical judgment has been made that the sexual dysfunction is clinically significant, the next task is to determine its underlying etiology. The possible etiologies include psychological factors, nonpsychiatric medical conditions, the side effects of many prescribed medications, and the consequence of drug abuse. This evaluation can be difficult because very often more than one etiology contributes to the sexual dysfunction. Before deciding that a sexual dysfunction is mediated entirely by psychological factors, the clinician needs to consider the possible contribution of a nonpsychiatric medical condition or substance (including medication side effects), especially because these etiologies often have specific treatment implications (e.g., discontinuation of the offending medication). Also, the clinician needs to remember that the identification of a specific etiological nonpsychiatric medical condition, medication, or drug of abuse does not negate the important contribution of psychological factors to the etiology of the sexual dysfunction.

Sexual problems are also commonly associated with a number of mental disorders (e.g., Depressive Disorders, Anxiety Disorders, Schizophrenia Spectrum and Other Psychotic Disorders). An additional diagnosis of a sexual dysfunction is not given if the sexual problems are better explained by the mental disorder. For example, low sexual desire occurring only during a Major Depressive Episode would not justify a separate diagnosis of Female Sexual Interest/Arousal Disorder. Both diagnoses can be given only if the low sexual desire is judged to be independent of the Depressive Disorder (i.e., it precedes the onset of the Major Depressive Episode or persists long after the depression has remitted). Similarly, sexual dysfunction that is better explained as a consequence of severe relationship distress would be diagnosed as a relational problem rather than a sexual dysfunction unless evidence demonstrated that the sexual dysfunction occurred independently of the relational problem.

After substances, nonpsychiatric medical conditions, and relationship distress have been considered and ruled out, the focus then goes to the primary sexual dysfunctions themselves. In DSM-5-TR (unchanged from DSM-5), the female version of the DSM-IV-TR category Hypoactive Sexual Desire Disorder and the DSM-IV-TR category Female Sexual Arousal Disorder have been combined into a single diagnostic category called Female Sexual Interest/Arousal Disorder, reflecting evidence that sexual desire and sexual arousal are often not separable concepts in woman. Thus, Female Sexual Interest/Arousal Disorder covers a wide variety of problems, including reduced interest in sexual activity, reduced frequency of erotic thoughts or fantasies, reduced frequency of initiation of sexual activity, reduced sexual excitement or pleasure during sexual activity, reduced interest or arousal in response to erotic cues, and reduced genital and nongenital sensations during sexual activity. Female Orgasmic Disorder includes marked delay in achieving orgasm, marked infrequency or absence of orgasm, or markedly reduced intensity of orgasmic sensations. Unchanged from DSM-5, the DSM-5-TR category Genito-Pelvic Pain/Penetration Disorder combines two DSM-IV-TR categories (i.e., Vaginismus and Dyspareunia) and includes difficulties with having vaginal intercourse or penetration; marked vulvovaginal or pelvic pain during intercourse or penetration attempts; marked fear or anxiety about vulvovaginal or pelvic pain in anticipation of, during, or as a result of vaginal penetration; or marked tensing or tightening of the pelvic floor muscles during attempted vaginal penetration.

If a sexual dysfunction does not meet criteria for one of the sexual dysfunctions described above (perhaps because of inadequate frequency or duration) and it is judged to be a maladaptive response to a psychosocial stressor, a diagnosis of an Adjustment Disorder may be appropriate. Otherwise, if it is judged to be clinically significant and that it represents a psychological or biological dysfunction in the individual, then Other Specified/Unspecified Sexual Dysfunction may be diagnosed.

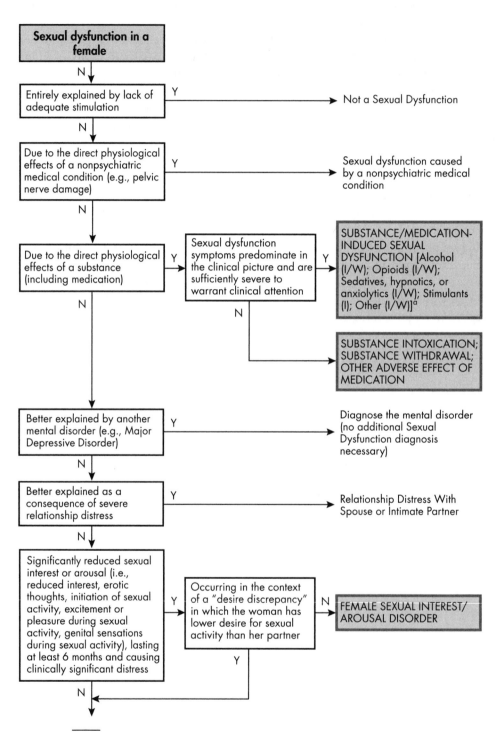

^{a}I = occurring during Substance Intoxication; I/W = occurring during
Substance Intoxication or Substance Withdrawal, as indicated in DSM-5-TR,
Table 1: "Diagnoses associated with substance class," p. 545.

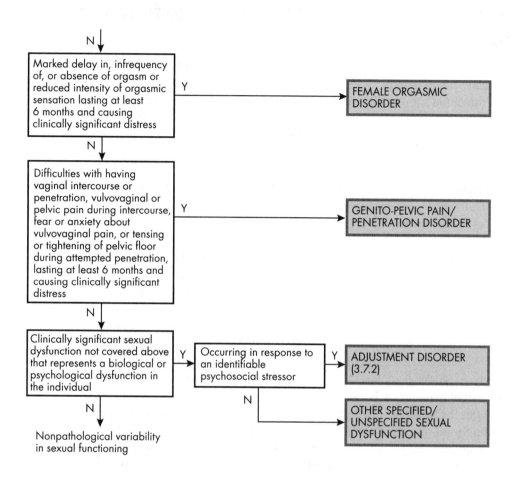

2.24 Decision Tree for Sexual Dysfunction in a Male

The major difficulty in evaluating sexual dysfunctions in both men and women is that there are no accepted guidelines for determining what is "normal" sexual functioning. The threshold for normal sexual functioning varies with the man's age and prior sexual experience, the availability and novelty of partners, and the expectations and standards characteristic of the man's cultural, ethnic, or religious group. Successful arousal and orgasm require a level of sexual stimulation that is adequate in focus, intensity, and duration. A diagnosis of Erectile Disorder or Delayed Ejaculation therefore requires a clinical judgment that the man has experienced adequate stimulation. Moreover, occasional sexual dysfunction is an inherent part of human sexuality and is not indicative of a disorder unless the symptoms have persisted for at least approximately 6 months and result in marked distress or interpersonal difficulty.

Once the clinical judgment has been made that the sexual dysfunction is clinically significant, the next task is to determine its underlying etiology. The possible etiologies include psychological factors, nonpsychiatric medical conditions, the side effects of many prescribed medications, and the consequence of drug abuse. This evaluation can be difficult because very often more than one etiology contributes to the sexual dysfunction. For example, it is not uncommon for someone who develops mild erectile dysfunction as a result of a nonpsychiatric medical condition (e.g., vascular problems) to develop other sexual dysfunctions (e.g., low desire) as a psychological consequence. Before deciding that any sexual dysfunction is mediated strictly by psychological factors, the clinician needs to consider the possible contribution of a nonpsychiatric medical condition or substance (including medication side effects), especially because these etiologies often have specific treatment implications (e.g., discontinuation of the offending medication). Also, the clinician needs to remember that the identification of a specific etiological nonpsychiatric medical condition, medication, or drug of abuse does not negate the important contribution of psychological factors to the etiology of the dysfunction.

Sexual problems are also commonly associated with a number of mental disorders (e.g., Depressive Disorders, Anxiety Disorders, Schizophrenia Spectrum and Other Psychotic Disorders). An additional diagnosis of a sexual dysfunction is not given if the sexual problems are better explained by the mental disorder. For example, low sexual desire occurring only during a Major Depressive Episode would not warrant a separate diagnosis of Male Hypoactive Sexual Desire Disorder. Both diagnoses can be given only if the low sexual desire is judged to be independent of the Depressive Disorder (i.e., it precedes the onset of the Major Depressive Episode or persists long after the depression has remitted). Similarly, sexual dysfunction that is better explained as a consequence of severe relationship distress would be diagnosed as a relational problem rather than a sexual dysfunction unless evidence demonstrated that the sexual dysfunction occurred independently of the relational problem.

Primary sexual dysfunctions in males are organized on the basis of when the problem occurs during the sexual response cycle. Male Hypoactive Sexual Desire Disorder is related to the initial phase, sexual desire. Erectile Disorder is related to the second phase, sexual arousal. Delayed Ejaculation and Premature (Early) Ejaculation are for problems that occur in the third phase, orgasm. Not infrequently, problems occur in more than one phase of the sexual response cycle. Because the phases of the sexual response cycle occur in sequence, successful functioning in one phase generally requires successful functioning in the previous phases (e.g., orgasm requires some level of arousal, which requires some level of desire). However, anticipation of the recurrence of problems in a later phase (e.g., difficulty ejaculating) often leads to problems in an earlier phase (e.g., consequent erectile dysfunction or low sexual desire).

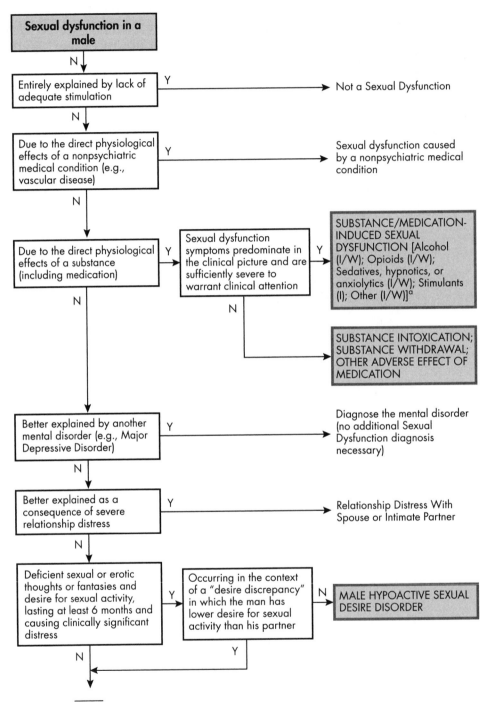

I = occurring during Substance Intoxication; I/W = occurring during
Substance Intoxication or Substance Withdrawal, as indicated in DSM-5-TR,
Table 1: "Diagnoses associated with substance class," p. 545.

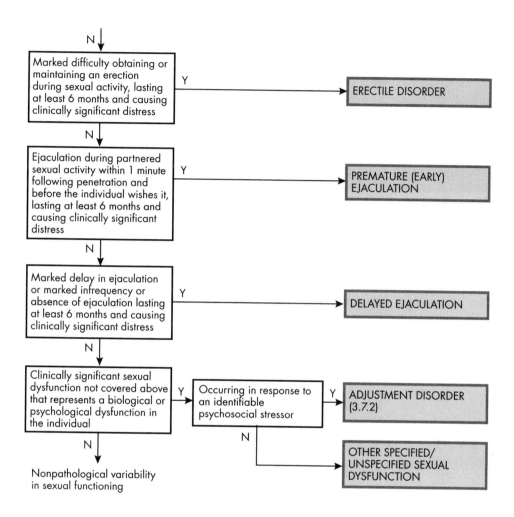

2.25 Decision Tree for Aggressive Behavior

Although aggressive behavior is a defining feature in the diagnostic criteria of only a handful of DSM-5-TR disorders (i.e., Intermittent Explosive Disorder, Conduct Disorder, Antisocial Personality Disorder, and Disruptive Mood Dysregulation Disorder), it is a complication of a number of other DSM-5-TR mental disorders. An important note is that most violent behavior occurs for reasons very far afield from the domain of mental illness (e.g., material gain, status, sadistic pleasure, revenge, furthering a political or religious cause). This consideration is reflected in the last decision in the tree, in which aggressive behavior that does not represent a psychological or biological dysfunction in the individual is considered to be nonpsychiatric antisocial behavior. Moreover, even when the aggressive behavior is associated with a mental disorder, this fact does not by itself absolve the individual of criminal responsibility.

Among the DSM-5-TR disorders, the Substance-Related and Addictive Disorders are by far the most frequent cause of aggressive behavior. Aggression can also result from the cognitive impairment and reduction in impulse control that is characteristic of Delirium and Major or Mild Neurocognitive Disorder Due to Another Medical Condition.

When the aggressive behavior is a direct physiological consequence of a nonpsychiatric medical condition but occurs in the absence of cognitive impairment, Personality Change Due to Another Medical Condition should be diagnosed. One issue that sometimes arises in the diagnosis of Personality Change Due to Another Medical Condition is whether to consider nonspecific medical findings (e.g., neurological soft signs, diffuse slowing on electroencephalogram) as definitive evidence of a causative nonpsychiatric medical condition. The DSM-5-TR convention is to diagnose Personality Change Due to Another Medical Condition only if the findings constitute a diagnosable nonpsychiatric medical condition. However, when clinical judgment strongly suggests that a central nervous system dysfunction is present and responsible for the personality change, but no specific diagnosis can be made, the nonpsychiatric medical condition Unspecified Condition of Brain can be indicated as the causative disorder and coded as an additional disorder (ICD-10-CM: G93.9).

Although the association is much less prominent, episodes of aggressive behavior may occur at somewhat elevated rates in individuals with Schizophrenia Spectrum and Other Psychotic Disorders and in those with Bipolar and Related Disorders.

The presence of a long-standing pattern of aggressive behavior suggests that the behavior is part of a Personality Disorder (e.g., Antisocial Personality Disorder, Borderline Personality Disorder).

Aggressive behavior in children can occur in the context of a number of disorders. When aggressive behavior occurs as part of a pattern of antisocial behavior in a child, the diagnosis of Conduct Disorder applies. If the aggressive behavior occurs in the context of severe temper outbursts that are grossly out of proportion in intensity or duration to the situation or provocation, with persistent anger and irritability between the outbursts, the DSM-5-TR diagnosis Disruptive Mood Dysregulation Disorder should be considered. Much less commonly, aggressive behavior can be associated with other childhood disorders, including Oppositional Defiant Disorder, Attention-Deficit/Hyperactivity Disorder, Separation Anxiety Disorder, Autism Spectrum Disorder, and Intellectual Developmental Disorder (Intellectual Disability).

Recurrent episodes of aggressive behavior (i.e., verbal aggression or physical aggression against people, animals, or property) that is not accounted for by any other mental disorder (including a Personality Disorder) may qualify the individual for a diagnosis of Intermittent Explosive Disorder if the minimum requirements are met for the frequency of behavioral outbursts (twice weekly for 3 months for verbal or physical aggression that does not result in injury or destruction of property, or three outbursts in a 12-month period for physical aggression resulting in injury to others or damage to property).

Aggressive behavior can also occur in response to an identifiable psychosocial stressor. If the stressor is of a particularly traumatic nature (i.e., exposure to actual or threatened death, serious injury, or sexual violence), the aggressive behavior might be part of the syndrome of Posttraumatic Stress Disorder (or Acute Stress Disorder if the duration is 1 month or less). Otherwise, aggressive behavior can be a manifestation of an Adjustment Disorder.

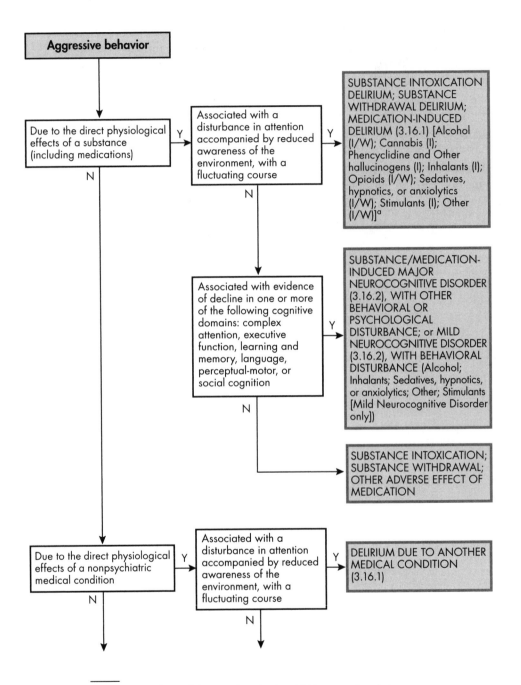

a I = occurring during Substance Intoxication; I/W = occurring during
Substance Intoxication or Substance Withdrawal, as indicated in DSM-5-TR,
Table 1: "Diagnoses associated with substance class," p. 545.

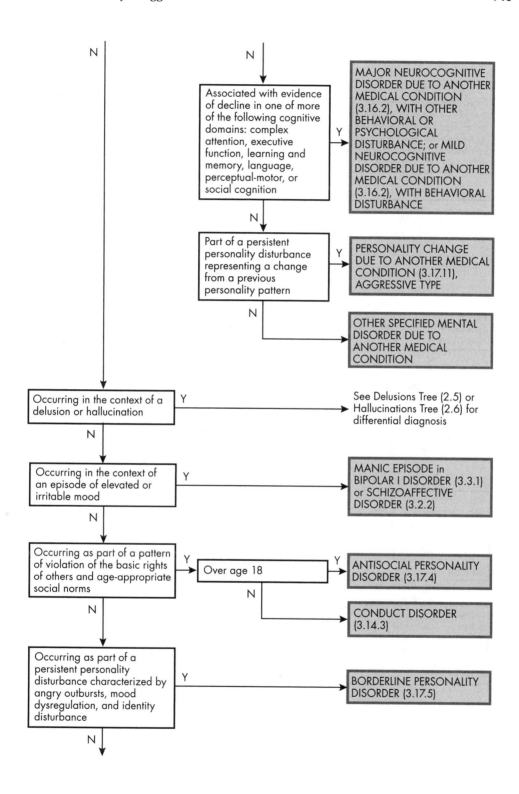

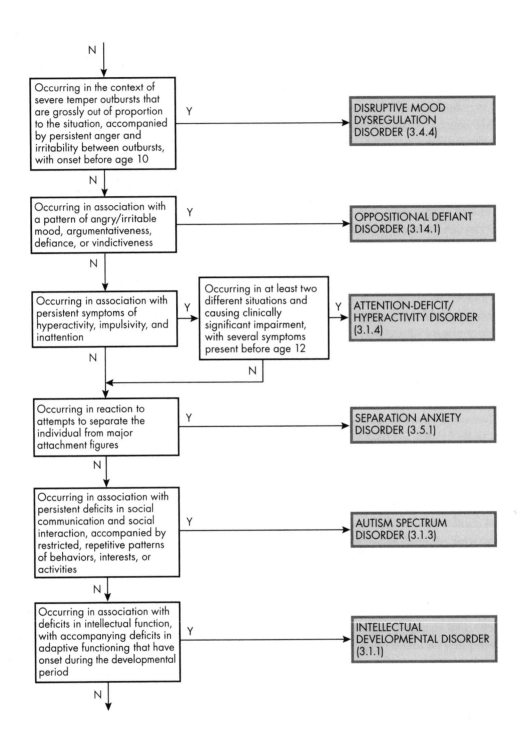

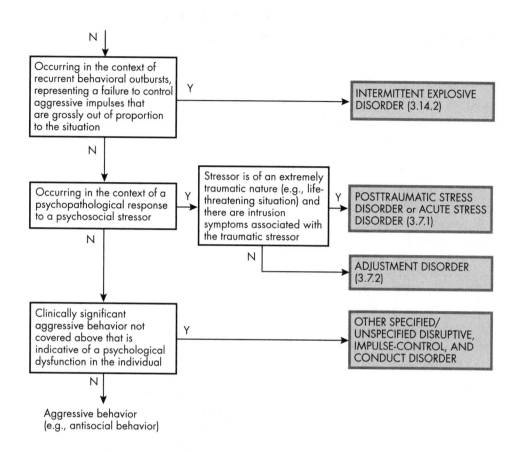

N

Occurring in the context of recurrent behavioral outbursts, representing a failure to control aggressive impulses that are grossly out of proportion to the situation

Y → INTERMITTENT EXPLOSIVE DISORDER (3.14.2)

N

Occurring in the context of a psychopathological response to a psychosocial stressor

Y → Stressor is of an extremely traumatic nature (e.g., life-threatening situation) and there are intrusion symptoms associated with the traumatic stressor

Y → POSTTRAUMATIC STRESS DISORDER or ACUTE STRESS DISORDER (3.7.1)

N → ADJUSTMENT DISORDER (3.7.2)

N

Clinically significant aggressive behavior not covered above that is indicative of a psychological dysfunction in the individual

Y → OTHER SPECIFIED/ UNSPECIFIED DISRUPTIVE, IMPULSE-CONTROL, AND CONDUCT DISORDER

N

Aggressive behavior (e.g., antisocial behavior)

2.26 Decision Tree for Impulsivity or Impulse-Control Problems

Decision Tree 2.26 covers two related symptoms: the trait of impulsivity and the problem of diminished impulse control. Impulsivity involves the tendency to act on a whim, displaying behavior characterized by little or no forethought, reflection, or consideration of consequences. A number of DSM-5-TR disorders are characterized by excessive impulsivity. Other disorders are characterized by problems in controlling certain impulses (e.g., the person's impulse to pull out their hair in Trichotillomania, the impulse to binge in Binge-Eating Disorder). Both excessive impulsivity and impairment in controlling specific impulses can lead to impulsive behavior that can be both self-destructive and harmful to others.

Substance use is a common cause of impulsivity and must be considered as a possible sole or contributory factor in every presentation of impulsive behavior. Nonpsychiatric medical conditions can also result in the disinhibition of impulse control, which is often accompanied by poor judgment and other cognitive symptoms warranting a diagnosis of Delirium or Major or Mild Neurocognitive Disorder. When a nonpsychiatric medical condition results in persistent impulsivity that occurs in the absence of clinically significant cognitive impairment, the diagnosis is Personality Change Due to Another Medical Condition (usually of the Disinhibited or Aggressive Type).

Certain disorders are characterized by impulsivity that is confined exclusively to the episode of the disturbance. Once substance use and a nonpsychiatric medical condition are ruled out, the next step is to determine whether the presentation includes symptoms that would lead to a diagnosis of a Bipolar Disorder, Depressive Disorder, Posttraumatic Stress Disorder, or Acute Stress Disorder. Generalized impulsivity that has an early onset and persistent course is most likely to be associated with Attention-Deficit/Hyperactivity Disorder, Conduct Disorder, Antisocial Personality Disorder, or Borderline Personality Disorder.

A wide range of DSM-5-TR disorders are characterized by specific behaviors that can be conceptualized as manifestations of impaired impulse control. These include Gambling Disorder, in which the person's ability to control gambling behavior is impaired; Bulimia Nervosa and Binge-Eating Disorder, which are characterized by out-of-control binge eating; Pyromania and Kleptomania, which are characterized by an inability to resist impulses to set fires and to steal objects of little value, respectively; and Intermittent Explosive Disorder, which is characterized by an intermittent inability to resist aggressive impulses. Trichotillomania and Excoriation Disorder are characterized by the individual's recurrent pulling out of their hair or picking their skin, respectively, along with repeated attempts to decrease or stop their hair pulling or skin picking. Trichotillomania was classified as Impulse-Control Disorders Not Elsewhere Classified up through DSM-IV and reclassified as Obsessive-Compulsive and Related Disorders in DSM-5 (continuing in DSM-5-TR) after a review of the literature suggested that Trichotillomania had more in common with the other Obsessive-Compulsive and Related Disorders than with the Impulse-Control Disorders (e.g., many cases of Trichotillomania lack an increasing sense of tension before the act, which is characteristic of Pyromania and Kleptomania).

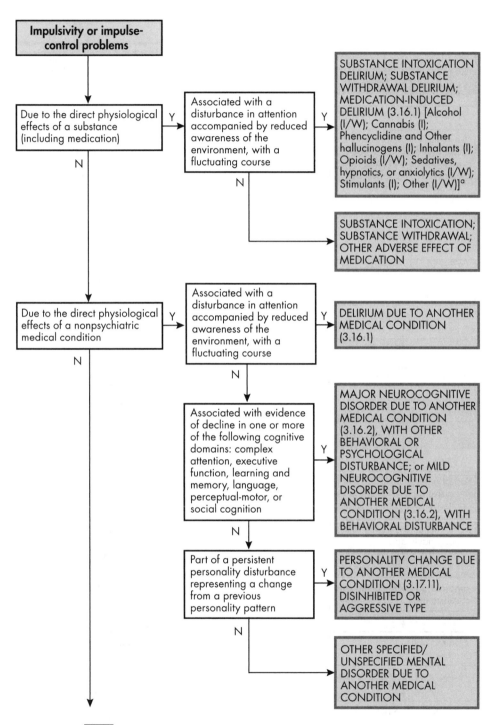

ª I = occurring during Substance Intoxication; I/W = occurring during
Substance Intoxication or Substance Withdrawal, as indicated in DSM-5-TR,
Table 1: "Diagnoses associated with substance class," p. 545.

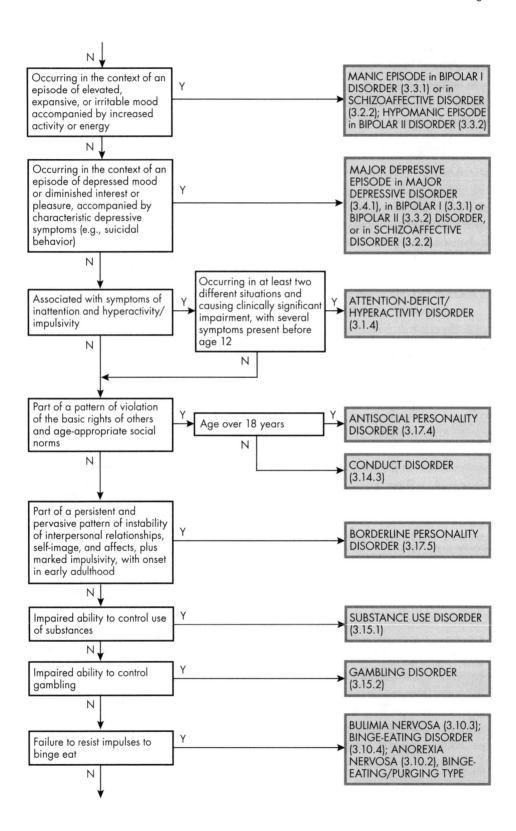

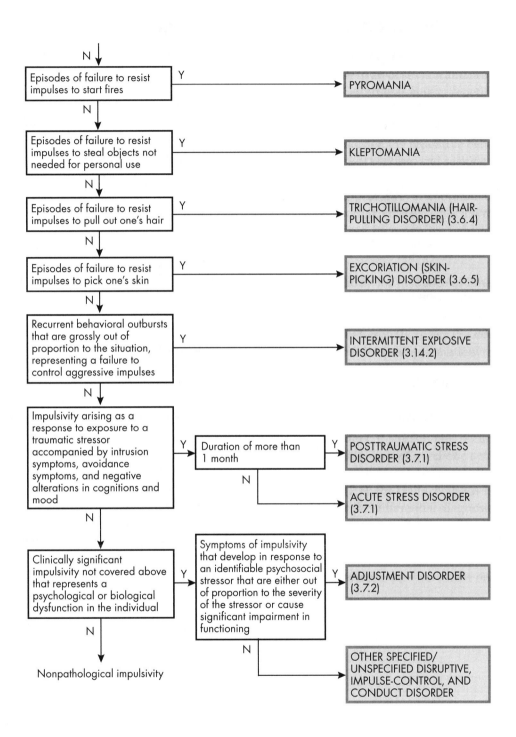

2.27 Decision Tree for Self-Injurious Behavior

Self-injurious behaviors include the person cutting, burning, hitting, head banging, hair pulling, skin picking, and self-biting various parts of their own body. Notably, motivations for self-injurious behaviors vary in the diagnoses for which the behavior is a complication. The diagnosis most frequently associated with self-injury is Borderline Personality Disorder. For some patients with this disorder, the self-injurious behavior often occurs as a means of "treating" dissociative states, wherein the patient returns to feeling alive only when experiencing pain or seeing blood. In other patients with Borderline Personality Disorder, self-injury is a means of "treating" intense dysphoria or counteracting intense anger. The likelihood of self-injurious episodes is greatly increased by Substance Intoxication or Substance Withdrawal. The motivation for self-injury in psychotic patients is usually a delusional belief (e.g., the need to punish evil spirits) or a response to a command hallucination. In Delirium and Major Neurocognitive Disorder, the self-injury sometimes occurs as a by-product of the confusion (e.g., struggling against restraints). The self-injurious behavior that infrequently occurs as a complication of Obsessive-Compulsive Disorder results from the inability to resist the constant need to perform a compulsive act (e.g., cleaning hands raw as a result of a hand-washing compulsion). In Trichotillomania, there is an inability of the individual to resist the impulse to pull out their hair, which may result in patches of hair loss. Similarly, the individual's failure to resist impulses to pick their skin in Excoriation Disorder leads to noticeable skin lesions. In Sexual Masochism Disorder, the motivation for the self-injurious behavior is sexual pleasure.

Stereotypies, which can result in self-injury, are the central component of Stereotypic Movement Disorder. When Stereotypic Movement Disorder results in clinically significant self-injury, this can be indicated by specifying "with self-injurious behavior." Stereotypies are not infrequent in Intellectual Developmental Disorder (Intellectual Disability) and should be diagnosed separately as Stereotypic Movement Disorder only if they are not better explained by the underlying cause of the Intellectual Developmental Disorder.

Self-injurious behavior is sometimes a manifestation of Factitious Disorder or Malingering. The patient learns that cutting or burning will result in a desired hospitalization or prevents an undesired discharge. Factitious Disorder and Malingering are differentiated on the basis of whether the feigned behavior occurs in the absence of obvious external rewards. If there is an absence of obvious external rewards, the diagnosis is Factitious Disorder. If the feigned self-injurious behavior occurs only in the presence of obvious external rewards, Malingering is diagnosed instead.

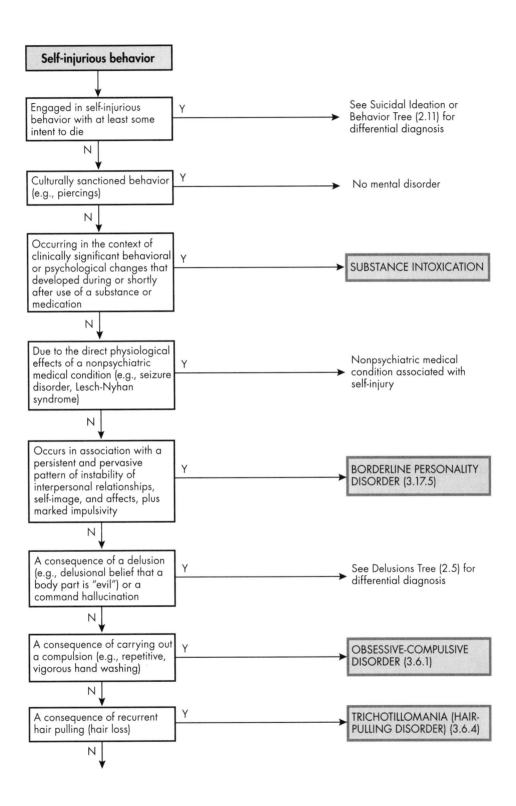

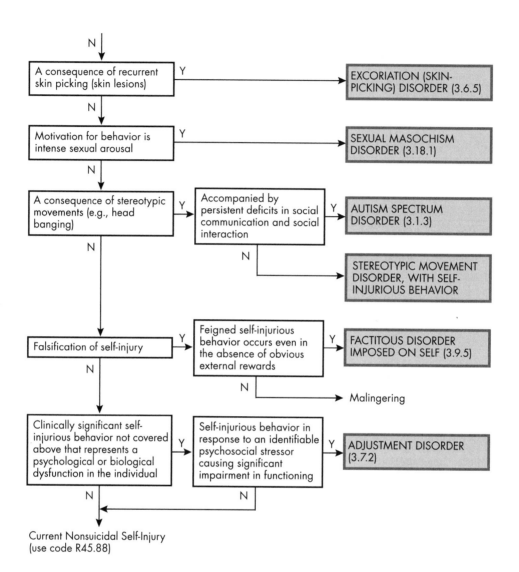

Current Nonsuicidal Self-Injury
(use code R45.88)

2.28 Decision Tree for Excessive or Problematic Substance Use

Many individuals can take substances without having any clinically significant problems that would warrant a DSM-5-TR diagnosis. However, substance-related disorders are among the most common and impairing of the mental disorders. Because substance-related presentations are so frequently encountered in mental health care, substance use disorder treatment, and primary care settings, a Substance-Related Disorder must be considered in every differential diagnosis.

In DSM-5-TR, the term *substance-related* refers to disorders associated with drugs of abuse, the side effects of medication, and toxin-induced states. There are two types of substance-related diagnoses in DSM-5-TR: the Substance Use Disorders, which describe a pattern of problematic substance use, and the Substance-Induced Disorders (comprising Substance Intoxication, Substance Withdrawal, and Substance/Medication-Induced Mental Disorders), which describe behavioral syndromes that are caused by the direct effect of a substance on the central nervous system (CNS). More often than not, Substance-Induced Disorders occur in the context of an accompanying Substance Use Disorder, and in such situations, both diagnoses should be given. However, in contrast to the standard ICD-10-CM recording procedure used throughout DSM-5-TR, in which each diagnosis is assigned its own diagnostic code, the ICD-10-CM convention for coding a comorbid Substance Use Disorder and Substance-Induced Disorder assigns a single ICD-10-CM code for the combination. For example, Cocaine-Induced Depressive Disorder, With Onset During Withdrawal, occurring in an individual with Severe Cocaine Use Disorder, receives a single combination diagnosis and code: F14.24 Severe Cocaine Use Disorder, With Cocaine-Induced Depressive Disorder, With Onset During Withdrawal. See the recording procedures for the individual Substance/Medication-Induced Mental Disorders in DSM-5-TR for more information. For this reason, the decision tree starts off with a decision point that highlights the fact that Substance Use Disorders and Substance-Induced Disorders are often comorbid, and clearly indicates that if a Substance Use Disorder is present and there is evidence that the substance has caused psychiatric symptoms because of its direct effect on the CNS, the remainder of the tree must be reviewed to determine the differential diagnosis of the relevant Substance/Medication-Induced Disorder.

Substance Intoxication and Substance Withdrawal can be characterized by psychopathology that mimics other disorders contained in DSM-5-TR and must always be considered in the differential diagnosis of every condition (see Step 2 in Chapter 1). The Substance/Medication-Induced Mental Disorders (i.e., Substance/Medication-Induced Psychotic Disorder, Substance/Medication-Induced Bipolar and Related Disorder, and so forth) have been included in DSM-5-TR for presentations in which a particular symptom (e.g., delusions, hallucinations, mania) predominates in the clinical picture and warrants clinical attention. For example, virtually every individual withdrawing from cocaine will experience some dysphoric mood, and in most situations a diagnosis of Cocaine Withdrawal will suffice. However, were the individual to become suicidally depressed, the diagnosis of Cocaine-Induced Depressive Disorder, With Onset During Withdrawal, may be more appropriate. Often, more than one substance-induced symptom (e.g., depressed mood and anxiety) may be prominent enough to be a focus of clinical attention. In such situations, it is generally preferable to give just one substance/medication-induced diagnosis, depending on the predominating symptom.

The psychiatric sequelae to substance/medication use can develop in any of four contexts: 1) during or soon after substance intoxication; 2) during or soon after withdrawal from a substance; 3) after exposure to or withdrawal from a medication; and 4) substance-induced symptoms that persist and remain stable (or improve) after a period of abstinence (e.g., Persistent Alcohol-Induced Major Neurocognitive Disorder).

Delirium Due to Multiple Etiologies and Major or Mild Neurocognitive Disorder Due to Multiple Etiologies have been included in DSM-5-TR (and in this decision tree) to emphasize that very often these conditions have multiple interacting etiologies, including substances. A common (and sometimes devastating) error is for clinicians to assume that their job is finished once they have identified a substance as a contributing etiology to the Delirium or the Major or Mild Neurocognitive Disorder—and thus miss the associated contribution of head trauma or another medical condition.

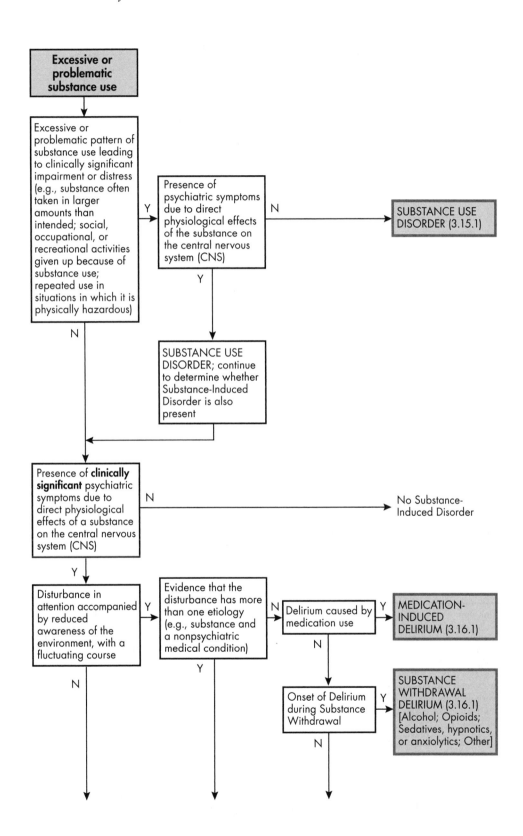

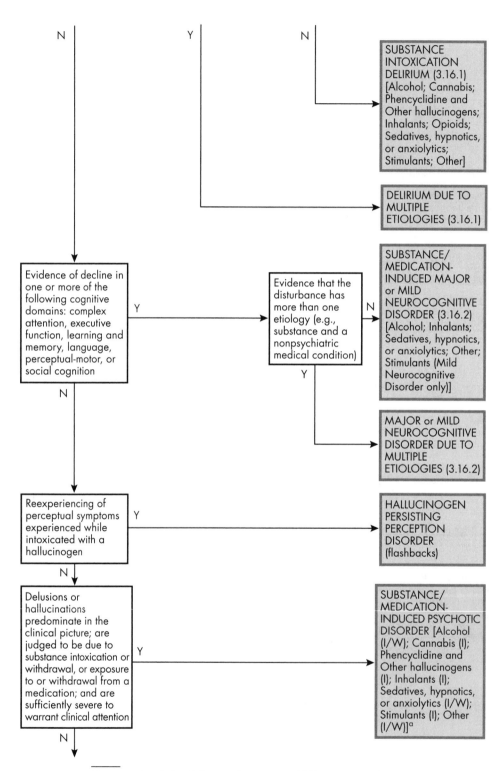

[a] I = occurring during Substance Intoxication; I/W = occurring during Substance Intoxication or Substance Withdrawal, as indicated in DSM-5-TR, Table 1: "Diagnoses associated with substance class," p. 545.

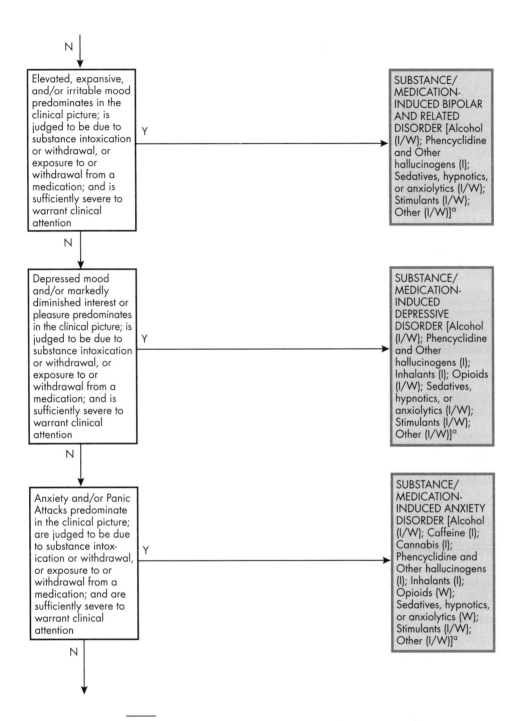

---

^a I = occurring during Substance Intoxication; I/W = occurring during Substance Intoxication or Substance Withdrawal; W = occurring during Substance Withdrawal, as indicated in DSM-5-TR, Table 1: "Diagnoses associated with substance class," p. 545.

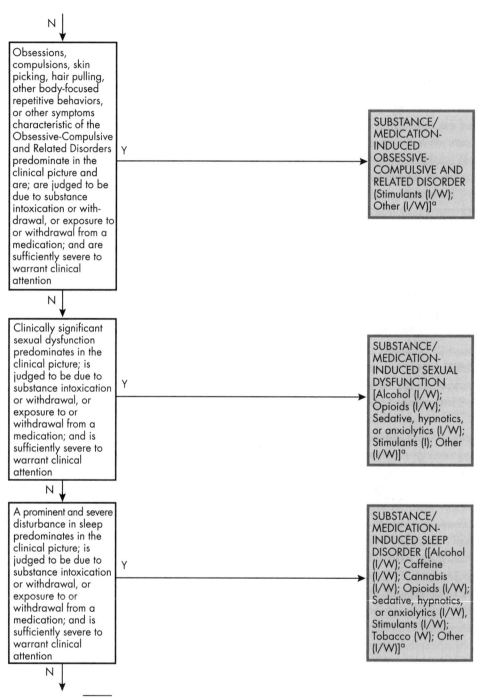

ᵃI = occurring during Substance Intoxication; I/W = occurring during
Substance Intoxication or Substance Withdrawal; W = occurring during
Substance Withdrawal, as indicated in DSM-5-TR, Table 1: "Diagnoses
associated with substance class," p. 545.

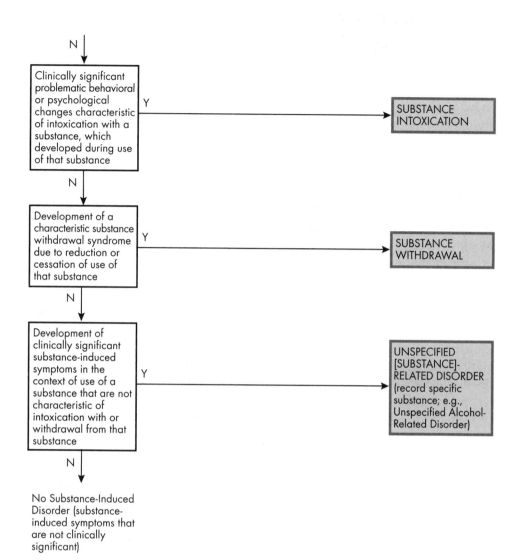

2.29 Decision Tree for Memory Loss or Memory Impairment

DSM-5-TR defines the Neurocognitive Disorders in terms of impairments in six defined cognitive domains: 1) learning and memory; 2) complex attention; 3) executive function; 4) language; 5) perceptual-motor functions; and 6) social cognition functions. Although Neurocognitive Disorders usually involve impairments in several of these domains, this decision tree should be used for the differential diagnosis of impairment in learning or memory in the absence of impairments in other cognitive domains. Refer to the Cognitive Impairment Tree (2.30) for presentations involving 1) impairments in memory due to a specific etiology (e.g., nonpsychiatric medical condition), along with impairments in other cognitive domains; and 2) presentations of other types of cognitive impairment, without impairments in memory or learning.

Memory impairment or memory loss can be characterized by difficulty in laying down new memories (learning) and/or in the recall of previous memories (memory loss). The various aspects of memory functioning may be tested separately. These include 1) registration (the ability of the patient to repeat numbers or words immediately after hearing them), 2) short-term recall (the ability of the patient to repeat the names of three unrelated objects after a period of several minutes), 3) recognition (the ability of the patient to retrieve previously forgotten names if provided with clues), and 4) remote memory (the ability of the patient to recall important personal or historical events). The differential decisions in this tree concern whether the etiology of the memory loss is the direct physiological effect on the central nervous system of substance/medication use or a nonpsychiatric medical condition, whether it is an associated feature of another mental disorder, or whether the memory loss is a dissociative phenomenon (e.g., as in Posttraumatic Stress Disorder or a Dissociative Disorder).

In the context of this decision tree, Major and Mild Neurocognitive Disorders are defined as a decline in learning and memory in the absence of other cognitive impairments. (These learning and memory declines would have been diagnosed as Amnestic Disorder in DSM-IV and earlier DSM editions and still are diagnosed as Amnestic Disorder in ICD-11.) Major Neurocognitive Disorder is differentiated from Mild Neurocognitive Disorder in this decision tree on the basis of the severity of the memory impairment and its impact on functioning. Major Neurocogntive Disorder is characterized by a significant decline in memory and learning that is so severe that it interferes with independence, whereas in Mild Neurocognitive Disorder, the decline in memory and learning is limited to a "modest" level of severity.

Memory impairment associated with substance use can be either temporary (as in Substance Intoxication, Substance Withdrawal, or Other Adverse Effect of Medication) or persistent (as in Substance/Medication-Induced Major or Mild Neurocognitive Disorder, which requires the impairments in memory and learning to persist beyond the usual duration of acute intoxication or withdrawal).

Memory impairment is also a common associated feature of a number of mental disorders. For example, memory impairment occurring in the context of a Major Depressive Episode can be severe enough to resemble an irreversible dementing process ("pseudodementia"). Frequently, it is only when the memory impairment resolves after successful treatment that it becomes clear that there was in fact no comorbid Major Neurocognitive Disorder. This differential is further complicated by medication (e.g., lithium) being taken by the patient that may also contribute to memory problems.

Dissociation is a disruption in the usually integrated functions of consciousness, memory, identity, or perception of the environment. Memory loss, especially for traumatic events, is a feature of Dissociative Amnesia and Dissociative Identity Disorder, as well as of Posttraumatic Stress Disorder and Acute Stress Disorder. Particularly when someone has been exposed to an event that is both physically and psychologically traumatic (e.g., car accident), it can be difficult to tease apart whether the memory loss is a psychological reaction to the events or is a result of head trauma. Moreover, especially in forensic situations, feigned claims of memory loss may be used in an attempt to deny responsibility. In such cases, the diagnosis is either Factitious Disorder or Malingering, with Factitious Disorder diagnosed when the feigned memory loss is evident even in the absence of obvious external rewards. Otherwise, Malingering (which is not considered to be a mental disorder) is diagnosed.

It should also be noted that virtually everyone wishes that their memory were better than it is and that this longing usually becomes more poignant as people get older and begin having more difficulty with recall. Before considering the disorders in this decision tree, the clinician must determine that the individual's memory loss is sufficiently severe to be clinically significant and that it is more severe than might be expected given the individual's previous memory functioning and the norms for their age. If the clinician determines that the decline in memory is due to the aging process and is within normal limits given the individual's age, a symptom code may be given for Age-Related Cognitive Decline (in the DSM-5-TR chapter "Other Conditions That May Be a Focus of Clinical Attention").

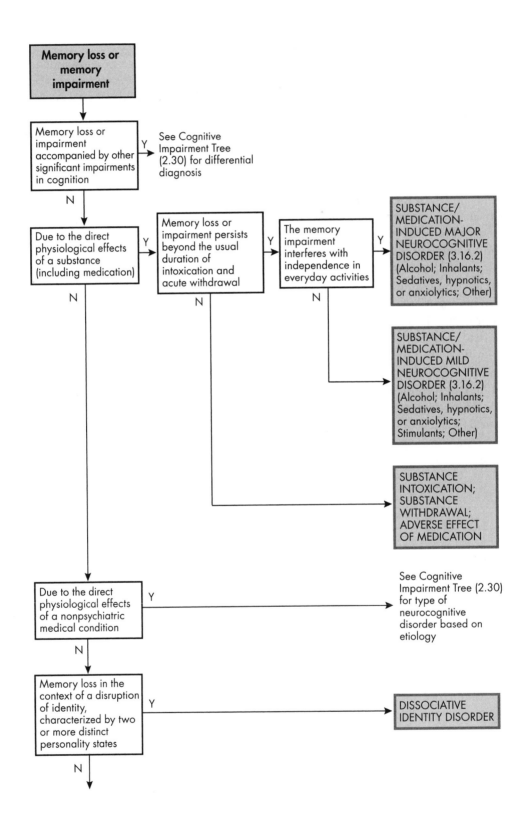

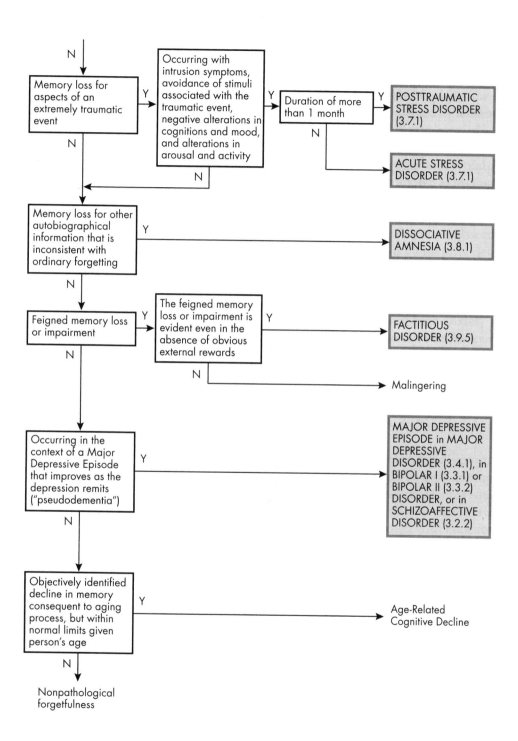

2.30 Decision Tree for Cognitive Impairment

Although *cognitive impairment* is a broad term that can include impairment in virtually any cognitive function, in the context of this decision tree, the term is referring to impairment in one of the six cognitive domains listed in the criteria for Major or Mild Neurocognitive Disorder (NCD): complex attention, executive function, learning and memory, language, perceptual-motor, or social cognition. If cognitive impairment is restricted to memory loss, refer to the Memory Loss or Memory Impairment Tree (2.29) for the differential diagnosis.

Each of the cognitive domains describes aspects of cognitive function. The domain of *complex attention* includes the ability to sustain attention over a period of time, to divide attention to more than one task at a time, and to maintain attention despite distractions; this domain also includes processing speed. The domain of *executive function* involves the ability to plan ahead and make decisions, to hold information for a brief period and manipulate that information (e.g., adding up a list of numbers), and to benefit from feedback; this domain also includes cognitive flexibility (e.g., the ability to shift between two concepts). The domain of *learning and memory* includes recent memory, semantic memory (memory for facts), autobiographical memory (memory for personal events or people), and procedural memory (learning of skills). The *language* domain includes expressive language (including naming, word finding, fluency, grammar, and syntax) and receptive language (comprehension). The *perceptual-motor* domain includes visual perception, visuoconstructional abilities (e.g., assembly of items requiring hand-eye coordination), the ability to integrate perception with purposeful movement, the integrity of learned movements (praxis), and recognition of faces and colors (gnosis). The domain of *social cognition* involves recognition of emotions in others and the ability to consider another person's mental state.

The pattern of cognitive impairments that defines the Delirium syndrome is rather specific. The hallmark of Delirium is a clouding of consciousness characterized by a disturbance in attention (i.e., a reduced ability to direct, focus, sustain, and shift attention), accompanied by reduced awareness of the environment that develops over a short period of time and fluctuates in severity during the course of a day. The definition of Delirium also requires an accompanying disturbance in cognition (which can take the form of memory impairment, language, visuospatial ability, or perception). Once the syndrome of Delirium is established, the actual DSM-5-TR diagnosis depends on its etiology; Delirium can be due to the direct physiological effects of a substance or medication (Substance Intoxication Delirium, Substance Withdrawal Delirium, Medication-Induced Delirium) or to the direct physiological effects of a nonpsychiatric medical condition (Delirium Due to Another Medical Condition).

Beyond Delirium, NCDs in the tree are classified according to etiology largely based on clinical factors such as course, symptom profile, and temporal association with a nonpsychiatric medical condition: insidious onset and gradual progression of impairment in the setting of established Parkinson's disease for NCD Due to Parkinson's Disease; cognitive impairment developing after head trauma in NCD Due to Traumatic Brain Injury; cognitive impairment in the context of HIV in NCD Due to HIV Infection; insidious onset, gradual progression, and evidence that symptoms are a direct consequence of

Huntington's disease in NCD Due to Huntington's Disease; insidious onset, rapid progression, and biomarker evidence of prion disease in NCD Due to Prion Disease; insidious onset, gradual progression, and behavioral symptoms (such as disinhibition, loss of empathy, compulsive behavior) or decline in language ability with sparing of learning and memory in Frontotemporal NCD; gradual progression with fluctuating cognition, visual hallucinations, spontaneous features of parkinsonism, REM sleep behavior disorder, or neuroleptic sensitivity in NCD With Lewy Bodies; cerebrovascular disease and features consistent with vascular etiology in Vascular NCD; gradual onset and gradual progression of impairment in at least two cognitive domains in NCD Due to Alzheimer's Disease; and the physiological effects of a substance or medication that persist beyond the usual duration of substance intoxication or substance withdrawal in Substance/Medication-Induced NCD. Each NCD is diagnosed as either Major Neurocognitive Disorder (if cognitive decline leads to substantial impairment in cognitive functions that interferes with independence) or Mild Neurocognitive Disorder (if cognitive decline is modest and insufficiently severe to interfere with the capacity for independence in everyday activities. Moreover, for a number of the NCDs due to specific nonpsychiatric medical conditions, different criteria are provided depending on whether the presence of the presumed causative nonpsychiatric medical condition is "probable" or "possible" (i.e., Alzheimer's disease, frontotemporal degeneration, Lewy body disease) and on whether causal relationship between the NCD and an already established nonpsychiatric medical condition is "probable" or "possible" (i.e., Parkinson's disease, vascular disease).

Significant cognitive impairment can also occur in the context of various mental disorders. Because such cognitive impairment is considered to be an associated feature of the mental disorder, no additional diagnosis is given. In Schizophrenia, cognitive symptoms—especially decrements in declarative and working memory, language function, and other executive functions—are extremely common and are a major contributor to poor long-term functioning. Similarly, although many individuals in the midst of a Manic Episode feel more confident in their cognitive abilities, in between mood episodes there may be significant cognitive impairment that has a negative impact on long-term functioning. Depressive Disorders, such as Major Depressive Disorder and Persistent Depressive Disorder, are characterized by a diminished ability to think or concentrate, which in some cases can be severe enough to resemble a dementing illness ("pseudodementia"). Difficulty with concentration is common during the dysphoric periods in Premenstrual Dysphoric Disorder, and is also part of the symptomatic pictures of Posttraumatic Stress Disorder, Acute Stress Disorder, and Generalized Anxiety Disorder. Inattention and distractibility are defining features of Attention-Deficit/Hyperactivity Disorder.

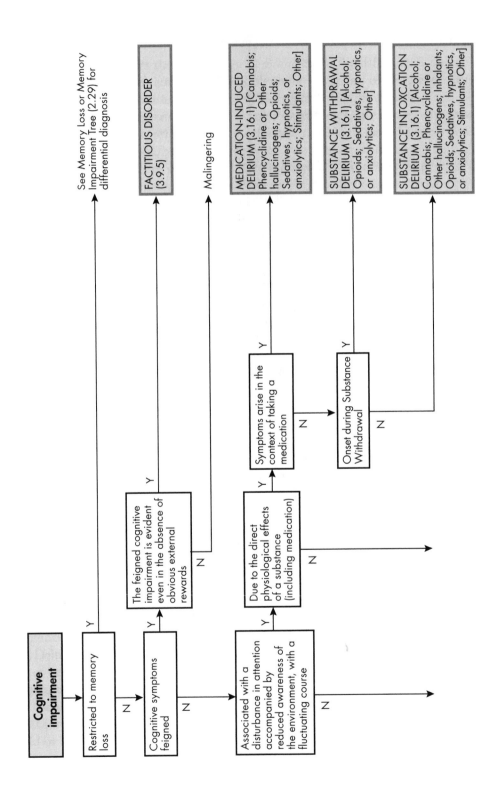

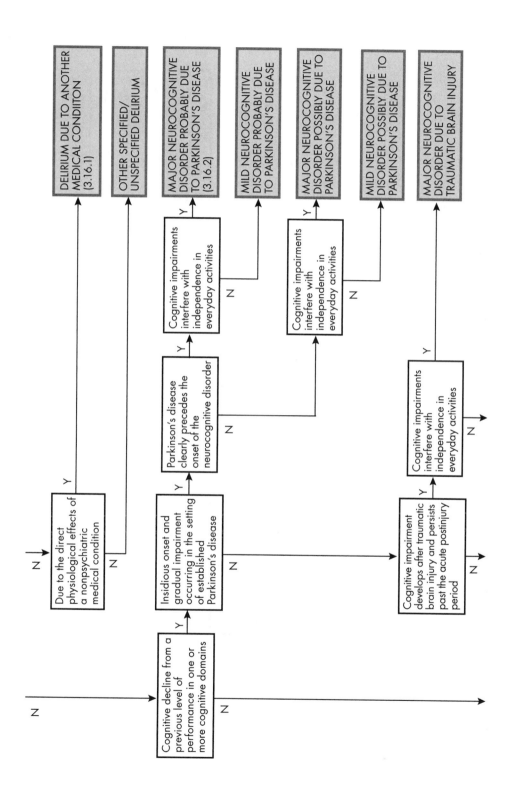

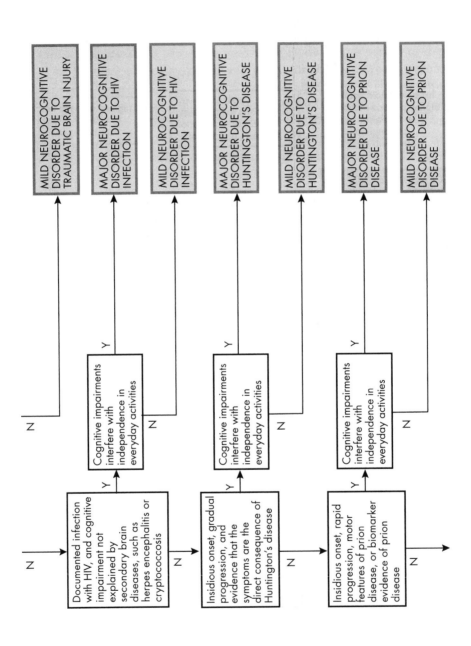

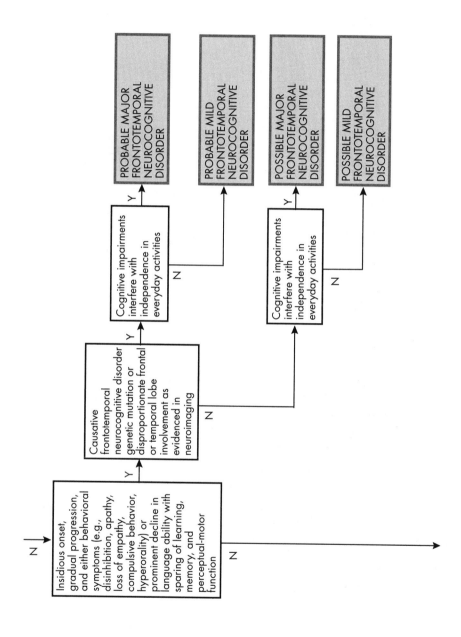

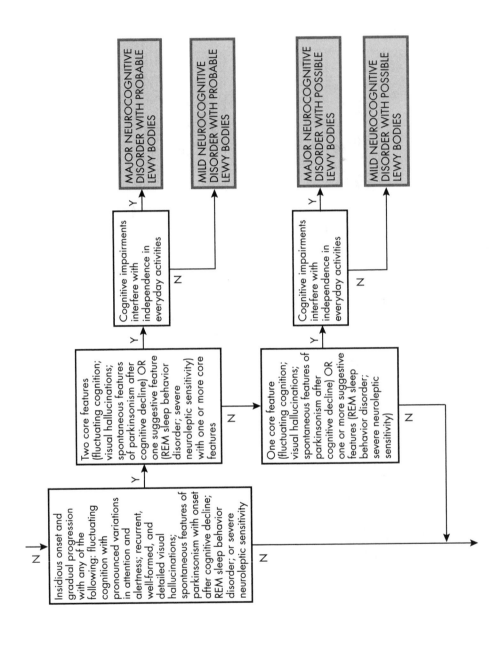

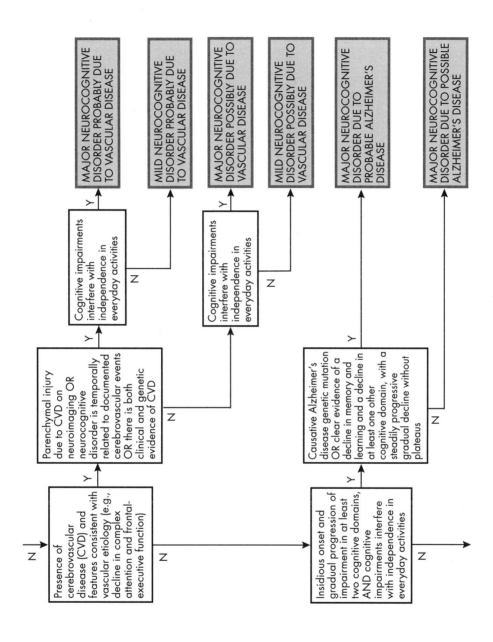

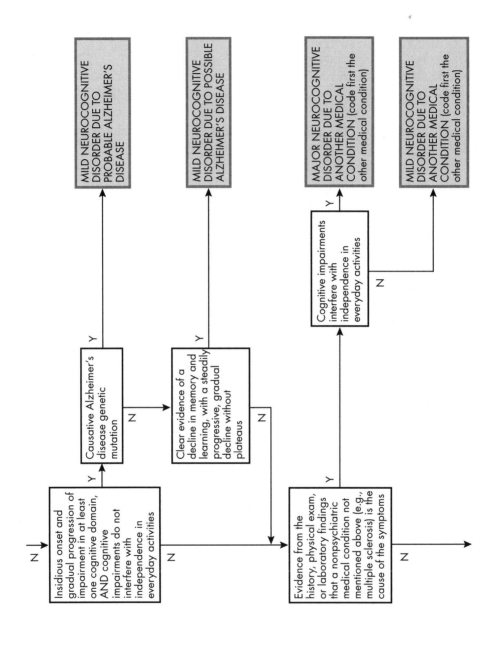

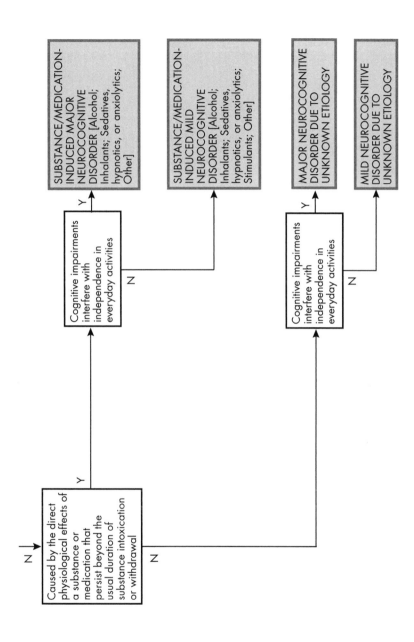

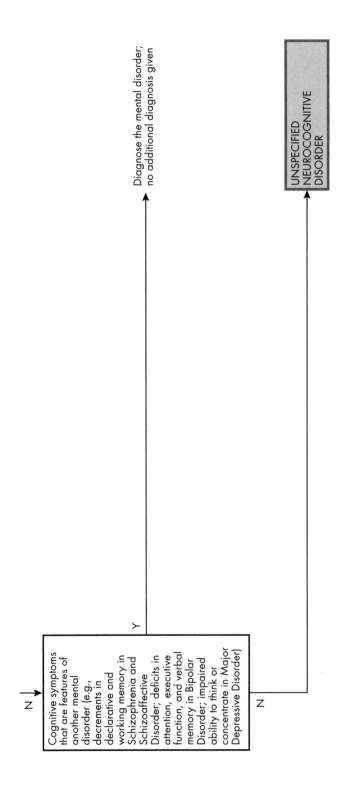

Cognitive symptoms that are features of another mental disorder (e.g., decrements in declarative and working memory in Schizophrenia and Schizoaffective Disorder; deficits in attention, executive function, and verbal memory in Bipolar Disorder; impaired ability to think or concentrate in Major Depressive Disorder)

Y → Diagnose the mental disorder; no additional diagnosis given

N → UNSPECIFIED NEUROCOGNITIVE DISORDER

3

Differential Diagnosis by the Tables

In contrast to the 30 decision trees included in Chapter 2, which use presenting symptoms as their starting points, the entry points to the 67 differential diagnosis tables included in this chapter are the DSM-5-TR disorders themselves. Although the practice of quickly arriving at a working diagnosis based on the gestalt of the patient has its pitfalls in terms of prematurely closing the clinician's mind to other equally valid possible diagnostic contenders, this is likely the method most often used by experienced clinicians. To help ensure that the clinician's working diagnosis is in fact the best diagnostic fit for the patient's clinical presentation, the disorder-oriented differential diagnosis tables can be invaluable in providing a comprehensive listing of those DSM-5-TR disorders that share important features with the initial working diagnosis so that these disorders can be considered and ruled out.

The first step is to locate the differential diagnosis table(s) corresponding to the working diagnosis (or diagnoses, if multiple diagnoses initially seem likely). In the list included at the end of this introduction, the differential diagnosis tables are grouped according to DSM-5-TR diagnostic class so that the relevant differential diagnosis table is easier to find. (An alphabetical index of differential diagnosis tables is also available at the end of this handbook.) Each disorder-oriented differential diagnosis table in this chapter includes two columns. The first left-hand entry in each table summarizes the definition of the index disorder to facilitate its differentiation from the other disorders in the table. The left-hand column lists those disorders (or nonpathological conditions) that share diagnostic features with the index disorder and thus need to be considered and ruled out as part of the differential diagnosis of the index disorder. For each such disorder or nonpathological condition in the differential diagnosis, the entry in the right-hand column indicates the diagnostic feature that differentiates it from the index disorder. For example, the differential diagnosis table for Separation Anxiety Disorder (Table 3.5.1) includes Agoraphobia in the differential diagnosis, because both Separation Anxiety Disorder and Agoraphobia have anxiety and avoidance as shared diagnostic features. If a clinician is considering a diagnosis of Separation Anxiety Disorder on the basis of a clinical presentation of severe anxiety that occurs upon leaving the home, Agoraphobia should also be considered as a possible explanatory disorder and thus is included in the table. The corresponding entry in the right-hand column explains how Separation Anxiety Disorder and Agoraphobia can be differentiated "[Agoraphobia] is characterized by anxiety about being trapped or incapacitated in places or situations from which escape is perceived as difficult in the event of panic-like or other incapacitating symptoms. In Separation Anxiety Disorder, the focus of the fear is on separation from major attachment figures."

Sometimes it may not be immediately obvious which diagnostic features the other disorders have in common with the index disorder that would justify their inclusion in the differential diagnosis table. In such cases, the entry in the right-hand column begins by stating what the putatively shared diagnostic feature is. For example, the differential diagnosis table for Avoidant/Restrictive Food Intake Disorder (ARFID; Table 3.10.1) includes Autism Spectrum Disorder, which may seem mysterious, given that restrictive eating behavior is not part of the definition of Autism Spectrum Disorder. The entry in the right-hand column therefore begins by noting that Autism Spectrum Disorder "may be characterized by rigid eating behaviors and heightened sensory sensitivities," which is also a feature of ARFID, and then goes on to differentiate the two disorders by noting that "these symptoms often do not result in the level of impairment…that would be required for a diagnosis of ARFID."

Multiple disorders are grouped in some tables to reduce the number of differential diagnosis tables. In some tables, such as Table 3.2.1, Schizophrenia or Schizophreniform Disorder, and Table 3.7.1, Posttraumatic Stress Disorder or Acute Stress Disorder, the disorders have been grouped together because they share virtually all the same diagnostic features except duration (which is noted in an accompanying footnote) and therefore share the same differential diagnosis list. In other tables, such as Table 3.1.2, Communication Disorders, a single differential diagnosis table is provided that covers all the disorders in that diagnostic grouping as if that were a single disorder. In these types of tables, if a disorder is included in the differential diagnosis list that pertains to only one of the disorders within that diagnostic grouping, it will be indicated in a parenthetical phrase. For example, in Table 3.1.2, although most of the differential diagnostic entries listed apply to all of the Communication Disorders, the entry for Autism Spectrum Disorder ("Is characterized by restricted, repetitive patterns of behavior, interests, or activities in addition to social communication deficits, whereas in Social [Pragmatic] Communication Disorder, restricted, repetitive patterns of behavior, interests, or activities are absent") applies only to Social (Pragmatic) Communication Disorder. Therefore, the phrase "(as distinguished from Social [Pragmatic] Communication Disorder)" is included in that row of the table to indicate that this differentiation applies only to that disorder within the group of Communication Disorders.

Some caveats should be kept in mind regarding the use of the tables. First, although the entries in the tables focus on the features that differentiate between disorders, given that only a minority of DSM-5-TR disorders (e.g., Bipolar I Disorder and Major Depressive Disorder) are by definition mutually exclusive, diagnostic comorbidity is the default position. Thus, unless otherwise stated, if the criteria are fully met for both the index disorder and a disorder in the table, both should be diagnosed.

Second, although the pertinent Other Specified and Unspecified categories are not included in the differential diagnosis tables, they are an important consideration in the differential diagnosis for every disorder. Every experienced clinician knows that the complexity of practice offers many presentations that fall between the neatly defined DSM-5-TR disorders. Many patients do not present a clear picture that comfortably approximates the prototype for any of the disorders described in the DSM-5-TR criteria sets. Instead, patients often have clinical features that appear to be at the boundary between criteria sets or that satisfy the criteria for a number of possibly related disorders. It is important to recognize that a boundary patient is indeed a boundary patient and should not be shoehorned into a diagnosis that does not fit well. Such patients may require serial trials of treatment to help clarify the most appropriate diagnosis and plan of management.

Third, the differential diagnosis tables tend to focus on cross-sectional symptom presentations because these are the easiest to define and evaluate. Other factors that may be useful in guiding differential diagnosis include the patient's previous history, family history of psychopathology, course, biological test results, and responses to previous treatment trials. Especially in doubtful cases, these factors may tip the differential diagnostic balance one way or the other.

Differential diagnostic tables grouped by DSM-5-TR diagnostic class

Neurodevelopmental Disorders
3.1.1   Intellectual Developmental Disorder (Intellectual Disability)
3.1.2   Communication Disorders
3.1.3   Autism Spectrum Disorder
3.1.4   Attention-Deficit/Hyperactivity Disorder
3.1.5   Specific Learning Disorder
3.1.6   Tic Disorders

Schizophrenia Spectrum and Other Psychotic Disorders
3.2.1   Schizophrenia or Schizophreniform Disorder
3.2.2   Schizoaffective Disorder
3.2.3   Delusional Disorder
3.2.4   Brief Psychotic Disorder
3.2.5   Unspecified Catatonia

Bipolar and Related Disorders
3.3.1   Bipolar I Disorder
3.3.2   Bipolar II Disorder
3.3.3   Cyclothymic Disorder

Differential diagnostic tables grouped by DSM-5-TR diagnostic class *(continued)*

Depressive Disorders
3.4.1   Major Depressive Disorder
3.4.2   Persistent Depressive Disorder
3.4.3   Premenstrual Dysphoric Disorder
3.4.4   Disruptive Mood Dysregulation Disorder

Anxiety Disorders
3.5.1   Separation Anxiety Disorder
3.5.2   Selective Mutism
3.5.3   Specific Phobia
3.5.4   Social Anxiety Disorder
3.5.5   Panic Disorder
3.5.6   Agoraphobia
3.5.7   Generalized Anxiety Disorder

Obsessive-Compulsive and Related Disorders
3.6.1   Obsessive-Compulsive Disorder
3.6.2   Body Dysmorphic Disorder
3.6.3   Hoarding Disorder
3.6.4   Trichotillomania (Hair-Pulling Disorder)
3.6.5   Excoriation (Skin-Picking) Disorder

Trauma- and Stressor-Related Disorders
3.7.1   Posttraumatic Stress Disorder or Acute Stress Disorder
3.7.2   Adjustment Disorder
3.7.3   Prolonged Grief Disorder

Dissociative Disorders
3.8.1   Dissociative Amnesia
3.8.2   Depersonalization/Derealization Disorder

Somatic Symptom and Related Disorders
3.9.1   Somatic Symptom Disorder
3.9.2   Illness Anxiety Disorder
3.9.3   Functional Neurological Symptom Disorder (Conversion Disorder)
3.9.4   Psychological Factors Affecting Other Medical Conditions
3.9.5   Factitious Disorder

Feeding and Eating Disorders
3.10.1   Avoidant/Restrictive Food Intake Disorder
3.10.2   Anorexia Nervosa
3.10.3   Bulimia Nervosa
3.10.4   Binge-Eating Disorder

Sleep-Wake Disorders
3.11.1   Insomnia Disorder
3.11.2   Hypersomnolence Disorder

Neurodevelopmental Disorders

3.1.1 Differential Diagnosis for Intellectual Developmental Disorder (Intellectual Disability)

Intellectual Developmental Disorder, which is characterized by global deficits in intellectual functions (such as reasoning, problem solving, planning, abstract thinking, judgment, academic learning, and learning from experience) and deficits in adaptive functioning that result in failure to meet developmental and sociocultural standards for personal independence and social responsibility, must be differentiated from…	In contrast to Intellectual Developmental Disorder…
Specific Learning Disorder	Is characterized by an impairment confined to a specific area of academic achievement (e.g., reading, spelling, written expression, arithmetic calculation, mathematical reasoning). There are no deficits in intellectual and adaptive behavior.
Communication Disorders (i.e., Language Disorder, Speech Sound Disorder, Childhood-Onset Fluency Disorder [Stuttering], Social [Pragmatic] Communication Disorder)	Are characterized by impairments that are confined to speech or language problems. There are no deficits in intellectual and adaptive behavior.
Autism Spectrum Disorder	Is defined by the presence of persistent deficits in social communication and social interaction, along with restricted, repetitive patterns of behaviors, interests, or activities. Although there may be some impairment in social communicative skills in Intellectual Developmental Disorder, it is on par with deficits in other intellectual skills. Intellectual Developmental Disorder is frequently comorbid with Autism Spectrum Disorder, and if criteria are met for both, both diagnoses should be given.

3.1.1 Differential Diagnosis for Intellectual Developmental Disorder (Intellectual Disability) *(continued)*

Major Neurocognitive Disorder	Is characterized by a significant cognitive decline from a previous level of performance in one or more cognitive domains, such as executive function, learning, memory, and language. Both Major Neurocognitive Disorder and Intellectual Developmental Disorder can be diagnosed if the onset of intellectual and adaptive deficits is during the developmental period.
Borderline intellectual functioning	Is characterized by a lesser degree of intellectual impairment (typically IQ around 70) or no problems in adaptive functioning if there are significant intellectual impairments (e.g., IQ is below 70).

3.1.2 Differential Diagnosis for Communication Disorders

Communication Disorders (i.e., Language Disorder, Speech Sound Disorder, Childhood-Onset Fluency Disorder [Stuttering], Social [Pragmatic] Communication Disorder) must be differentiated from…	In contrast to Communication Disorders…
Intellectual Developmental Disorder	Involves an overall impairment in intellectual functioning as opposed to only language impairment. A Communication Disorder can also be diagnosed if the language problems are in excess of those usually associated with Intellectual Developmental Disorder.
Communication difficulties related to hearing impairment, a neurological deficit (e.g., Landau-Kleffner syndrome), a motor disorder (e.g., dysarthria), or a structural defect (e.g., cleft palate)	Are attributable to hearing impairment, a neurological deficit, a motor disorder, or a structural defect and are not in excess of that expected given the sensory or speech-motor deficit. A Communication Disorder can be diagnosed if the problems in communication are in excess of those usually associated with the deficits or disorders.
Selective Mutism	Is characterized by a lack of speech in some settings (e.g., in school, with strangers), whereas the child speaks normally in "safe" settings (e.g., at home). In a Communication Disorder, the communication problems are consistent across all settings. Some children with a Communication Disorder may develop Selective Mutism because of embarrassment about their speech deficits.
Tourette's Disorder (as distinguished from Childhood-Onset Fluency Disorder)	Is characterized by vocal tics and repetitive vocalizations that differ in nature and timing from the repetitive sounds of Childhood-Onset Fluency Disorder, which are characterized by broken words (i.e., pauses within a word), audible or silent blocking (i.e., filled or unfilled pauses in speech), circumlocutions (i.e., word substitutions to avoid problematic words), words produced with an excess of physical tension, and monosyllabic whole-word repetitions (e.g., "I-I-I-I see him").

3.1.2 Differential Diagnosis for Communication Disorders *(continued)*

Autism Spectrum Disorder (as distinguished from Social [Pragmatic] Communication Disorder)	Is characterized by restricted, repetitive patterns of behavior, interests, or activities in addition to social communication deficits, whereas in Social (Pragmatic) Communication Disorder, restricted, repetitive patterns of behavior, interests, or activities are absent.
Social Anxiety Disorder (as distinguished from Social [Pragmatic] Communication Disorder)	Is characterized by the lack of use of appropriately developed social communication skills because of anxiety, fear, or distress about social interactions. In Social (Pragmatic) Communication Disorder, these skills have never been present.
Normal dysfluencies or articulation difficulties in young children	Are developmentally appropriate.

3.1.3 Differential Diagnosis for Autism Spectrum Disorder

Autism Spectrum Disorder, which is characterized by persistent deficits in social communication and social interaction across multiple contexts, accompanied by restricted, repetitive patterns of behavior, interests, or activities that were present during the early developmental period, must be differentiated from…	In contrast to Autism Spectrum Disorder…
Schizophrenia	Childhood-onset Schizophrenia usually develops after a period of normal, or near-normal, development. The Schizophrenia prodromal state may include social impairment and atypical interests and beliefs, which could be confused with the social deficits seen in Autism Spectrum Disorder. Hallucinations and delusions, which are defining features of Schizophrenia, are not seen in Autism Spectrum Disorder.
Selective Mutism	Is characterized by normal early development and by appropriate social communication functioning in certain "safe" contexts and settings (e.g., at home with parents).
Language Disorder	Is characterized by a lack of qualitative impairment in social interaction, and the individual's range of interests and behaviors is not restricted.
Social (Pragmatic) Communication Disorder	Is characterized by impairment in social communication and social interactions without the restricted and repetitive behaviors or interests characteristic of Autism Spectrum Disorder.

3.1.3 Differential Diagnosis for Autism Spectrum Disorder *(continued)*

Intellectual Developmental Disorder	Involves general impairment in intellectual functioning; there is no discrepancy between the level of the social communicative skills and other intellectual skills. A diagnosis of Autism Spectrum Disorder in an individual with Intellectual Developmental Disorder is appropriate when social communication and interaction are significantly impaired relative to the developmental level of the individual's nonverbal skills.
Stereotypic Movement Disorder	Occurs in the absence of impairment of social interaction and language development. Stereotypic Movement Disorder is generally not diagnosed if the stereotypy is part of Autism Spectrum Disorder; however, when stereotypies cause self-injury and become a focus of treatment, both diagnoses may be appropriate.

3.1.4 Differential Diagnosis for Attention-Deficit/Hyperactivity Disorder

Attention-Deficit/Hyperactivity Disorder (ADHD), which is characterized by symptoms of inattention and/or hyperactivity-impulsivity that are inconsistent with developmental level and that negatively impact social and academic/occupational activities, must be differentiated from…	In contrast to Attention-Deficit/ Hyperactivity Disorder…
Normative behaviors in active children	Are consistent with developmental level.
Understimulating environments	Lead to inattention that is related to boredom.
Oppositional Defiant Disorder	May be characterized by resistance to work or school tasks because of a refusal to submit to others' demands, which is accompanied by negativity, hostility, and defiance. In ADHD, however, the aversion to school or mentally demanding tasks is due to difficulty in sustaining mental effort, forgetting instructions, and impulsivity.
Intermittent Explosive Disorder	Is also characterized by high levels of impulsive behavior, but unlike ADHD, there are episodes of serious aggression toward others. An additional diagnosis of Intermittent Explosive Disorder can be made if the recurrent impulsive aggressive outbursts are in excess of those usually seen in ADHD and warrant independent clinical attention.
Conduct Disorder	May be characterized by high levels of impulsivity, but there is also a pattern of antisocial behavior.
Stereotypic Movement Disorder	Is characterized by repetitive motor behavior that may resemble the increased motor behavior in ADHD. In contrast to ADHD, however, the motor behavior is generally fixed and repetitive (e.g., body rocking, self-biting), whereas the fidgetiness and restlessness in ADHD are typically generalized.

3.1.4 Differential Diagnosis for Attention-Deficit/Hyperactivity Disorder *(continued)*

Specific Learning Disorder	May be characterized by inattentive behavior because of frustration, lack of interest, or limited ability. However, inattention in individuals with Specific Learning Disorder who do not have ADHD is not impairing outside of schoolwork.
Intellectual Developmental Disorder	May be characterized by symptoms of inattention and/or hyperactivity-impulsivity among children placed in academic settings that are inappropriate for their intellectual ability. Individuals with Intellectual Developmental Disorder without ADHD do not have symptoms during nonacademic tasks. A diagnosis of ADHD in individuals with Intellectual Developmental Disorder requires that the inattention or hyperactivity be excessive for the individual's mental age.
Autism Spectrum Disorder	May be characterized by social disengagement and social isolation due to deficits in social communication, as well as temper tantrums due to an inability to tolerate a change from the expected course of events, whereas social dysfunction and peer rejection in ADHD are related to symptoms of inattention and hyperactivity, and misbehavior and temper tantrums are related to impulsivity or poor self-control.
Disinhibited Social Engagement Disorder	Is characterized by social disinhibition, but not the full ADHD symptom cluster. Children with Disinhibited Social Engagement Disorder also have a history of extremes of insufficient care.
Disruptive Mood Dysregulation Disorder	Is characterized by pervasive irritability and intolerance of frustration. Given that most children and adolescents with Disruptive Mood Dysregulation Disorder also have symptoms that meet criteria for ADHD, an additional diagnosis may be made.

3.1.4 Differential Diagnosis for Attention-Deficit/Hyperactivity Disorder *(continued)*

Anxiety Disorders	May be characterized by symptoms of inattention due to fear, worry, and rumination. In ADHD, the inattention is due to attraction to external stimuli or new activities, or preoccupation with enjoyable activities.
Major Depressive Disorder	May be characterized by an inability to concentrate; however, the poor concentration is prominent only during Major Depressive Episodes.
Bipolar I or Bipolar II Disorder	May be characterized by increased activity, poor concentration, increased impulsivity, and distractibility, but these features are episodic, occurring several days to weeks at a time. Moreover, the symptoms are accompanied by elevated or irritable mood, grandiosity, and other specific bipolar features. Although individuals with ADHD may show significant changes in mood within the same day, such lability is distinct from a Manic or Hypomanic Episode, which must be sustained and last at least a week (or 4 days for a Hypomanic Episode) to be a clinical indicator of Bipolar I or Bipolar II Disorder.
Borderline, Antisocial, and Narcissistic Personality Disorders	Share the features of disorganization, social intrusiveness, emotional dysregulation, and cognitive dysregulation. These disorders are distinguished from ADHD by the presence of additional maladaptive features, such as self-injury, antisocial behavior, fear of abandonment, and lack of empathy. If criteria are met for both ADHD and a Personality Disorder, both may be diagnosed.

3.1.4 Differential Diagnosis for Attention-Deficit/Hyperactivity Disorder *(continued)*

Medication-induced symptoms of ADHD	Are characterized by symptoms of inattention and/or hyperactivity-impulsivity caused by medications (e.g., bronchodilators, isoniazid, antipsychotic medications and other dopamine receptor blocking agents [resulting in akathisia], thyroid replacement medication) and remit when the medications are stopped. ADHD is not diagnosed if the symptoms occur only during medication use.
Neurocognitive Disorders	May be characterized by cognitive impairments similar to those in ADHD; they are distinguished by their typically later age at onset.

3.1.5 Differential Diagnosis for Specific Learning Disorder

Specific Learning Disorder, which is characterized by difficulties in learning and using academic skills (e.g., reading, spelling, written expression, arithmetic calculation, mathematical reasoning), must be differentiated from…

In contrast to Specific Learning Disorder…

Normal variations in academic attainment	Do not result in clinically significant interference with academic achievement, occupational performance, or activities of daily living that require these academic skills; the affected academic skills are not substantially and quantifiably below those expected for the individual's chronological age (on the basis of appropriate standardized measures); or the difficulties abate with the provision of interventions that target the difficulties.
Poor academic performance due to lack of opportunity, poor teaching, or learning in a second language	Represents factors external to the individual and thus not indicative of an internal dysfunction. To justify a diagnosis of Specific Learning Disorder, the learning difficulties must persist in the presence of adequate educational opportunity, exposure to the same instruction as the peer group, and competency in the language of instruction.
Poor academic performance due to impaired vision or hearing or other neurological deficit	Is at a level that would be expected given the nature of the sensory or neurological deficit. Specific Learning Disorder can still be diagnosed if the academic difficulties are not adequately accounted for by the sensory or neurological deficit.
Intellectual Developmental Disorder	Consists of an overall impairment in intellectual functioning that is not confined to a particular academic skill. Specific Learning Disorder can be diagnosed along with Intellectual Developmental Disorder, as long as the learning difficulties are in excess of those usually associated with Intellectual Developmental Disorder.

3.1.5 Differential Diagnosis for Specific Learning Disorder *(continued)*

Autism Spectrum Disorder	Includes persistent deficits in social communication and social interaction, along with restricted, repetitive patterns of behaviors, interests, or activities; these deficits and patterns are not confined to a particular academic skill.
Communication Disorders	Involves impairments in speech or language skills that are not restricted to particular academic skills, such as reading or writing.
Major Neurocognitive Disorder	The difficulties are manifested as a marked decline from a former state, whereas in Specific Learning Disorder, the difficulties occur during the developmental period and do not represent a loss of previously acquired skills.
Attention-Deficit/Hyperactivity Disorder	Is characterized by problems that reflect difficulties in performing academic skills due to inattention, hyperactivity, and/or impulsivity rather than specific difficulties learning academic skills.
Schizophrenia	Associated academic and cognitive processing difficulties may result in an often rapid decline in academic functioning that has its onset in adolescence or early adulthood, whereas the learning difficulties in Specific Learning Disorder become apparent during the elementary school years when children are required to learn to read, spell, write, and do mathematics.

3.1.6 Differential Diagnosis for Tic Disorders

Tic Disorders (i.e., Tourette's Disorder, Persistent [Chronic] Motor or Vocal Tic Disorder, Provisional Tic Disorder), which are characterized by sudden, rapid, recurrent, nonrhythmic motor movements or vocalizations, must be differentiated from…	In contrast to Tic Disorders…
Choreiform movements associated with neurological or other medical conditions	Are characterized by rapid, random, continual, abrupt, irregular, unpredictable, nonstereotyped actions that are usually bilateral and affect all parts of the body (i.e., face, trunk, and limbs).
Dystonic movements associated with neurological or other medical conditions	Are characterized by the simultaneous sustained contracture of both agonist and antagonist muscles, resulting in distorted posture or movement of parts of the body.
Myoclonus	Is characterized by sudden unidirectional movements that are often nonrhythmic and may be worsened by movement and occur during sleep. Myoclonus is differentiated from tics by its rapidity, lack of suppressibility, and absence of a premonitory urge.
Tics caused by substances or medications	Remit when the substance or medication (e.g., stimulant) is stopped and are diagnosed as Unspecified [Substance]-Related Disorder (e.g., Unspecified Amphetamine-Related Disorder) or Other Medication-Induced Movement Disorder.
Stereotypic Movement Disorder, or stereotypies in Autism Spectrum Disorder	Are characterized by nonfunctional, usually rhythmic, seemingly driven behaviors that are generally more complex than tics.

3.1.6 Differential Diagnosis for Tic Disorders *(continued)*

Compulsions in Obsessive-Compulsive Disorder	Occur in response to an obsession or according to rigidly applied rules.
Schizophrenia	May be characterized by disorganized or bizarre vocalizations or behaviors that are accompanied by the other characteristic symptoms (e.g., delusions, negative symptoms) and have a characteristic course (e.g., marked decline in functioning).

Schizophrenia Spectrum and Other Psychotic Disorders

3.2.1 Differential Diagnosis for Schizophrenia or Schizophreniform Disorder[a]

Schizophrenia and Schizophreniform Disorder, which are characterized by a disturbance lasting for months (at least 6 months for Schizophrenia and between 1 and 6 months for Schizophreniform Disorder) that significantly impairs functioning and that includes at least 1 month of active-phase psychotic symptoms, must be differentiated from…	In contrast to Schizophrenia or Schizophreniform Disorder…
Psychotic Disorder Due to Another Medical Condition, Delirium Due to Another Medical Condition, or Major Neurocognitive Disorder Due to Another Medical Condition	Requires the presence of an etiological nonpsychiatric medical condition. Schizophrenia or Schizophreniform Disorder is not diagnosed if the psychotic symptoms are all due to the direct physiological effects of a nonpsychiatric medical condition.
Substance/Medication-Induced Psychotic Disorder, Substance/Medication-Induced Neurocognitive Disorder, Substance Intoxication Delirium, Substance Withdrawal Delirium, Medication-Induced Delirium, Substance Intoxication, or Substance Withdrawal	Requires that the psychotic symptoms be initiated and maintained by substance use (including medication side effects). Schizophrenia or Schizophreniform Disorder is not diagnosed if the psychotic symptoms are all due to the direct physiological effects of a substance (including medication).
Schizoaffective Disorder	Is characterized by symptoms that meet criteria for a Major Depressive Episode (specifically Criterion A1, depressed mood) or a Manic Episode concurrent with Criterion A of Schizophrenia,[b] and the mood episodes are present for the majority of the total duration of the active and residual portion of the illness. In Schizophrenia or Schizophreniform Disorder, the mood episodes have been present for only a minority of the total duration of the active and residual periods of the illness.

3.2.1 Differential Diagnosis for Schizophrenia or Schizophreniform Disorder[a] *(continued)*

Major Depressive Disorder, With Psychotic Features; Bipolar I or Bipolar II Disorder, With Psychotic Features; Catatonia Associated With Major Depressive Disorder; or Catatonia Associated With Bipolar I or Bipolar II Disorder	Is characterized by psychotic or catatonic symptoms that occur exclusively during Manic or Major Depressive Episodes.
Brief Psychotic Disorder	Is characterized by a total duration of psychotic symptoms of at least 1 day but less than 1 month.
Delusional Disorder	Is characterized by delusions occurring in the absence of the other characteristic symptoms of Schizophrenia (i.e., prominent auditory or visual hallucinations, disorganized speech, grossly disorganized or catatonic behavior, negative symptoms).
Posttraumatic Stress Disorder	May be characterized by flashbacks that have a hallucinatory quality and hypervigilance that may reach paranoid proportions, but it is distinguished by the requirement of exposure to a traumatic event with a characteristic cluster of intrusion, avoidance, and other symptoms.
Autism Spectrum Disorder	Is characterized by an early onset (e.g., before age 3 years) and an absence of prominent delusions or hallucinations. A diagnosis of Schizophrenia or Schizophreniform Disorder may be warranted in individuals with a preexisting diagnosis of Autism Spectrum Disorder only if prominent hallucinations or delusions have been present for at least 1 month.

3.2.1 Differential Diagnosis for Schizophrenia or Schizophreniform Disorder[a] *(continued)*

Schizotypal, Schizoid, and Paranoid Personality Disorders	Are characterized by personality features that are subthreshold versions of many of the symptoms of Schizophrenia (e.g., odd beliefs, perceptual distortions, odd thinking and speech, social anxiety).

[a]Schizophrenia and Schizophreniform Disorder have essentially the same differential diagnosis and thus have been combined for the purposes of this differential diagnosis table. They are differentiated primarily on the basis of the duration of the disturbance. In Schizophreniform Disorder, the duration is between 1 and 6 months. In Schizophrenia, the duration is 6 months or longer.
[b]Two or more of the following symptoms during a 1-month period: delusions, hallucinations, disorganized speech, grossly disorganized or catatonic behavior, and negative symptoms, with at least one symptom being delusions, hallucinations, or disorganized speech.

3.2.2 Differential Diagnosis for Schizoaffective Disorder

Schizoaffective Disorder, which is characterized by times in which Major Depressive Episodes (specifically Criterion A1, depressed mood) or Manic Episodes occur concurrently with symptoms that meet Criterion A of Schizophrenia,[a] and times in which there are delusions or hallucinations without mood symptoms, must be differentiated from...

In contrast to Schizoaffective Disorder...

Psychotic Disorder Due to Another Medical Condition, Delirium Due to Another Medical Condition, or Major Neurocognitive Disorder Due to Another Medical Condition	Requires the presence of an etiological nonpsychiatric medical condition. Schizoaffective Disorder is not diagnosed if the psychotic or mood symptoms are all due to the direct physiological effects of a nonpsychiatric medical condition.
Substance/Medication-Induced Psychotic Disorder, Substance/Medication-Induced Neurocognitive Disorder, Substance Intoxication Delirium, Substance Withdrawal Delirium, Medication-Induced Delirium, Substance Intoxication, or Substance Withdrawal	Requires that the psychotic and mood symptoms be due to substance use (including medication side effects). Schizoaffective Disorder is not diagnosed if the psychotic or mood symptoms are all due to the direct physiological effects of a substance (including medication).
Schizophrenia	Is characterized either by the absence of mood episodes or, if there are mood episodes, they have been present for only a minority of the total duration of the active and residual periods of the illness.
Bipolar I or Bipolar II Disorder, With Psychotic Features; Major Depressive Disorder, With Psychotic Features	Is characterized by psychotic symptoms that occur exclusively during a Manic or Major Depressive Episode.
Delusional Disorder	Is characterized by delusions that persist for at least 1 month, occurring in the absence of a period that meets Criterion A for Schizophrenia.[a]

[a]Two or more of the following symptoms during a 1-month period: delusions, hallucinations, disorganized speech, grossly disorganized or catatonic behavior, and negative symptoms, with at least one symptom being delusions, hallucinations, or disorganized speech.

3.2.3 Differential Diagnosis for Delusional Disorder

Delusional Disorder, which is characterized by persistent delusions and the absence of a symptomatic period that meets Criterion A of Schizophrenia,[a] must be differentiated from...	In contrast to Delusional Disorder...
Psychotic Disorder Due to Another Medical Condition, Delirium Due to Another Medical Condition, or Major Neurocognitive Disorder Due to Another Medical Condition	Requires the presence of an etiological nonpsychiatric medical condition. Delusional Disorder is not diagnosed if the delusions are all due to the direct physiological effects of a nonpsychiatric medical condition.
Substance/Medication-Induced Psychotic Disorder, Substance/Medication-Induced Neurocognitive Disorder, Substance Intoxication Delirium, Substance Withdrawal Delirium, Medication-Induced Delirium, Substance Intoxication, or Substance Withdrawal	Requires that the psychotic symptoms be due to substance use (including medication side effects). Delusional Disorder is not diagnosed if the delusions are all due to the direct physiological effects of a substance (including medication).
Schizophrenia or Schizophreniform Disorder	Is characterized by at least one period of symptoms that meet Criterion A of Schizophrenia.[a]
Bipolar I or Bipolar II Disorder, With Psychotic Features; Major Depressive Disorder, With Psychotic Features	Is characterized by delusions that occur exclusively during Manic or Major Depressive Episodes. When there is a history of Manic or Major Depressive Episodes, Delusional Disorder can be diagnosed only if the total duration of all mood episodes remains brief relative to the total duration of the delusional disturbance. If not, then the appropriate diagnosis is Other Specified Schizophrenia Spectrum and Other Psychotic Disorder.
Brief Psychotic Disorder	Is characterized by psychotic symptoms that last for less than 1 month. In Delusional Disorder, the minimum duration of the delusions is 1 month.

3.2.3 Differential Diagnosis for Delusional Disorder *(continued)*

Obsessive-Compulsive Disorder	If an individual with Obsessive-Compulsive Disorder is completely convinced that their Obsessive-Compulsive Disorder beliefs are true (and thus has a delusional belief), then the diagnosis should be Obsessive-Compulsive Disorder, With Absent Insight/Delusional Beliefs, rather than Delusional Disorder.
Body Dysmorphic Disorder	In situations in which an individual with Body Dysmorphic Disorder is completely convinced that their beliefs are true (i.e., that their appearance is defective), they have a delusional belief, and the diagnosis should be Body Dysmorphic Disorder, With Absent Insight/Delusional Beliefs, rather than Delusional Disorder.
Paranoid Personality Disorder or Schizotypal Personality Disorder	Is characterized by paranoid ideation without clear-cut or persisting delusional beliefs.

[a]Two or more of the following symptoms during a 1-month period: delusions, hallucinations, disorganized speech, grossly disorganized or catatonic behavior, and negative symptoms, with at least one symptom being delusions, hallucinations, or disorganized speech.

3.2.4 Differential Diagnosis for Brief Psychotic Disorder

Brief Psychotic Disorder, which is characterized by psychotic symptoms lasting less than 1 month, must be differentiated from...	In contrast to Brief Psychotic Disorder...
Psychotic Disorder Due to Another Medical Condition, Delirium Due to Another Medical Condition, or Major Neurocognitive Disorder Due to Another Medical Condition	Requires the presence of an etiological nonpsychiatric medical condition. Brief Psychotic Disorder is not diagnosed if the psychotic symptoms are all due to the direct physiological effects of a nonpsychiatric medical condition.
Substance/Medication-Induced Psychotic Disorder	Requires that the psychotic symptoms be due to substance use (including medication side effects). Brief Psychotic Disorder is not diagnosed if the psychotic symptoms are all due to the direct physiological effects of a substance (including medication).
Bipolar I, Bipolar II, or Major Depressive Disorder, With Psychotic Features	Is characterized by psychotic symptoms occurring exclusively during mood episodes. Brief Psychotic Disorder is not diagnosed if the psychotic symptoms are better accounted for by Bipolar I, Bipolar II, or Major Depressive Disorder, With Psychotic Features.
Schizophreniform Disorder, Schizophrenia, or Delusional Disorder	Is characterized by psychotic symptoms that last 1 month or longer.
Psychotic symptoms occurring in the context of some Personality Disorders (e.g., Borderline Personality Disorder)	Are usually transient and last less than 1 day. If clinically significant, they may be diagnosed as Other Specified/Unspecified Schizophrenia Spectrum and Other Psychotic Disorder. If psychotic symptoms persist for at least 1 day, the additional diagnosis of Brief Psychotic Disorder may be warranted.

3.2.5 Differential Diagnosis for Unspecified Catatonia

Unspecified Catatonia, which describes presentations in which clinically significant symptoms of Catatonia are present and either the nature of the underlying mental disorder or nonpsychiatric medical condition is unclear or the full criteria for the syndrome of Catatonia are not met, must be differentiated from...	In contrast to Uspecified Catatonia...
Catatonic Disorder Due to Another Medical Condition	Is characterized by the full syndrome of Catatonia that is due to the direct physiological effects of a nonpsychiatric medical condition, especially neurological conditions (e.g., neoplasms, head trauma, cerebrovascular disease, encephalitis) and metabolic conditions (e.g., hypercalcemia, hepatic encephalopathy, homocystinuria, diabetic ketoacidosis).
Mutism or posturing in Delirium Due to Another Medical Condition	Is characterized by catatonic symptoms occurring in the context of a disturbance in attention (i.e., reduced ability to direct, focus, sustain, and shift attention), and is accompanied by reduced awareness of the environment. If catatonia symptoms occur exclusively during the course of Delirium, they are considered to be symptoms of the Delirium, and neither Unspecified Catatonia nor Catatonic Disorder Due to Another Medical Condition is diagnosed.
Akinesia, rigidity, or posturing in medication-induced movement disorders (including neuroleptic malignant syndrome)	Is due to the direct physiological effects of a medication, including antipsychotic medications and other dopamine receptor blocking agents.
Catatonia Associated With [any of the following] Schizophrenia, Schizoaffective Disorder, Schizophreniform Disorder, or Brief Psychotic Disorder	Is characterized by the full syndrome of Catatonia that is accompanied by other characteristic symptoms of the relevant psychotic disorder.

3.2.5 Differential Diagnosis for Unspecified Catatonia *(continued)*

Catatonia Associated With Bipolar I, Bipolar II, or Major Depressive Disorder	Is characterized by the full syndrome of Catatonia that occurs exclusively during Manic or Major Depressive Episodes.
Catatonia Associated With Autism Spectrum Disorder	Is characterized by the full syndrome of Catatonia that is accompanied by the characteristic symptoms of Autism Spectrum Disorder (e.g., social communication difficulties, restricted repertoire of interests and behaviors).

Bipolar and Related Disorders

3.3.1 Differential Diagnosis for Bipolar I Disorder

Bipolar I Disorder, which is characterized by at least one Manic Episode that may have been preceded by or followed by Hypomanic or Major Depressive Episodes, must be differentiated from...	In contrast to Bipolar I Disorder...
Bipolar and Related Disorder Due to Another Medical Condition	Requires the presence of an etiological nonpsychiatric medical condition. Bipolar I Disorder is not diagnosed if the Manic Episodes are all due to the direct physiological effects of a nonpsychiatric medical condition.
Substance/Medication-Induced Bipolar and Related Disorder	Is due to the direct physiological effects of a substance (including medication). A full Manic Episode that emerges during antidepressant treatment (e.g., with a selective serotonin reuptake inhibitor) but persists at a fully syndromal level beyond the direct physiological effect of that treatment meets criteria for a Manic Episode and, therefore, a Bipolar I Disorder diagnosis is most appropriate.
Major Depressive Disorder	Is characterized by the absence of both Manic Episodes and Hypomanic Episodes. Given that the presence of some manic or hypomanic symptoms (i.e., fewer symptoms or a shorter duration of symptoms than required for mania or hypomania) may still be compatible with a diagnosis of Major Depressive Disorder (and would warrant use of the specifier With Mixed Features), it is important to ascertain whether the symptoms meet full criteria for a Manic or Hypomanic Episode to determine whether it is more appropriate to make the diagnosis of a Bipolar Disorder.
Bipolar II Disorder	Is characterized by the presence of Hypomanic and Major Depressive Episodes and the absence of Manic Episodes. Bipolar II Disorder cannot be diagnosed if criteria have ever been met for Bipolar I Disorder.

3.3.1 Differential Diagnosis for Bipolar I Disorder *(continued)*

Cyclothymic Disorder	Is characterized by numerous periods of hypomanic symptoms that do not meet criteria for a Manic or Hypomanic Episode and by periods of depressive symptoms that do not meet criteria for a Major Depressive Episode. For the diagnosis of Cyclothymic Disorder to apply, criteria must never have been met for Manic, Hypomanic, or Major Depressive Episode.
Schizophrenia, Delusional Disorder, or Schizophreniform Disorder	Is characterized by psychotic symptoms that occur at times other than just during Manic or Major Depressive Episodes. If all Manic Episodes have been superimposed on Schizophrenia, Delusional Disorder, or Schizophreniform Disorder, the presence of such Manic Episodes can be indicated by giving an additional diagnosis of Other Specified Bipolar and Related Disorder. The diagnosis is Bipolar I Disorder, With Psychotic Features, if the psychotic symptoms have occurred exclusively during Manic or Major Depressive Episodes.
Schizoaffective Disorder	Is characterized by periods in which Manic Episodes and/or Major Depressive Episodes (specifically Criterion A1, depressed mood) are concurrent with the active-phase symptoms of Schizophrenia, periods in which delusions or hallucinations occur for at least 2 weeks in the absence of a Manic or Major Depressive Episode during the lifetime course of the illness, and symptoms that meet criteria for a Manic or Major Depressive Episode are present for a majority of the total duration of the active and residual portions of the illness. The diagnosis is Bipolar I Disorder, With Psychotic Features, if the psychotic symptoms have occurred exclusively during Manic and Major Depressive Episodes.
Attention-Deficit/Hyperactivity Disorder	Is characterized by persistent symptoms of inattention and/or hyperactivity-impulsivity, which may resemble the symptoms of a Manic Episode (e.g., distractibility, increased activity, impulsive behavior) and have their onset before age 12, whereas the symptoms of mania in Bipolar I Disorder occur in distinct episodes and typically begin in late adolescence or early adulthood.

3.3.1 Differential Diagnosis for Bipolar I Disorder *(continued)*

Disruptive Mood Dysregulation Disorder	Is characterized by severe recurrent temper outbursts manifested verbally and/or behaviorally, which are accompanied by persistently irritable or angry mood most of the day, nearly every day, in between the outbursts. In contrast, the irritability in Bipolar I Disorder occurs in distinct episodes that last at least 1 week, is clearly different from the individual's baseline, and is accompanied by the characteristic associated symptoms of mania (e.g., grandiosity, decreased need for sleep).
Personality Disorders (especially Borderline Personality Disorder)	May be characterized by symptoms such as mood lability and impulsivity that are persistent and have their onset by early adulthood. In contrast, the mood symptoms in Bipolar I Disorder occur in distinct episodes that represent a noticeable change from normal baseline functioning.

3.3.2 Differential Diagnosis for Bipolar II Disorder

Bipolar II Disorder, which is characterized by at least one Hypomanic Episode and one Major Depressive Episode, must be differentiated from...	In contrast to Bipolar II Disorder...
Bipolar and Related Disorder Due to Another Medical Condition	Requires the presence of an etiological nonpsychiatric medical condition. Bipolar II Disorder is not diagnosed if the Hypomanic and Major Depressive Episodes are all due to the direct physiological effects of a nonpsychiatric medical condition.
Substance/Medication-Induced Bipolar and Related Disorder	Is characterized by Hypomanic and Major Depressive Episodes that are due to the direct physiological effects of a substance (including medication). A full Hypomanic Episode that emerges during antidepressant treatment (e.g., with a selective serotonin reuptake inhibitor) but persists at a fully syndromal level beyond the direct physiological effect of that treatment meets criteria for a Hypomanic Episode, and therefore, potentially a Bipolar II Disorder diagnosis if there has also been a history of Major Depressive Episodes.
Major Depressive Disorder	Is characterized by the absence of both Manic Episodes and Hypomanic Episodes. Given that the presence of some manic or hypomanic symptoms (i.e., fewer symptoms or a shorter duration of symptoms than required for mania or hypomania) may still be compatible with a diagnosis of Major Depressive Disorder (and would warrant use of the specifier With Mixed Features), it is important to ascertain whether the symptoms meet criteria for a Hypomanic Episode to determine whether it is more appropriate to make the diagnosis of Bipolar II Disorder.
Bipolar I Disorder	Is characterized by the presence of at least one Manic Episode. Bipolar II Disorder cannot be diagnosed if criteria have ever been met for a Manic Episode.

3.3.2 Differential Diagnosis for Bipolar II Disorder *(continued)*

Cyclothymic Disorder	Is characterized by numerous periods of hypomanic symptoms that do not meet criteria for a Manic or Hypomanic Episode and by periods of depressive symptoms that do not meet criteria for a Major Depressive Episode. For the diagnosis of Cyclothymic Disorder to apply, criteria must never have been met for a Hypomanic or Major Depressive Episode.
Schizophrenia, Delusional Disorder, or Schizophreniform Disorder	Is characterized by psychotic symptoms, which occur at times other than just during Major Depressive Episodes. If all Major Depressive Episodes have been superimposed on Schizophrenia, Delusional Disorder, or Schizophreniform Disorder, the presence of such Major Depressive Episodes can be indicated by giving an additional diagnosis of Other Specified Depressive Disorder. The diagnosis is Bipolar II Disorder, With Psychotic Features, if the psychotic symptoms have occurred exclusively during Major Depressive Episodes.
Schizoaffective Disorder	Is characterized by periods in which Major Depressive Episodes (specifically Criterion A1, depressed mood) are concurrent with the active-phase symptoms of Schizophrenia, periods in which delusions or hallucinations occur for at least 2 weeks in the absence of a Major Depressive Episode during the lifetime course of the illness, and symptoms that meet criteria for a Major Depressive Episode are present for a majority of the total duration of the active and residual portions of the illness. The diagnosis is Bipolar II Disorder, With Psychotic Features, if the psychotic symptoms have occurred exclusively during Major Depressive Episodes.
Attention-Deficit/Hyperactivity Disorder	Is characterized by persistent symptoms of inattention and/or hyperactivity-impulsivity, which may resemble the symptoms of a Hypomanic Episode (e.g., distractibility, increased activity, impulsive behavior) and have their onset before age 12. In contrast, the symptoms of hypomania in Bipolar II Disorder occur in distinct episodes and typically begin in late adolescence or early adulthood.

3.3.2 Differential Diagnosis for Bipolar II Disorder *(continued)*

Disruptive Mood Dysregulation Disorder	Is characterized by severe recurrent temper outbursts manifested verbally and/or behaviorally, which are accompanied by persistently irritable or angry mood most of the day, nearly every day, in between the outbursts. In contrast, the irritability in Bipolar II Disorder occurs in distinct episodes that last at least 4 days, is clearly different from the individual's baseline, and is accompanied by the characteristic associated symptoms of hypomania (e.g., grandiosity, decreased need for sleep).
Personality Disorders (especially Borderline Personality Disorder)	May be characterized by symptoms such as mood lability and impulsivity that are persistent and have their onset by early adulthood. In contrast, the mood symptoms in Bipolar II Disorder occur in distinct episodes that represent a noticeable change from normal baseline functioning.

3.3.3 Differential Diagnosis for Cyclothymic Disorder

Cyclothymic Disorder, which is characterized by numerous periods with hypomanic symptoms that do not meet criteria for a Hypomanic Episode and numerous periods with depressive symptoms that do not meet criteria for a Major Depressive Episode, must be differentiated from…

In contrast to Cyclothymic Disorder…

Bipolar I or Bipolar II Disorder, With Rapid Cycling

Is characterized by four or more mood episodes (each of which meets full criteria for a Manic, Hypomanic, or Major Depressive Episode) occurring in a 12-month period. Cyclothymic Disorder is characterized by numerous periods of hypomanic and depressive symptoms that do not meet criteria for a Hypomanic or Major Depressive Episode. If criteria have ever been met for a Manic, Hypomanic, or Major Depressive Episode, Cyclothymic Disorder is not diagnosed.

Borderline Personality Disorder

Is characterized by additional personality features (e.g., identity disturbance, self-mutilating behavior) besides affective lability. If criteria are met for Cyclothymic Disorder and Borderline Personality Disorder, both can be diagnosed.

Bipolar and Related Disorder Due to Another Medical Condition

Requires the presence of an etiological nonpsychiatric medical condition. Cyclothymic Disorder is not diagnosed if the mood symptoms are all due to the direct physiological effects of a nonpsychiatric medical condition.

Substance/Medication-Induced Bipolar and Related Disorder

Is due to the direct physiological effects of a substance. Cyclothymic Disorder is not diagnosed if the mood symptoms are all due to the direct physiological effects of a substance (including medication).

Depressive Disorders

3.4.1 Differential Diagnosis for Major Depressive Disorder

Major Depressive Disorder, which is characterized by episodes of depressed mood or diminished interest or pleasure most of the day, nearly every day, for at least 2 weeks and that are accompanied by characteristic associated symptoms (e.g., changes in sleep, appetite, or activity level; fatigue; difficulty concentrating; feelings of worthlessness or excessive guilt; suicidal ideation or behavior), must be differentiated from…

In contrast to Major Depressive Disorder…

Bipolar I or Bipolar II Disorder	Includes one or more Manic or Hypomanic Episodes. Major Depressive Disorder cannot be diagnosed if a Manic or Hypomanic Episode has ever been present. A diagnosis of Major Depressive Disorder may be compatible with the presence of some manic or hypomanic symptoms (i.e., fewer symptoms or a shorter duration of symptoms than required for mania or hypomania) and might warrant the use of the specifier With Mixed Features.
Depressive Disorder Due to Another Medical Condition	Requires the presence of an etiological medical condition. Major Depressive Disorder is not diagnosed if the major depressive–like episodes are all due to the direct physiological effects of a nonpsychiatric medical condition.
Substance/Medication-Induced Depressive Disorder	Is due to the direct physiological effects of a substance or medication. Major Depressive Disorder is not diagnosed if the major depressive–like episodes are all due to the direct physiological effects of a substance (including medication).
Persistent Depressive Disorder	Is characterized by depressed mood, more days than not, for at least 2 years. If criteria are met for both Major Depressive Disorder and Persistent Depressive Disorder, both should be diagnosed.

3.4.1 Differential Diagnosis for Major Depressive Disorder *(continued)*

Premenstrual Dysphoric Disorder	Is characterized by dysphoric mood that is present in the final week before the onset of menses and that starts to improve within a few days after the onset of menses, and becomes minimal or absent in the week postmenses. In contrast, the onset and offset of Major Depressive Disorder Episodes are not temporally connected to the menstrual cycle.
Disruptive Mood Dysregulation Disorder	Is characterized by severe, recurrent temper outbursts manifested verbally and/or behaviorally, accompanied by a persistently irritable or angry mood most of the day, nearly every day, in between the outbursts. In contrast, in Major Depressive Disorder, irritability is confined to the Major Depressive Episodes.
Schizophrenia, Delusional Disorder, or Schizophreniform Disorder	Is characterized by psychotic symptoms that occur at times other than just during Major Depressive Episodes. If all Major Depressive Episodes have been superimposed on Schizophrenia, Delusional Disorder, or Schizophreniform Disorder, the presence of such Major Depressive Episodes can be indicated by giving an additional diagnosis of Other Specified Depressive Disorder. The diagnosis is Major Depressive Disorder, With Psychotic Features, if the psychotic symptoms have occurred exclusively during Major Depressive Episodes.

3.4.1 Differential Diagnosis for Major Depressive Disorder *(continued)*

Schizoaffective Disorder	Is characterized by periods in which Major Depressive Episodes (specifically Criterion A1, depressed mood) are concurrent with the active-phase symptoms of Schizophrenia, periods in which delusions or hallucinations occur for at least 2 weeks in the absence of a Major Depressive Episode during the lifetime course of the illness, and symptoms that meet criteria for a Major Depressive Episode are present for a majority of the total duration of the active and residual portions of the illness. The diagnosis is Major Depressive Disorder, With Psychotic Features, if the psychotic symptoms have occurred exclusively during Major Depressive Episodes.
Major or Mild Neurocognitive Disorder Due to Another Medical Condition, With Mood Symptoms; or Substance/Medication-Induced Major or Mild Neurocognitive Disorder, With Mood Symptoms	Is characterized by evidence of decline from a previous level of performance in one or more cognitive domains, in addition to the depression that is due to the direct physiological effects of the nonpsychiatric medical condition causing the neurocognitive disorder or the persisting effects of medication or substance use.
Adjustment Disorder, With Depressed Mood	Is characterized by depressive symptoms that occur in response to an identifiable psychosocial stressor and do not meet criteria for a Major Depressive Episode.

3.4.1 Differential Diagnosis for Major Depressive Disorder *(continued)*

Prolonged Grief Disorder	Is a persistent, pervasive grief response that continues to cause clinically significant distress or impairment for more than 12 months after the death of someone close. It can be differentiated from a Major Depressive Episode by the requirement of intense yearning or longing for, or preoccupation with, the deceased. For a diagnosis of Prolonged Grief Disorder, other required symptoms (such as emotional pain, marked reduction in emotional experiences, feeling that life is meaningless, and having difficulty reintegrating socially or feeling engaged in ongoing activities) are judged to result from the significant interpersonal loss. Although these symptoms may be consistent with a diagnosis of Major Depressive Disorder, by contrast, in a Major Depressive Episode, there is a more generalized depressed mood that is not specifically related to the loss. Both Prolonged Grief Disorder and Major Depressive Disorder should be diagnosed if criteria for both are met.
Bereavement	Occurs in response to the loss of a loved one and is generally less severe than a Major Depressive Episode. The predominant affects in grief are feelings of emptiness and loss, whereas in Major Depressive Episode they are persistent depressed mood and a diminished ability to experience pleasure. Moreover, the dysphoric mood in grief is likely to decrease in intensity over days to weeks and occurs in waves that tend to be associated with thoughts or reminders of the deceased, whereas the depressed mood in a Major Depressive Episode is more persistent and not tied to specific thoughts or preoccupations.
Nonpathological periods of sadness	Are characterized by short duration, few associated symptoms, and lack of significant functional impairment or distress.

3.4.2 Differential Diagnosis for Persistent Depressive Disorder

Persistent Depressive Disorder, which is characterized by depressed mood for most of the day, for more days than not, for at least 2 years, must be differentiated from…

In contrast to Persistent Depressive Disorder…

Major Depressive Disorder

Requires one or more Major Depressive Episodes, which are characterized by a period of depressed mood or diminished interest or pleasure for most of the day, nearly every day, for at least 2 weeks, accompanied by at least five characteristic symptoms (e.g., sleep changes, appetite changes, changes in level of activity, fatigue, feelings of worthlessness or excessive guilt, difficulty concentrating, suicidal ideation or behavior). Persistent Depressive Disorder has a lower symptom threshold (i.e., only two symptoms plus depressed mood) and a lower persistence threshold (i.e., more days than not vs. most of the day, nearly every day) but requires at least a 2-year duration. Thus, a Major Depressive Episode lasting at least 2 years will also meet criteria for Persistent Depressive Disorder. If criteria are met for both Major Depressive Disorder and Persistent Depressive Disorder, both should be diagnosed.

Chronic psychotic disorders (i.e., Schizophrenia, Delusional Disorder, Schizoaffective Disorder)

May be characterized by associated chronic depressed mood. A separate diagnosis of Persistent Depressive Disorder is not made if the symptoms occur only during the course of the psychotic disorder (including residual phases).

3.4.2 Differential Diagnosis for Persistent Depressive Disorder *(continued)*

Depressive Disorder Due to Another Medical Condition	Requires the presence of an etiological nonpsychiatric medical condition. Persistent Depressive Disorder is not diagnosed if the depressive symptoms are all due to the direct physiological effects of a chronic nonpsychiatric medical condition. Chronic mild depression is a common associated feature of many chronic medical conditions (e.g., diabetes), and the depressive symptoms may be a psychological consequence of the chronic psychological stress related to having the medical condition, rather than an etiological consequence of the nonpsychiatric medical condition, as required by the diagnosis of Depressive Disorder Due to Another Medical Condition.
Substance/Medication-Induced Depressive Disorder	Is due to the direct physiological effects of a substance (including medication). Persistent Depressive Disorder is not diagnosed if the depressive symptoms are judged to be due to the direct physiological effects of chronic substance or medication use.
Bipolar I and Bipolar II Disorders	Are characterized by Manic Episodes and Hypomanic Episodes, respectively. Persistent Depressive Disorder cannot be diagnosed if a Manic or Hypomanic Episode has ever been present.
Cyclothymic Disorder	Is characterized by hypomanic periods in addition to depressive periods. Persistent Depressive Disorder cannot be diagnosed if the criteria for Cyclothymic Disorder have ever been met.
Personality Disorder	Is characterized by an enduring pattern of inner experience and behavior that deviates markedly from the expectations of the individual's culture, with onset by adolescence or early adulthood. Personality disorders commonly co-occur with Persistent Depressive Disorder. If criteria are met for Persistent Depressive Disorder and a Personality Disorder, both may be diagnosed.

3.4.3 Differential Diagnosis for Premenstrual Dysphoric Disorder

Premenstrual Dysphoric Disorder (characterized by marked affective lability, irritability, anger, or increased interpersonal conflicts; marked depressed mood, feelings of hopelessness, or self-deprecating thoughts; or marked anxiety, tension, and/or feelings of being "keyed up" or "on edge"—which develops in the final week before the onset of menses, starts to improve within a few days after the onset of menses, and becomes minimal or absent in the week postmenses) must be differentiated from...

In contrast to Premenstrual Dysphoric Disorder...

Premenstrual syndrome (PMS)	Is characterized by symptoms that occur during the premenstrual period of the menstrual cycle and that fall short of the required threshold of five symptoms for Premenstrual Dysphoric Disorder. Moreover, Premenstrual Dysphoric Disorder, unlike PMS, requires that at least one of these symptoms be mood related (e.g., depression, irritability, anxiety, or mood lability), whereas in PMS, there is no requirement that there be affective symptoms during the premenstrual period.
Dysmenorrhea	Is characterized by menstrual pain that begins with the onset of menses. In contrast, Premenstrual Dysphoric Disorder begins before the onset of menses and is characterized by affective changes.
Depressive Disorder Due to Another Medical Condition	Is characterized by dysphoric symptoms that are due to the direct physiological effects of a nonpsychiatric medical condition (e.g., hyperthyroidism).
Substance/Medication-Induced Depressive Disorder (including hormonal treatments)	Is characterized by dysphoric symptoms that are due to the direct physiological effects of a substance or medication. Moderate to severe premenstrual symptoms may develop after initiation of exogenous hormone use. If the woman stops taking hormones and the symptoms disappear, this is consistent with Substance/Medication-Induced Depressive Disorder.

3.4.3 Differential Diagnosis for Premenstrual Dysphoric Disorder *(continued)*

Bipolar I Disorder, Bipolar II Disorder, or Major Depressive Disorder	Is characterized by Manic, Hypomanic, and Major Depressive Episodes that are temporally unrelated to the menstrual cycle. However, because the onset of menses constitutes a memorable event, some women may report that mood symptoms seem to occur only during the premenstrual period or that symptoms worsen premenstrually. Prospective daily symptom ratings during at least two symptomatic cycles are therefore important for documenting the time of onset and offset of mood symptoms.
Premenstrual exacerbation of another mental disorder (e.g., Depressive Disorders, Bipolar and Related Disorders, Anxiety Disorders, Bulimia Nervosa, Substance Use Disorders) or a nonpsychiatric medical condition (e.g., migraine, asthma, allergies, seizure disorders)	The symptom in question (e.g., depression, anxiety, binge eating) does not abate during the postmenstrual interval. In contrast, the diagnosis of Premenstrual Dysphoric Disorder requires that symptoms become minimal or absent in the week postmenses.

3.4.4 Differential Diagnosis for Disruptive Mood Dysregulation Disorder

Disruptive Mood Dysregulation Disorder, which is characterized by severe recurrent temper outbursts manifested verbally and/or behaviorally that are grossly out of proportion in intensity to the provocation and that are accompanied by a persistently irritable or angry mood most of the day, nearly every day, in between the outbursts, must be differentiated from…	In contrast to Disruptive Mood Dysregulation Disorder…
Depressive Disorder Due to Another Medical Condition	Is characterized by dysphoric symptoms that are due to the direct physiological effects of a nonpsychiatric medical condition.
Substance/Medication-Induced Depressive Disorder	Is characterized by dysphoric symptoms that are due to the direct physiological effects of a substance or medication.
Bipolar I and Bipolar II Disorders	Are episodic disorders with discrete periods of mood perturbation that are distinguishable from the child's baseline. In addition, the change in mood during Manic or Hypomanic Episodes is accompanied by increased energy and activity as well as associated cognitive, behavioral, and somatic symptoms (e.g., distractibility, rapid speech, decreased need for sleep). In contrast, the irritability of Disruptive Mood Dysregulation Disorder is persistent and present chronically over many months.
Oppositional Defiant Disorder	Is characterized by a pattern of angry/irritable mood or argumentative/defiant behavior. In contrast, Disruptive Mood Dysregulation Disorder is characterized by the presence of severe and frequently recurrent outbursts and a persistent disruption in mood between outbursts. If full criteria are met for both disorders, only Disruptive Mood Dysregulation Disorder is diagnosed.

3.4.4 Differential Diagnosis for Disruptive Mood Dysregulation Disorder *(continued)*

Major Depressive Disorder	May be characterized by irritable mood accompanying the episodes of depressed mood or diminished interest or pleasure. Children whose irritability is present only in the context of a Major Depressive Episode should receive a diagnosis of Major Depressive Disorder rather than Disruptive Mood Dysregulation Disorder. If the irritability extends outside the Major Depressive Episodes, both diagnoses may be appropriate.
Anxiety Disorders	May be characterized by irritable mood occurring in anxiety-provoking situations. Children whose irritability manifests only in anxiety-provoking contexts should receive the relevant Anxiety Disorder diagnosis rather than a diagnosis of Disruptive Mood Dysregulation Disorder. If the irritability extends outside the anxiety-provoking situations, diagnoses of both Disruptive Mood Dysregulation Disorder and the Anxiety Disorder may be appropriate.
Autism Spectrum Disorder	May be characterized by temper outbursts, especially when routines are disturbed. If the temper outbursts are better explained by Autism Spectrum Disorder, then Disruptive Mood Dysregulation Disorder is not diagnosed.
Intermittent Explosive Disorder	Is characterized by aggressive outbursts that can resemble the severe temper tantrums in Disruptive Mood Dysregulation Disorder; however, there is no persistent irritable or angry mood between outbursts as in Disruptive Mood Dysregulation Disorder. In addition, Intermittent Explosive Disorder requires only 3 months of active symptoms, in contrast to the 12-month requirement for Disruptive Mood Dysregulation Disorder. Intermittent Explosive Disorder is not diagnosed if criteria are met for Disruptive Mood Dysregulation Disorder.

Anxiety Disorders

3.5.1 Differential Diagnosis for Separation Anxiety Disorder

Separation Anxiety Disorder, which is characterized by developmentally inappropriate and excessive anxiety concerning separation from major attachment figures, must be differentiated from…	In contrast to Separation Anxiety Disorder…
Generalized Anxiety Disorder	Is characterized by anxiety and worry about a number of different events or activities and is not limited to issues of separation from family.
Panic Disorder	Is characterized by recurrent unexpected Panic Attacks. In contrast, individuals with Separation Anxiety Disorder may experience Panic Attacks, but only when threatened with separation from major attachment figures.
Agoraphobia	Is characterized by anxiety about being trapped or incapacitated in places or situations from which escape is perceived as difficult in the event of panic-like or other incapacitating symptoms. In Separation Anxiety Disorder, the focus of the fear is on separation from major attachment figures.
Posttraumatic Stress Disorder	May be characterized by fear of separation from loved ones after traumatic events such as disasters, particularly when periods of separation from loved ones were experienced during the traumatic event. However, in Posttraumatic Stress Disorder, the main symptoms involve reexperiencing memories or avoiding situations associated with the traumatic event itself, whereas in Separation Anxiety Disorder, the worries and avoidance concern the well-being of attachment figures and fears of being separated from them.
Prolonged Grief Disorder	Involves distress about separation from a deceased person, whereas Separation Anxiety Disorder is characterized by anxiety about separation from current attachment figures.

3.5.1 Differential Diagnosis for Separation Anxiety Disorder *(continued)*

Social Anxiety Disorder	May be characterized by school refusal that is due to the fear of being judged negatively by peers or teachers. In contrast, school refusal in Separation Anxiety Disorder is due to worries about being separated from major attachment figures.
Illness Anxiety Disorder	May be characterized by the individual's worry about specific illnesses they may have, but the main concern is the medical diagnosis itself. In Separation Anxiety Disorder, the focus of illness concern is on the possibility that the illness might result in the person's being separated from major attachment figures.
Conduct Disorder	May be characterized by school avoidance (truancy), but anxiety about separation from attachment figures is not responsible for the school absences, and the child or adolescent usually stays away from, rather than returns to, the home.
Oppositional Defiant Disorder	Is characterized by persistent oppositional behavior unrelated to the anticipation or occurrence of separation. In contrast, some children and adolescents with Separation Anxiety Disorder may be oppositional in the context of being forced to separate from attachment figures.
Depressive disorders	May be associated with reluctance to leave home that is due to loss of interest, fatigue, or concern about crying in public rather than worry or fear of untoward events befalling attachment figures.
Dependent Personality Disorder	Is characterized by an indiscriminate tendency to rely on others. In contrast, in Separation Anxiety Disorder, the concern is about the proximity and safety of main attachment figures.

3.5.1 Differential Diagnosis for Separation Anxiety Disorder *(continued)*

Borderline Personality Disorder	Is characterized by fear of abandonment by loved ones, but there are also problems with identity, self-direction, interpersonal functioning, and impulsivity. If criteria are met for both Separation Anxiety Disorder and Borderline Personality Disorder, both may be diagnosed.
Developmentally appropriate separation anxiety	Is part of normal early development and may indicate the development of secure attachment relationships, such as when infants around age 1 year experience stranger anxiety.

3.5.2 Differential Diagnosis for Selective Mutism

Selective Mutism, which is characterized by consistent failure to speak in specific social situations in which there is an expectation for speaking, must be differentiated from…	In contrast to Selective Mutism…
Communication Disorders	Are characterized by speech disturbances (e.g., dysfluencies, speech sound problems) that occur consistently regardless of the situation that the individual is in. In contrast, in Selective Mutism, the speech difficulties occur only in certain situations (e.g., social situations with children and adults) but not others (e.g., with immediate family).
Autism Spectrum Disorder	May also be characterized by difficulty speaking in social situations, but unlike Selective Mutism, these difficulties are evident even when the individual is speaking with immediate family members.
Social Anxiety Disorder	Is characterized by fear and anxiety occurring in social situations in which the person is exposed to possible scrutiny by others, whereas a diagnosis of Selective Mutism specifically describes a pattern of inability to speak in certain situations, which are typically social. In situations where the failure to speak is associated with feelings of social anxiety, both Selective Mutism and Social Anxiety Disorder may be diagnosed.

3.5.3 Differential Diagnosis for Specific Phobia

Specific Phobia, which is characterized by marked fear or anxiety about a specific object or situation, must be differentiated from...	In contrast to Specific Phobia...
Agoraphobia	Is characterized by fear and avoidance of situations from two or more agoraphobic clusters (i.e., public transportation, open spaces, enclosed places, standing in line or being in a crowd, being outside of the home alone). In Specific Phobia, Situational Type, the fear and avoidance is confined to only one situation (e.g., heights) or several situations, all of which fall within the same cluster of phobic stimuli (e.g., elevators and airplanes, both within the public transportation cluster).
Social Anxiety Disorder	Is characterized by fear and avoidance restricted to social situations, including performing in front of others.
Posttraumatic Stress Disorder or Acute Stress Disorder	Is characterized by fear and avoidance confined to stimuli that remind the individual of a previously experienced life-threatening event.
Obsessive-Compulsive Disorder	May be characterized by fear and avoidance of specific situations that might trigger an obsession (e.g., avoidance of dirt by an individual with a contamination obsession).
Separation Anxiety Disorder	Is characterized by fear or avoidance of situations in which the individual would be separated from major attachment figures.
Psychotic Disorders	May be characterized by avoidance that occurs as a consequence of a delusional belief (e.g., avoidance of flying by an individual with a persecutory delusional system who is unjustifiably convinced that they are going to be the target of a terrorist attack).
Anorexia Nervosa, Avoidant/Restrictive Food Intake Disorder, Bulimia Nervosa, and Binge-Eating Disorder	May be characterized by avoidance behavior, but it is exclusively related to avoiding food and food-related cues.

3.5.3 Differential Diagnosis for Specific Phobia *(continued)*

Nonpathological avoidance of circumscribed objects or situations	Either represents a realistic level of avoidance given the actual danger (e.g., avoidance of skydiving from an airplane) or is not severe enough to cause clinically significant impairment or distress, often because of the ease of avoiding the phobic stimulus (e.g., a person living in Manhattan fears snakes but would be unlikely to encounter one).
Transient fears in childhood	Are common and short-lived, lasting for less than 6 months.

3.5.4 Differential Diagnosis for Social Anxiety Disorder

Social Anxiety Disorder, which is characterized by marked fear or anxiety about social situations in which the individual is exposed to possible scrutiny by others, must be differentiated from…

In contrast to Social Anxiety Disorder…

Panic Disorder	Is characterized by Panic Attacks that at least initially, are unexpected (i.e., occur "out of the blue"). In contrast, Panic Attacks in someone with Social Anxiety Disorder are exclusively cued by social situations in which the individual is exposed to possible scrutiny by others.
Agoraphobia	May be characterized by fear and avoidance of social situations (e.g., going to a crowded party), but the individual's fear is that escape might be difficult or help might not be available in the event of incapacitation or panic-like symptoms. In Social Anxiety Disorder, the focus of the fear is scrutiny by others.
Generalized Anxiety Disorder	May be characterized by social worries, but the focus is more on the nature of ongoing relationships than on fear of negative evaluation. For example, individuals with Generalized Anxiety Disorder, particularly children, may be excessively worried about the quality of their social performance, but they also worry about the quality of their performance in nonsocial situations where social evaluation by others is not the issue (e.g., getting a good grade on a test). In Social Anxiety Disorder, the worries are exclusively focused on social performance and the scrutiny of others.
Specific Phobia	May be characterized by fear of embarrassment or humiliation related to the individual's intense reaction to exposure to phobic stimuli (e.g., embarrassment about fainting when having blood drawn), but there is not a general fear of negative evaluation in other social situations.

3.5.4 Differential Diagnosis for Social Anxiety Disorder *(continued)*

Separation Anxiety Disorder	May be characterized by avoidance of social settings (including school refusal), but the avoidance is due to concerns about being separated from attachment figures or concerns about being embarrassed by needing to leave prematurely to return to attachment figures. Individuals with Social Anxiety Disorder tend to be uncomfortable even in social situations in which attachment figures are present.
Selective Mutism	Is characterized by a failure to speak in some situations due to a fear of negative evaluation, but unlike Social Anxiety Disorder, there is no fear of negative evaluation in social situations where no speaking is required (e.g., nonverbal play).
Oppositional Defiant Disorder	May be characterized by a refusal to speak to teachers or other authority figures. Individuals with Social Anxiety Disorder may be afraid to speak due to fear of negative evaluation.
Autism Spectrum Disorder	Is characterized by social anxiety and social communication deficits that typically result in a lack of age-appropriate social relationships. Although individuals with Social Anxiety Disorder may appear impaired when first interacting with unfamiliar peers or adults, they typically have adequate age-appropriate social relationships and social communication capacity.
Avoidant Personality Disorder	Is conceptualized as a Personality Disorder but describes many of the same individuals who have generalized Social Anxiety Disorder. If criteria are met for Social Anxiety Disorder and Avoidant Personality Disorder, both diagnoses may be given.

3.5.4 Differential Diagnosis for Social Anxiety Disorder *(continued)*

Major Depressive Disorder	Is characterized by negative self-esteem that may be accompanied by concerns about being negatively evaluated by others, but these concerns extend beyond social situations. Individuals with Social Anxiety Disorder are worried about being negatively evaluated because of certain social behaviors, physical symptoms, or appearance, and generally do not experience negative self-esteem outside of social situations.
Body Dysmorphic Disorder	Is characterized by the relatively fixed belief that particular aspects of their physical appearance render the individual misshapen or ugly, which may result in social anxiety and avoidance of social situations. A separate diagnosis of Social Anxiety Disorder is generally not warranted if the social fears and avoidance are restricted to body dysmorphic concerns.
Delusional Disorder	May be characterized by a delusion involving the belief that the individual has a defect in physical appearance or is emitting a foul or offensive odor, resulting in the person being socially rejected. Although some individuals with Social Anxiety Disorder may harbor such concerns, these are not held with delusional intensity.
Medical conditions	May produce symptoms that may be socially embarrassing (e.g., trembling in Parkinson's disease, reddening in rosacea). An additional diagnosis of Social Anxiety Disorder is given only when the fear of negative evaluation by others because of those symptoms is judged to be excessive.

3.5.4 Differential Diagnosis for Social Anxiety Disorder *(continued)*

Social anxiety and avoidance associated with other mental disorders, such as Eating Disorders or Schizophrenia	Are characterized by anxiety that occurs only during the course of the other mental disorder. If the anxiety is judged to be better accounted for by the other mental disorder, an additional diagnosis of Social Anxiety Disorder is not given. For example, social fears and discomfort can occur as part of Schizophrenia, but other evidence for psychotic symptoms will also be present. Social anxiety may co-occur with Eating Disorders, but if the fear of negative evaluation about symptoms (e.g., purging and vomiting) is the sole source of social anxiety, an additional diagnosis of Social Anxiety Disorder is generally not warranted.
Nonpathological shyness	Is a common personality trait that for most shy people does not lead to a clinically significant adverse impact on functioning.

3.5.5 Differential Diagnosis for Panic Disorder

Panic Disorder, which is characterized by recurrent unexpected Panic Attacks followed by 1 month or more of worry or a change in behavior related to the attacks, must be differentiated from…	In contrast to Panic Disorder…
Anxiety Disorder Due to Another Medical Condition	Requires the presence of an etiological medical condition (e.g., hyperthyroidism). Panic Disorder is not diagnosed if the Panic Attacks are all due to the direct physiological effects of the nonpsychiatric medical condition on the central nervous system.
Substance/Medication-Induced Anxiety Disorder	Is due to the direct physiological effects of a substance or medication. Panic Disorder is not diagnosed if the Panic Attacks are all due to the direct physiological effects of a substance (including medication).
Panic Attacks occurring as part of another mental disorder	Many mental disorders (e.g., Social Anxiety Disorder, Specific Phobia, Separation Anxiety Disorder, Obsessive-Compulsive Disorder, Hoarding Disorder, Posttraumatic Stress Disorder, Major Depressive Disorder) may be characterized by Panic Attacks occurring in situations in which the individual is already experiencing some degree of anxiety related to that disorder. For example, a person with Social Anxiety Disorder may become so anxious in a social situation that a Panic Attack is triggered, or an individual with contamination concerns in Obsessive-Compulsive Disorder may develop extreme distress when exposed to germs or dirt, which culminates in a Panic Attack. In such cases, the specifier With Panic Attacks may be noted. In contrast, the Panic Attacks in individuals with Panic Disorder are unexpected (i.e., the Panic Attacks occur "out of the blue"), at least during the initial phase of the disorder.

3.5.5 Differential Diagnosis for Panic Disorder *(continued)*

Exposure to an extremely anxiety-provoking experience	May be characterized by the development of a Panic Attack (e.g., an individual having a Panic Attack while being held up at gunpoint). In contrast, the Panic Attacks in individuals with Panic Disorder are unexpected (i.e., occur out of the blue), at least during the initial phase of the disorder.
Isolated Panic Attack	Is characterized by a single Panic Attack, which may or may not occur out of the blue and by itself is not indicative of psychopathology. A diagnosis of Panic Disorder requires at least two unexpected Panic Attacks.
Limited-symptom attacks	Are characterized by panic-like attacks that have fewer than the minimum of four symptoms required for a Panic Attack.

3.5.6 Differential Diagnosis for Agoraphobia

Agoraphobia, which is characterized by fear or avoidance of multiple situations due to thoughts that escape might be difficult or help might not be available in the event of developing panic-like symptoms, must be differentiated from…	In contrast to Agoraphobia…
Social Anxiety Disorder	Is characterized by avoidance specifically of social situations in which the person will be exposed to the scrutiny of others.
Specific Phobia, Situational Type	Is characterized by avoidance of a specific feared situation, such as closed spaces, as opposed to fear and avoidance of multiple situations across two or more of the agoraphobic clusters (i.e., public transportation, open spaces, enclosed places, standing in line or being in a crowd, being outside of the home alone).
Posttraumatic Stress Disorder or Acute Stress Disorder	May be characterized by avoidance of people, places, activities, or situations that arouse upsetting memories, thoughts, or feelings about the traumatic event.
Major Depressive Disorder	Some individuals with Major Depressive Disorder may be housebound due to feelings of apathy, fatigue, loss of capacity to experience pleasure, or concerns about crying in public. In contrast, the unwillingness of some individuals with Agoraphobia to leave their homes is a result of extreme fears that help might be unavailable if they develop panic-like symptoms and become incapacitated.
Psychotic Disorder featuring delusions (e.g., Delusional Disorder; Schizophrenia; Major Depressive Disorder, With Psychotic Features)	May be characterized by avoidance that is a consequence of delusional fears (e.g., the individual's avoidance of going outside the house because of the conviction that they are being followed).
Obsessive-Compulsive Disorder	May be characterized by avoidance behavior that is intended to prevent triggering an obsession or compulsion (e.g., avoidance of "dirty" objects related to fears of contamination, avoidance of kitchen knives by someone who is having obsessive thoughts of stabbing their spouse).

3.5.6 Differential Diagnosis for Agoraphobia *(continued)*

Separation Anxiety Disorder	Is characterized by avoidance of situations that involve being away from major attachment figures, including refusing to go out of one's house because of a fear of separation.
Avoidance related to potentially disabling medical conditions	May be characterized by avoidance that results from realistic concerns (e.g., about fainting for an individual with an arrhythmia). However, in contrast to the avoidance in Agoraphobia, avoidance related to a disabling condition is appropriate given the nature of the medical condition.

3.5.7 Differential Diagnosis for Generalized Anxiety Disorder

Generalized Anxiety Disorder, which is characterized by excessive anxiety and worry lasting at least 6 months, must be differentiated from…	In contrast to Generalized Anxiety Disorder…
Anxiety Disorder Due to Another Medical Condition	Requires the presence of an etiological medical condition (e.g., pheochromocytoma). Generalized Anxiety Disorder is not diagnosed if the generalized anxiety is due to the direct physiological effects of a nonpsychiatric medical condition.
Substance/Medication-Induced Anxiety Disorder	Is due to the direct physiological effects of a substance or medication and may have its onset during intoxication with or withdrawal from an abused substance, or occur in the context of taking or withdrawing from a medication. Generalized Anxiety Disorder is not diagnosed if the generalized anxiety is due to the direct physiological effects of a substance on the central nervous system, such as during Cocaine Intoxication or Opioid Withdrawal.
Panic Disorder	Is characterized by anxiety and worry about having additional Panic Attacks. An additional diagnosis of Generalized Anxiety Disorder should be made only if there is additional anxiety and worry about events, situations, or activities unrelated to the Panic Attacks.
Social Anxiety Disorder	Is characterized by excessive anxiety and worry focused exclusively on social situations. An additional diagnosis of Generalized Anxiety Disorder should be made only if there is anxiety and worry focused on nonsocial situations (e.g., work or school performance).

3.5.7 Differential Diagnosis for Generalized Anxiety Disorder *(continued)*

Somatic Symptom Disorder or Illness Anxiety Disorder	May be characterized by excessive anxiety and worry focused exclusively on health, becoming ill, or the seriousness of somatic symptoms (e.g., worry that a headache is indicative of a brain tumor). An additional diagnosis of Generalized Anxiety Disorder should be made only if there is anxiety and worry focused on non-health-related situations.
Separation Anxiety Disorder	Is characterized by excessive anxiety and worry focused exclusively on concerns about separation from major attachment figures. An additional diagnosis of Generalized Anxiety Disorder should be made only if there is anxiety and worry focused on situations that are unrelated to separation concerns.
Posttraumatic Stress Disorder or Acute Stress Disorder	Is characterized by anxiety occurring in relation to exposure to internal or external cues that symbolize or resemble an aspect of the traumatic event or occurring as part of the generalized hyperarousal and reactivity associated with having been exposed to the traumatic event. An additional diagnosis of Generalized Anxiety Disorder should be made only if there is anxiety and worry focused on situations that are unrelated to the traumatic event.
Anorexia Nervosa	May be characterized by anxiety or worry associated with the fear of gaining weight. An additional diagnosis of Generalized Anxiety Disorder should be made only if there is anxiety and worry unrelated to issues about weight.

3.5.7 Differential Diagnosis for Generalized Anxiety Disorder *(continued)*

Obsessive-Compulsive Disorder	Is usually characterized by repetitive anxiety-provoking thoughts that are experienced as intrusive, unwanted, inappropriate, and ego-dystonic, and that are usually accompanied by compulsions that serve to reduce the anxiety. In contrast, the worries in Generalized Anxiety Disorder typically arise from everyday routine life, such as job responsibilities, the health of family members, finances, or minor matters such as household chores or being late for appointments.
Body Dysmorphic Disorder	May be characterized by anxiety and worry about perceived defects in appearance being observed by others. An additional diagnosis of Generalized Anxiety Disorder should be made only if there is anxiety and worry unrelated to physical appearance.
Adjustment Disorder, With Anxiety	Is characterized by clinically significant anxiety symptoms that do not meet the criteria for any specific anxiety disorder (including Generalized Anxiety Disorder) and that develop in response to an identifiable psychosocial stressor.
Manic Episode, With Anxious Distress; Hypomanic Episode, With Anxious Distress; or Major Depressive Episode, With Anxious Distress	Is characterized by prominent symptoms related to anxiety (feeling tense, feeling restless, having difficulty concentrating, feelings of dread) that occur during the majority of days of the mood episode.
Psychotic Disorders	May be accompanied by anxiety related to the content of delusional beliefs and include other psychotic symptoms characteristic of the particular Psychotic Disorder. An additional diagnosis of Generalized Anxiety Disorder should be made only if there is anxiety and worry focused on situations that are unrelated to the psychosis.
Nonpathological anxiety	Is characterized by worries that are more controllable or are not severe enough to cause clinically significant distress or impairment in functioning.

Obsessive-Compulsive and Related Disorders

3.6.1 Differential Diagnosis for Obsessive-Compulsive Disorder

Obsessive-Compulsive Disorder (OCD), which is characterized by obsessions (i.e., recurrent thoughts, urges, or images that are experienced as intrusive and unwanted that the person attempts to ignore or suppress) and/or compulsions (i.e., repetitive behaviors or mental acts that the person feels driven to perform in response to an obsession or according to rules that must be applied rigidly), must be differentiated from…

In contrast to Obsessive-Compulsive Disorder…

Obsessive-Compulsive and Related Disorder Due to Another Medical Condition	Requires the presence of an etiological nonpsychiatric medical condition. OCD is not diagnosed if the obsessions and compulsions are all due to the direct physiological effects of a nonpsychiatric medical condition.
Substance/Medication-Induced Obsessive-Compulsive and Related Disorder	Is due to the direct physiological effects of a substance or medication. OCD is not diagnosed if the obsessions and compulsions are all due to the direct physiological effects of a substance (including medication).
Hoarding Disorder	Is characterized by a persistent difficulty discarding or parting with possessions and an excessive accumulation of objects. However, for an individual with certain obsessions (e.g., concerns about incompleteness or harm) with associated hoarding compulsions (e.g., acquiring all objects in a set to attain a sense of completeness), a diagnosis of OCD should be given instead.
Body Dysmorphic Disorder	Is characterized by repetitive behaviors (e.g., mirror checking, excessive grooming) or mental acts (the individual comparing their appearance with that of others) in response to appearance concerns. A diagnosis of OCD should be considered only if there are additional obsessions and/or compulsions unrelated to appearance.

3.6.1 Differential Diagnosis for Obsessive-Compulsive Disorder *(continued)*

Eating Disorder

Is characterized by recurrent thoughts and behaviors that are limited to concerns about body weight and food.

Specific Phobia

Is characterized by fear and avoidance cued to specific circumscribed objects or situations. In OCD, the fear and avoidance of a specific object or situation is related to avoiding the triggering of an obsession or compulsion (e.g., avoidance of dirt in an individual with a contamination obsession).

Social Anxiety Disorder

Is characterized by fear and avoidance of social situations in which the person is exposed to possible scrutiny of others, and repetitive behaviors that involve seeking reassurance are focused on reducing the social fear.

Trichotillomania (Hair-Pulling Disorder) or Excoriation (Skin-Picking) Disorder

Is characterized by recurrent thoughts and actions limited to hair pulling or skin picking.

Illness Anxiety Disorder

Is characterized by recurrent thoughts exclusively related to the idea that one has a serious disease.

Major Depressive Episode

May be characterized by recurrent ruminations that are usually mood congruent and not necessarily experienced as intrusive or distressing.

Generalized Anxiety Disorder

Is characterized by recurrent thoughts (i.e., worries) about real-life concerns, and the thoughts are not accompanied by compulsions.

Delusional Disorder

Is characterized by persistent thoughts that are held with delusional conviction. Although some individuals with OCD may completely lack insight into the likelihood (or lack thereof) of a feared consequence of not performing their compulsion and thus would warrant the specifier With Absent Insight/Delusional Beliefs, these symptoms do not warrant a diagnosis of a Psychotic Disorder.

3.6.1 Differential Diagnosis for Obsessive-Compulsive Disorder *(continued)*

Schizophrenia	Is characterized by ruminative delusional thoughts and stereotyped behaviors that are accompanied by other characteristic symptoms of Schizophrenia (e.g., hallucinations, disorganized speech, negative symptoms).
Tic Disorders	Are characterized by sudden, rapid, recurrent, nonrhythmic motor movements or vocalizations (e.g., eye blinking, throat clearing) that are less complex than compulsions and are not aimed at neutralizing obsessions.
Stereotypic Movement Disorder	Is characterized by repetitive, seemingly driven, nonfunctional motor behaviors (e.g., head banging, body rocking, self-biting) that are less complex than compulsions and are not aimed at neutralizing obsessions.
Driven ("compulsive") behaviors associated with other mental disorders	Are associated with disorders such as Gambling Disorder, Paraphilic Disorders, and Substance Use Disorders, and are characterized by the person's deriving pleasure from the activity and wanting to resist it only because of its deleterious consequences. In contrast, the obsessions and compulsions in OCD are a source of intense anxiety and are not experienced as pleasurable.
Obsessive-Compulsive Personality Disorder	Involves an enduring and pervasive maladaptive pattern of excessive perfectionism and rigid control and is not characterized by the presence of obsessions or compulsions.
Nonpathological superstitions and repetitive behaviors	Are not time-consuming and do not result in clinically significant impairment or distress.

3.6.2 Differential Diagnosis for Body Dysmorphic Disorder

Body Dysmorphic Disorder, which is characterized by a preoccupation with perceived defects or flaws in physical appearance, must be differentiated from…	In contrast to Body Dysmorphic Disorder…
Normal dissatisfaction about appearance and concerns about clearly noticeable physical defects	Do not involve excessive appearance-related preoccupations and repetitive behaviors that are time-consuming, are usually difficult to resist or control, and cause marked distress or impairment.
Anorexia Nervosa and Bulimia Nervosa	Are characterized by concerns that are limited to body shape and weight. A comorbid diagnosis of Body Dysmorphic Disorder may be appropriate if appearance preoccupations go beyond overall body shape and weight (e.g., preoccupation with a perceived facial defect).
Gender Dysphoria	Is characterized by bodily concerns that are limited to wanting to get rid of primary or secondary sexual characteristics. Body Dysmorphic Disorder should be diagnosed only if appearance preoccupations go beyond physical manifestations of assigned gender.
Major Depressive Episode, Avoidant Personality Disorder, and Social Anxiety Disorder	Are often characterized by feelings of low self-esteem, self-consciousness, and defectiveness that may include concerns about body appearance. However, in Body Dysmorphic Disorder, the individual is preoccupied by their perceived defects in appearance and performs repetitive behaviors (e.g., mirror checking, excessive grooming, skin picking, reassurance seeking) or mental acts (e.g., comparing their appearance with that of others) in response to the appearance concerns.
Obsessive-Compulsive Disorder	Is characterized by intrusive thoughts and repetitive behaviors that are not limited to concerns about appearance.

3.6.2 Differential Diagnosis for Body Dysmorphic Disorder *(continued)*

Trichotillomania (Hair-Pulling Disorder)	Is characterized by the individual's recurrent pulling out of their hair, resulting in hair loss accompanied by repeated attempts to stop, and is not intended to improve perceived defects in the appearance of facial, head, or body hair. However, if the hair-pulling behavior occurs in conjunction with a preoccupation with a defect in appearance involving excessive body hair, a diagnosis of Body Dysmorphic Disorder may be appropriate.
Excoriation (Skin-Picking) Disorder	Is characterized by recurrent skin picking resulting in skin lesions, accompanied by repeated attempts to stop that are not motivated by a desire to improve the appearance of a perceived skin defect. If the skin-picking behavior occurs in conjunction with a preoccupation with a perceived skin defect, then a diagnosis of Body Dysmorphic Disorder may be more appropriate.
Delusional Disorder, Somatic Type	Is characterized by prominent delusions involving bodily functions or sensations. For some individuals with Body Dysmorphic Disorder, beliefs about a defect in appearance are held with delusional conviction (i.e., they are completely convinced that their view of their perceived defects is accurate). These individuals are diagnosed as having Body Dysmorphic Disorder, With Absent Insight, as opposed to having Delusional Disorder.
Histrionic Personality Disorder or Narcissistic Personality Disorder	May be characterized by overconcern with appearance that does not involve specific defects.
Body integrity identity disorder (preoccupation with the desire to become disabled, with onset in childhood)	May be characterized by a preoccupation with the desire to have a limb amputated to correct a perceived mismatch between the person's sense of bodily identity and their anatomical configuration, and not because the person considers the appearance of the limb to be ugly or defective.

3.6.3 Differential Diagnosis for Hoarding Disorder

Hoarding Disorder, which is characterized by persistent difficulty discarding or parting with possessions because of a perceived need to save the items, must be differentiated from...

In contrast to Hoarding Disorder...

Obsessive-Compulsive and Related Disorder Due to Another Medical Condition	Requires the presence of an etiological nonpsychiatric medical condition (e.g., traumatic brain injury, surgical resection for seizure control, cerebrovascular disease). Hoarding Disorder is not diagnosed if the hoarding behavior is due to the direct physiological effects of the nonpsychiatric medical condition.
Major Neurocognitive Disorder Due to a neurodegenerative condition, such as frontotemporal lobar degeneration or Alzheimer's disease	The onset of the accumulating behavior is gradual and follows the course of the Neurocognitive Disorder and may be accompanied by self-neglect and severe domestic squalor, alongside other neuropsychiatric symptoms. Hoarding Disorder is not diagnosed if the accumulation of objects is judged to be a direct consequence of a degenerative brain disorder.
Autism Spectrum Disorder	May include the excessive accumulation of objects related to a fixated interest that is abnormal in intensity (e.g., collecting matchbox covers), in which case a diagnosis of Hoarding Disorder is not made.

3.6.3 Differential Diagnosis for Hoarding Disorder *(continued)*

Obsessive-Compulsive Disorder	Is characterized by repetitive behaviors that the individual feels driven to perform in response to an obsession or according to rules that must be applied rigidly, and that are generally experienced by the individual as ego-dystonic. This is in contrast to the ego-syntonic accumulation of items in Hoarding Disorder. When an accumulation of objects occurs as a direct consequence of Obsessive-Compulsive Disorder (e.g., not discarding objects to avoid endless checking rituals), a diagnosis of Hoarding Disorder is not made. However, when severe hoarding appears concurrently with other typical symptoms of Obsessive-Compulsive Disorder but is judged to be independent from these symptoms, both Hoarding Disorder and Obsessive-Compulsive Disorder may be diagnosed.
Psychotic Disorder (e.g., Schizophrenia)	May be characterized by an accumulation of objects as a consequence of a delusional belief (e.g., collecting discarded pieces of aluminum foil to protect oneself from radiation) or a command hallucination, in which case a diagnosis of Hoarding Disorder is not made.
Major Depressive Episode	May be associated with a cluttered environment that occurs as a direct consequence of depressive symptoms such as fatigue, inertia, and psychomotor retardation, in which case a diagnosis of Hoarding Disorder is not made.
Nonpathological collecting behavior	Is organized and systematic, even if in some cases the actual amount of possessions may be similar to that accumulated by an individual with Hoarding Disorder. Moreover, it does not produce the clutter, distress, or impairment typical of Hoarding Disorder.

3.6.4 Differential Diagnosis for Trichotillomania (Hair-Pulling Disorder)

Trichotillomania, which is characterized by recurrent pulling out of one's hair, accompanied by repeated attempts to stop hair pulling, must be differentiated from…	In contrast to Trichotillomania…
Medical conditions that cause hair loss	Certain conditions such as scarring alopecia (e.g., alopecia areata) and non-scarring alopecia (e.g., chronic discoid lupus erythematosus) can fully account for the hair loss. Trichotillomania is not diagnosed if the hair pulling is attributable to one of these medical conditions.
Obsessive-Compulsive Disorder	Is characterized by behavior that is performed in response to an obsession or according to rules that must be applied rigidly. Trichotillomania is not diagnosed if the hair pulling is a direct consequence of an obsession or compulsion (e.g., individuals with symmetry concerns may pull out hairs as part of their symmetry rituals).
Body Dysmorphic Disorder	Is characterized by a preoccupation with an imagined defect in physical appearance that in some cases may result in a preoccupation with removing body hair that the individual perceives as ugly or abnormal. Trichotillomania is not diagnosed if the hair pulling is a direct consequence of the preoccupation with a perceived defect in appearance.
Psychotic Disorder (e.g., Schizophrenia)	May be characterized by hair pulling in response to delusions or hallucinations. Trichotillomania is not diagnosed if the hair pulling is better accounted for by a Psychotic Disorder.
Stereotypic Movement Disorder	Involves repetitive behaviors other than (or in addition to) hair pulling (e.g., hand shaking or waving, body rocking, head banging).

3.6.4 Differential Diagnosis for Trichotillomania (Hair-Pulling Disorder) *(continued)*

Hair pulling as a form of Nonsuicidal Self-Injury	Occurs in the absence of repeated attempts to decrease or stop hair pulling. If the behavior is sufficiently clinically significant, the code for Nonsuicidal Self-Injury may be given.
Normative hair removal or manipulation	Is characterized by hair removal that is performed solely for cosmetic reasons (i.e., to improve one's physical appearance) or by behavior that is confined to twisting, playing with, or biting one's hair. In such cases, distress or impairment in functioning is not significant and thus such presentations would not qualify for a diagnosis of Trichotillomania.

3.6.5 Differential Diagnosis for Excoriation (Skin-Picking) Disorder

Excoriation Disorder, which is characterized by recurrent skin picking resulting in skin lesions, accompanied by repeated attempts to stop, must be differentiated from…	In contrast to Excoriation Disorder…
Obsessive-Compulsive and Related Disorder Due to Another Medical Condition	The skin picking is due to the direct physiological effects of a nonpsychiatric medical condition. Excoriation Disorder is not diagnosed if the skin picking is attributable to the direct physiological effects of a dermatological condition (e.g., scabies).
Substance/Medication-Induced Obsessive-Compulsive and Related Disorder	The skin picking is due to the direct physiological effects of a substance (e.g., cocaine) or medication. Excoriation Disorder is not diagnosed if the skin picking is fully attributable to the substance (including medication).
Obsessive-Compulsive Disorder	May include skin lesions occurring as a consequence of severe washing compulsions. Excoriation Disorder is not diagnosed if the skin lesions are better explained by Obsessive-Compulsive Disorder.
Body Dysmorphic Disorder	May include skin-picking behavior to improve a perceived defect in appearance. Excoriation Disorder is not diagnosed if the skin picking is better explained by Body Dysmorphic Disorder.
Psychotic Disorder (e.g., Schizophrenia)	May include skin picking in response to a delusion (i.e., parasitosis) or tactile hallucination (i.e., formication). In such cases, Excoriation Disorder should not be diagnosed.
Stereotypic Movement Disorder	Involves repetitive behaviors other than (or in addition to) skin picking (e.g., hand shaking or waving, body rocking, head banging).

Trauma- and Stressor-Related Disorders

3.7.1 Differential Diagnosis for Posttraumatic Stress Disorder or Acute Stress Disorder[a]

Posttraumatic Stress Disorder (PTSD) and Acute Stress Disorder, which are characterized by exposure to actual or threatened death, serious injury, or sexual violence, followed by the development of intrusion symptoms, persistent avoidance of stimuli associated with the trauma, negative alterations of cognitions and mood, and marked alterations in arousal and reactivity, must be differentiated from…

In contrast to Posttraumatic Stress Disorder or Acute Stress Disorder…

Adjustment Disorder

Is characterized by the development of symptoms in response to an identifiable psychosocial stressor of any degree of severity that is not characterized by a specific type or pattern of symptoms. In contrast, the diagnoses of PTSD and Acute Stress Disorder require exposure to actual or threatened death, serious injury, or sexual violence, and are characterized by a specific response pattern (e.g., intrusion symptoms, avoidance symptoms, arousal symptoms). The diagnosis of Adjustment Disorder may be used when the response to an extreme stressor does not meet the criteria for PTSD or Acute Stress Disorder or when the full syndromal pattern of PTSD or Acute Stress Disorder develops in response to a psychosocial stressor (e.g., spouse leaving, being fired) that does not involve actual or threatened death, serious injury, or sexual violence.

3.7.1 Differential Diagnosis for Posttraumatic Stress Disorder or Acute Stress Disorder[a] (continued)

Prolonged Grief Disorder	Is characterized by the development of a grief response involving intense yearning or longing for the deceased, or preoccupation with thoughts or memories of the deceased, which persists for at least 12 months after the loss and causes clinically significant distress or impairment. In contrast to PTSD, where the intrusive thoughts and memories revolve around the traumatic events that caused the death of the loved one, intrusive memories in Prolonged Grief Disorder focus on many aspects of the deceased, including positive aspects of the relationship and distress over the loss of the loved one.
Other mental disorders that may develop after exposure to an extreme stressor	Are characterized by a response pattern that meets criteria for another mental disorder in DSM-5-TR (e.g., Brief Psychotic Disorder, Major Depressive Disorder).
Obsessive-Compulsive Disorder	Is usually characterized by recurrent intrusive thoughts, but these are experienced as inappropriate and are not related to a previously experienced traumatic event.
Panic Disorder	May be characterized by arousal and dissociative symptoms, but these occur during Panic Attacks and are not associated with a traumatic stressor.
Generalized Anxiety Disorder	May be characterized by persistent symptoms of irritability and anxiety, but unlike PTSD or Acute Stress Disorder, these symptoms are not associated with a traumatic stressor.
Dissociative Disorders	Are characterized by dissociative symptoms that are not necessarily related to exposure to a traumatic stressor (but often are). Dissociative symptoms occurring in the context of the full syndrome of PTSD might warrant use of the specifier With Dissociative Symptoms.

3.7.1 Differential Diagnosis for Posttraumatic Stress Disorder or Acute Stress Disorder[a] *(continued)*

Psychotic Disorders (e.g., Schizophrenia)	May be characterized by perceptual symptoms such as illusions or hallucinations. These should be differentiated from flashbacks in PSTD or Acute Stress Disorder, which are characterized by sensory intrusions comprising part of the traumatic event that can occur with complete loss of awareness of present surroundings. These episodes are typically brief but can be associated with prolonged distress and heightened arousal. The episodes are generally not considered psychotic phenomena.
Traumatic brain injury	Is characterized by neurocognitive symptoms (e.g., persistent disorientation and confusion) that develop after a traumatic brain injury (e.g., traumatic accident, bomb blast, acceleration/deceleration trauma). Because this traumatic event can also lead to the development of Acute Stress Disorder and PTSD, both diagnoses should be considered.
Malingering	Is characterized by feigning of symptoms and must always be ruled out when legal, financial, and other benefits play a role.

[a]PTSD and Acute Stress Disorder are differentiated on the basis of duration. The duration of the response pattern in Acute Stress Disorder is from 3 days to 1 month after exposure to the traumatic stressor. The duration of the response pattern in PTSD is more than 1 month.

3.7.2 Differential Diagnosis for Adjustment Disorder

Adjustment Disorder, which is characterized by the development of clinically significant emotional or behavioral symptoms that do not meet the criteria for another mental disorder, must be differentiated from…	In contrast to Adjustment Disorder…
All other specific DSM-5-TR mental disorders	Are characterized by a symptom pattern that meets diagnostic criteria for a specific DSM-5-TR-TR mental disorder, most of which do not require that the symptoms occur in response to an identifiable psychosocial stressor (with the exceptions of Posttraumatic Stress Disorder, Acute Stress Disorder, Prolonged Grief Disorder, Reactive Attachment Disorder, and Disinhibited Social Engagement Disorder). Adjustment Disorder is not diagnosed if the symptoms meet criteria for a specific mental disorder or represent an exacerbation of an existing disorder. Adjustment Disorder can be diagnosed in addition to another mental disorder if the latter does not fully explain the particular symptoms that occur in reaction to the stressor. For example, an individual may develop an Adjustment Disorder, With Depressed Mood, after losing a job, while at the same time having a diagnosis of Obsessive-Compulsive Disorder.
Posttraumatic Stress Disorder or Acute Stress Disorder	Requires that the stressor be extreme (i.e., exposure to actual or threatened death, serious injury, or sexual violence) and requires characteristic intrusion symptoms, persistent avoidance of stimuli associated with the trauma, negative alterations of cognitions and mood, and marked alterations in arousal and reactivity.
Other Specified or Unspecified categories (e.g., Other Specified Depressive Disorder)	Are diagnosed only when criteria are not met for any specific DSM-5-TR disorder (including Adjustment Disorder).

3.7.2 Differential Diagnosis for Adjustment Disorder *(continued)*

Psychological Factors Affecting Other Medical Conditions	Are characterized by specific psychological entities (e.g., psychological symptoms, behaviors, other factors) that precipitate, exacerbate, or put an individual at risk for medical illness, or worsen an existing nonpsychiatric medical condition. In contrast, when a nonpsychiatric medical condition acts as a psychosocial stressor leading to a psychological reaction, Adjustment Disorder is diagnosed.
Bereavement	Is characterized by a normal reaction to the loss of a loved one that is in keeping with what would be expected. Adjustment Disorder can be diagnosed only if the symptoms are judged to be out of proportion to what would be expected.
Prolonged Grief Disorder	Is characterized by the development of a grief response involving intense yearning or longing for the deceased, or preoccupation with thoughts or memories of the deceased, which causes clinically significant distress or impairment. In contrast to Adjustment Disorder, for which symptoms can persist for a maximum duration of 6 months once the stressor or its consequences have terminated, Prolonged Grief Disorder symptoms must persist for at least 12 months after the loss before the diagnosis is made.
Nonpathological reactions to stress	Are characterized by symptoms that are within what would be expected given the nature of the stressor and that do not lead to clinically significant distress or impairment.

3.7.3 Differential Diagnosis for Prolonged Grief Disorder

Prolonged Grief Disorder, which is characterized by the development of a grief response involving intense yearning or longing for the deceased, or preoccupation with thoughts or memories of the deceased, which persists for at least 12 months after the loss and causes clinically significant distress or impairment, must be differentiated from…

In contrast to Prolonged Grief Disorder…

Normal grief	Is time-limited and resolves in keeping with cultural, social, and religious norms.
Major Depressive Disorder or Persistent Depressive Disorder	Can develop in the context of the death of a loved one, but the symptoms reflect generalized low mood rather than being centered around feelings of loss and separation from the loved one.
Posttraumatic Stress Disorder (PTSD)	Requires exposure to actual or threatened death, serious injury, or sexual violence. Individuals who experience bereavement as a result of the violent or accidental death of a loved one may develop both PTSD and Prolonged Grief Disorder, both of which can involve avoidance of reminders of the death. Unlike avoidance in PTSD, which is manifested by avoidance of memories, thoughts, or feelings associated with the traumatic event that led to the death of the loved one (e.g., memories of the fatal automobile accident that killed the loved one), the avoidance in Prolonged Grief Disorder is of reminders that the loved one is no longer present (e.g., avoidance of activities experienced with the deceased). Moreover, reexperiencing memories in PTSD tend to be more perceptual, with the individual reporting that the memory feels like it is occurring in the "here and now," which tends not to be the case in Prolonged Grief Disorder. In Prolonged Grief Disorder, there is also a yearning for the deceased, which is absent in PTSD.

3.7.3 Differential Diagnosis for Prolonged Grief Disorder *(continued)*

Adjustment Disorder	Is characterized by symptoms that develop in response to an identifiable psychosocial stressor of any variety, not necessarily the loss of a loved one. Moreover, the symptoms cannot persist for more than an additional 6 months after the stressor and its consequences have terminated.
Separation Anxiety Disorder	Is characterized by anxiety about separation from current attachment figures, as opposed to distress about separation from a deceased person.

Dissociative Disorders

3.8.1 Differential Diagnosis for Dissociative Amnesia

Dissociative Amnesia, which is characterized by an inability to recall important autobiographical information, usually of a traumatic or stressful nature, must be differentiated from…	In contrast to Dissociative Amnesia…
Memory impairment in a Major or Mild Neurocognitive Disorder Due to Another Medical Condition	Is characterized by memory loss of personal information that is usually associated with cognitive, linguistic, affective, attentional, and behavioral disturbances. In Dissociative Amnesia, memory deficits are primarily for autobiographical information, and intellectual and other cognitive abilities are preserved.
Alcohol- or other substance-induced "blackouts"	Are characterized by a failure of memory storage secondary to the direct physiological effects of the substance on the central nervous system. Substance-induced memory loss usually cannot be reversed.
Posttraumatic amnesia due to brain injury	Is characterized by a history of a clear-cut physical trauma, a period of unconsciousness or amnesia, objective evidence of brain injury, and a brief retrograde amnesia for the time before the head injury. If the retrograde posttraumatic amnesia is so extensive that it is out of proportion to the brain injury, a comorbid diagnosis of Dissociative Amnesia may be appropriate.
Dissociative Identity Disorder	Is characterized by pervasive discontinuities in sense of self and agency, accompanied by many other dissociative symptoms. In individuals with Dissociative Amnesia, the amnesia tends to be localized, selective, and relatively stable. Dissociative Amnesia is not diagnosed if the memory gaps are better explained by Dissociative Identity Disorder.

3.8.1 Differential Diagnosis for Dissociative Amnesia *(continued)*

Posttraumatic Stress Disorder or Acute Stress Disorder	May be characterized by an inability to recall part or all of a specific traumatic event. Amnesia confined to the traumatic event and occurring in the context of Posttraumatic Stress Disorder would generally not warrant an additional diagnosis of Dissociative Amnesia. However, if the amnesia extends beyond the immediate time of the trauma, a comorbid diagnosis of Dissociative Amnesia may be warranted (e.g., for a rape victim who cannot recall most events for the entire day of the rape).
Malingering or Factitious Disorder	Is characterized by amnesia that is feigned. No test, battery of tests, or set of procedures, however, can reliably distinguish Dissociative Amnesia from feigned amnesia, and the same contextual factors associated with feigned amnesia (e.g., financial, sexual, or legal problems; or a wish to escape stressful circumstances) are also associated with Dissociative Amnesia.
Everyday memory loss, amnesia for dreams, amnesia for childhood experiences, posthypnotic amnesia, or age-related memory loss	Is characterized by difficulties in memory that are normative given the context.

3.8.2 Differential Diagnosis for Depersonalization/Derealization Disorder

Depersonalization/Derealization Disorder, which is characterized by persistent or recurrent experiences of depersonalization, must be differentiated from…	In contrast to Depersonalization/Derealization Disorder…
Dissociative symptoms due to a nonpsychiatric medical condition	Require the presence of an etiological nonpsychiatric medical condition, such as a seizure disorder, and would be diagnosed as Other Specified Mental Disorder Due to Another Medical Condition, With Dissociative Symptoms. Depersonalization/Derealization Disorder is not diagnosed if the symptoms are all due to the direct physiological effects of a nonpsychiatric medical condition on the central nervous system.
Substance Intoxication or Substance Withdrawal	May be characterized by dissociative symptoms along with the other symptoms of Substance Intoxication or Substance Withdrawal. The most common precipitating substances are cannabis, hallucinogens, ketamine, ecstasy, and salvia. Depersonalization/derealization symptoms attributable to the physiological effects of substances during acute intoxication or withdrawal are not diagnosed as Depersonalization/Derealization Disorder. However, substances can intensify the symptoms of a preexisting Depersonalization/Derealization Disorder.
Dissociative Identity Disorder	May be characterized by symptoms of depersonalization or derealization accompanying the pervasive discontinuities in sense of self and agency. Depersonalization/Derealization Disorder is not diagnosed if the symptoms are better explained by Dissociative Identity Disorder.

3.8.2 Differential Diagnosis for Depersonalization/Derealization Disorder *(continued)*

Panic Attacks	May be characterized by symptoms of depersonalization or derealization accompanying the other symptoms of the Panic Attack. Panic Attack symptoms have an abrupt onset and reach a peak within minutes. In contrast, episodes of depersonalization or derealization in Depersonalization/Derealization Disorder typically last for hours, weeks, or months. Depersonalization/Derealization Disorder is not diagnosed if the symptoms occur only during a Panic Attack.
Posttraumatic Stress Disorder or Acute Stress Disorder	Is characterized by exposure to actual or threatened death, serious injury, or sexual violence, followed by the development of intrusion symptoms, persistent avoidance of stimuli associated with the trauma, negative alterations of cognitions and mood, and marked alterations in arousal and reactivity. Some individuals with Posttraumatic Stress Disorder also develop persistent or recurrent symptoms of depersonalization and/or derealization in response to the stressor. In such cases, the specifier With Dissociative Symptoms should be used. Depersonalization/Derealization Disorder is not diagnosed if the symptoms are better explained by Posttraumatic Stress Disorder or Acute Stress Disorder.
Psychotic Disorders (e.g., Schizophrenia)	May be characterized by a delusion in which the individual believes that they are dead or that the world is not real. In contrast, reality testing about the depersonalization/derealization is intact in Depersonalization/Derealization Disorder (i.e., the person knows that they are not really dead and that the world is real).

3.8.2 Differential Diagnosis for Depersonalization/Derealization Disorder *(continued)*

Major Depressive Disorder	May be characterized by feelings of numbness, deadness, apathy, and being in a dream, along with the other characteristic symptoms of depression during Major Depressive Episodes. In Depersonalization/Derealization Disorder, feelings of numbness are associated with other symptoms of the disorder (e.g., a sense of detachment from one's self) and occur when the individual is not depressed.
Nonpathological symptoms of depersonalization or derealization	Are transient (i.e., lasting hours to days) and lack clinically significant impairment or distress. Approximately one-half of all adults have experienced at least one lifetime episode of depersonalization/derealization. Depersonalization/derealization symptoms meeting full criteria for this disorder are much less common, with a lifetime prevalence of approximately 1%–2%.

Somatic Symptom and Related Disorders

3.9.1 Differential Diagnosis for Somatic Symptom Disorder

Somatic Symptom Disorder, which is characterized by somatic symptoms that are distressing or result in significant disruption of daily life and are accompanied by excessive thoughts, feelings, or behaviors related to the somatic symptoms or associated health concerns, must be differentiated from…

In contrast to Somatic Symptom Disorder…

Distressing somatic symptoms characteristic of a nonpsychiatric medical condition	Are characterized by a lack of disproportionate and persistent thoughts about the seriousness of the individual's somatic symptoms, the absence of a persistently high level of anxiety about health or the somatic symptoms, and not devoting excessive time and energy to the somatic symptoms or health concerns. Having somatic symptoms of unclear etiology is not by itself sufficient for the diagnosis of Somatic Symptom Disorder, and having somatic symptoms of an established medical condition (e.g., diabetes or heart disease) does not exclude the diagnosis of Somatic Symptom Disorder if the criteria are otherwise met.
Illness Anxiety Disorder	Is characterized by extensive worries about health, but no or minimal somatic symptoms. In Somatic Symptom Disorder, the predominant focus is on the distressing somatic complaints.
Body Dysmorphic Disorder	Is characterized by a preoccupation with a perceived defect in physical appearance. In Somatic Symptom Disorder, the concern about somatic symptoms reflects concerns about underlying illness, not about a defect in appearance.

3.9.1 Differential Diagnosis for Somatic Symptom Disorder *(continued)*

Functional Neurological Symptom Disorder (Conversion Disorder)	Is characterized by one or more symptoms of altered voluntary motor or sensory function as the presenting symptom, whereas in Somatic Symptom Disorder the focus is on the distress that particular symptoms cause. Moreover, a diagnosis of Somatic Symptom Disorder requires the presence of accompanying excessive thoughts, feelings, or behaviors related to the somatic symptoms or associated health concerns. In contrast, Functional Neurological Symptom Disorder is often associated with "la belle indifference," a paradoxical absence of psychological distress, in a minority of individuals.
Generalized Anxiety Disorder	Is characterized by worry about multiple events, situations, or activities, which may include concerns about the individual's health. The main focus of worry in Somatic Symptom Disorder is on somatic symptoms and health concerns.
Panic Disorder	Is characterized by somatic symptoms occurring in the context of Panic Attacks and consequent worries about the health significance of the Panic Attacks. In Somatic Symptom Disorder, the anxiety and somatic symptoms are relatively persistent.
Obsessive-Compulsive Disorder	Is characterized by recurrent thoughts that are experienced as intrusive and unwanted and that the person attempts to ignore or suppress, and that are usually accompanied by repetitive behaviors that the individual feels driven to perform. In Somatic Symptom Disorder, the recurrent concerns about somatic symptoms or illness are less intrusive, and there are no associated repetitive behaviors that the person feels driven to perform.

3.9.1 Differential Diagnosis for Somatic Symptom Disorder *(continued)*

Depressive Disorders	Are commonly accompanied by somatic symptoms, but these are usually limited to episodes of depressed mood. Moreover, the somatic symptoms in the Depressive Disorders are accompanied by dysphoric mood and their characteristic associated symptoms.
Delusional Disorder, Somatic Type	Is characterized by the conviction that somatic symptoms are indicative of having a serious underlying illness. In contrast, in Somatic Symptom Disorder, the individual's beliefs that somatic symptoms might reflect serious underlying physical illness are not held with delusional intensity.
Factitious Disorder or Malingering	Is characterized by somatic symptoms that are intentionally produced or feigned.

3.9.2 Differential Diagnosis for Illness Anxiety Disorder

Illness Anxiety Disorder, which is characterized by a preoccupation with having or acquiring a serious illness without accompanying somatic symptoms, must be differentiated from…

In contrast to Illness Anxiety Disorder…

Expectable concerns regarding a nonpsychiatric medical condition

Concerns and distress about the medical condition are proportionate to its severity. A comorbid diagnosis of Illness Anxiety Disorder is appropriate only if the health-related anxiety and disease concerns are clearly disproportionate to the seriousness of the medical condition. Transient preoccupations related to a nonpsychiatric medical condition generally do not justify a diagnosis of Illness Anxiety Disorder.

Somatic Symptom Disorder

Is characterized by the presence of significant somatic symptoms. In contrast, individuals with Illness Anxiety Disorder have no or minimal somatic symptoms and are primarily concerned with the idea that they have a serious illness.

Specific Phobia of contracting a disease

Is characterized by a fear that one might contract a disease rather than a fear that one already has the disease as in Illness Anxiety Disorder.

Generalized Anxiety Disorder

Is characterized by anxiety and worry about multiple events, situations, or activities, only one of which may involve health.

Panic Disorder

May be characterized by anxiety or worry specifically regarding the idea that the Panic Attacks reflect the presence of a serious medical illness such as heart disease. Although individuals with Panic Disorder may have health anxiety, their anxiety is typically very acute and episodic. In contrast, the health anxiety and fears in Illness Anxiety Disorder are more chronic and enduring. Some individuals with Illness Anxiety Disorder experience Panic Attacks that are triggered by their illness concerns.

3.9.2 Differential Diagnosis for Illness Anxiety Disorder *(continued)*

Obsessive-Compulsive Disorder	May be characterized by intrusive thoughts that focus on fears of getting a disease in the future, and there usually are additional obsessions or compulsions involving other concerns. The intrusive thoughts of individuals with Illness Anxiety Disorder are about having a disease and may be accompanied by associated compulsive behaviors (e.g., seeking reassurance).
Body Dysmorphic Disorder	Is characterized by concerns that are limited to the individual's physical appearance, which is viewed as defective or flawed.
Adjustment Disorder	Is characterized by marked distress or impairment in functioning that develops in response to an identifiable psychosocial stressor (e.g., being diagnosed with a nonpsychiatric medical condition) and is time-limited (i.e., persisting for no longer than 6 months after the termination of the stressor). A diagnosis of Illness Anxiety Disorder requires the continuous persistence of disproportionate health-related anxiety for more than 6 months.
Major Depressive Disorder	May be characterized by ruminations about health and excessive worry about illness, along with the characteristic symptoms of a Major Depressive Episode (e.g., depressed mood, diminished interest or pleasure). A separate diagnosis of Illness Anxiety Disorder is not made if these concerns occur only during the Major Depressive Episodes. However, if excessive illness worry persists after remission of an episode of Major Depressive Disorder, the diagnosis of Illness Anxiety Disorder should be considered.

3.9.2 Differential Diagnosis for Illness Anxiety Disorder *(continued)*

Psychotic Disorders (e.g., Delusional Disorder)	May be characterized by somatic delusions (e.g., that an organ is rotting or dead) or delusional beliefs of having an illness. Concerns about illness in individuals with Illness Anxiety Disorder do not attain the rigidity and intensity seen in the somatic delusions occurring in Psychotic Disorders, and the person can acknowledge the possibility that the feared disease is not present.

3.9.3 Differential Diagnosis for Functional Neurological Symptom Disorder (Conversion Disorder)

Functional Neurological Symptom Disorder, which is characterized by symptoms of altered voluntary motor or sensory function that are incompatible with recognized neurological or medical conditions, must be differentiated from…	In contrast to Functional Neurological Symptom Disorder…
Occult neurological or other nonpsychiatric medical conditions, or substance/medication-induced disorders	Fully account for the deficits involving voluntary motor or sensory functioning. Functional Neurological Symptom Disorder can be diagnosed only if, after appropriate investigation, the symptom or deficit cannot be fully explained by a neurological or nonpsychiatric medical condition or by the direct physiological effects of a substance or medication.
Somatic Symptom Disorder	Is characterized by distressing somatic symptoms accompanied by excessive thoughts, feelings, or behaviors related to the somatic symptoms or associated health concerns, without regard to whether the somatic symptoms are adequately explained by a nonpsychiatric medical condition. In contrast, in Functional Neurological Symptom Disorder, clinical and/or laboratory findings must provide evidence that the neurological symptoms are incompatible with recognized neurological or other nonpsychiatric medical conditions.
Depressive Disorders	May be characterized by feelings of general "heaviness" of the limbs accompanied by core depressive symptoms, whereas the weakness of Functional Neurological Symptom Disorder is more focal and prominent.

3.9.3 Differential Diagnosis for Functional Neurological Symptom Disorder (Conversion Disorder) *(continued)*

Dissociative Disorders	Are characterized by a disruption of and/or discontinuity in the normal integration of consciousness, memory, identity, emotion, perception, body representation, motor control, and behavior, whereas in Functional Neurological Symptom Disorder, the symptoms involve disturbances in voluntary motor or sensory functioning (i.e., weakness or paralysis, abnormal movement, difficulties with swallowing or speech, seizures, sensory loss, and visual, olfactory, or hearing disturbance). Notably, the International Classification of Diseases considers Functional Neurological Symptom Disorder to be a Dissociative Disorder.
Factitious Disorder or Malingering	Is characterized by symptoms that are intentionally produced or feigned. In contrast, individuals with Functional Neurological Symptom Disorder have genuinely experienced symptoms, even though the presenting neurological symptoms are inconsistent with a bona fide neurological condition.

3.9.4 Differential Diagnosis for Psychological Factors Affecting Other Medical Conditions

Psychological Factors Affecting Other Medical Conditions, which are characterized by psychological factors that adversely affect the course or treatment of a nonpsychiatric medical condition, that constitute health risks for the individual, or that influence the underlying pathophysiology, must be differentiated from…	In contrast to Psychological Factors Affecting Other Medical Conditions…
Mental Disorder Due to Another Medical Condition (e.g., Depressive Disorder Due to a Another Medical Condition)	Is characterized by a temporal association between symptoms of a mental disorder and a nonpsychiatric medical condition. In a Mental Disorder Due to Another Medical Condition, the nonpsychiatric medical condition is judged to be causing the mental disorder through a direct physiological mechanism, whereas in Psychological Factors Affecting Other Medical Conditions, the psychological or behavioral factors adversely affect the course of the medical condition.
Adjustment Disorder	May be characterized by a clinically significant psychological response to a nonpsychiatric medical condition that can assume the role of the identifiable psychosocial stressor. For example, an individual with angina who develops maladaptive anticipatory anxiety would be diagnosed as having an Adjustment Disorder, With Anxiety, whereas an individual with angina that is precipitated whenever they become enraged would be diagnosed as having Psychological Factors Affecting Other Medical Conditions.

3.9.4 Differential Diagnosis for Psychological Factors Affecting Other Medical Conditions *(continued)*

Mental disorder causing or exacerbating a nonpsychiatric medical condition	Symptoms meeting full criteria for a mental disorder frequently result in medical complications. These mental disorders most notably include the Substance Use Disorders (e.g., Severe Alcohol Use Disorder, leading to alcoholic cirrhosis; Severe Tobacco Use Disorder, leading to emphysema). If an individual has a mental disorder that adversely affects or causes a nonpsychiatric medical condition, both the mental disorder and the nonpsychiatric medical condition are diagnosed; however, Psychological Factors Affecting Other Medical Conditions is diagnosed only when the psychological traits or behaviors do not meet criteria for a mental disorder.
Somatic Symptom Disorder	Is characterized by a combination of distressing somatic symptoms and excessive or maladaptive thoughts, feelings, and behaviors occurring in response to these symptoms, with the emphasis being on the maladaptive thoughts, feelings, and behaviors (e.g., an individual with angina who worries constantly that they will have a heart attack takes their blood pressure multiple times per day and restricts their activities). In Psychological Factors Affecting Other Medical Conditions, the emphasis is on the exacerbation of the nonpsychiatric medical condition (e.g., an individual with angina that is precipitated whenever they become anxious).
Illness Anxiety Disorder	Is characterized by high illness anxiety that is distressing or disruptive to daily life, with no or minimal somatic symptoms. In Psychological Factors Affecting Other Medical Conditions, anxiety may be a relevant psychological factor affecting a nonpsychiatric medical condition, but the clinical concern is the adverse effects on the medical condition.

3.9.5 Differential Diagnosis for Factitious Disorder[a]

Factitious Disorder, which is characterized by falsification of physical or psychological signs or symptoms or induction of injury or disease in oneself or another person, associated with identified deception, must be differentiated from...	In contrast to Factitious Disorder...
Somatic Symptom Disorder	May be characterized by excessive attention and treatment seeking for perceived medical concerns, but there is no evidence that the individual is providing false information or behaving deceptively.
Malingering	Is characterized by the intentional reporting or feigning of symptoms for personal gain (e.g., money, time off work), whereas the diagnosis of Factitious Disorder requires that the feigning behaviors persists even in the absence of obvious external incentives.
Functional Neurological Symptom Disorder (Conversion Disorder)	Is characterized by neurological symptoms that are inconsistent with neurological pathophysiology. Factitious Disorder with neurological symptoms is distinguished from Functional Neurological Symptom Disorder by evidence of deceptive falsification of symptoms.
Borderline Personality Disorder	May be characterized by deliberate physical self-harm in the absence of suicidal intent. Factitious Disorder requires that the induction of injury occurs in association with deception.

3.9.5 Differential Diagnosis for Factitious Disorder[a] *(continued)*

Child or elder abuse (as distinguished from Factitious Disorder Imposed on Another)	Is characterized by lying about abuse injuries in dependents solely to protect oneself from liability. Such individuals are not diagnosed with Factitious Disorder Imposed on Another because the deceptive behavior is motivated by an obvious external incentive (i.e., protection from criminal liability). Caregivers who are found to lie more extensively than needed for immediate self-protection may be diagnosed with Factitious Disorder Imposed on Another.

[a]Factitious Disorder comes in two forms: Factitious Disorder Imposed on Self, in which an individual feigns medical or psychiatric symptoms; and Factitious Disorder Imposed on Another, in which an individual falsifies a disease or injury in another, usually a dependent child or elder.

Feeding and Eating Disorders

3.10.1 Differential Diagnosis for Avoidant/Restrictive Food Intake Disorder

Avoidant/Restrictive Food Intake Disorder (ARFID), which is characterized by a feeding or eating disturbance associated with significant weight loss, significant nutritional deficiency, dependence on enteral feeding or nutritional supplements, or marked interference with psychosocial functioning, must be differentiated from…	In contrast to Avoidant/Restrictive Food Intake Disorder…
Nonpsychiatric medical conditions (e.g., gastrointestinal disease, food allergies and intolerances, occult malignancies)	May also result in restriction of food intake, especially in individuals with ongoing symptoms such as vomiting, loss of appetite, nausea, abdominal pain, or diarrhea. A diagnosis of ARFID may be appropriate if the disturbance in food intake exceeds that usually associated with the nonpsychiatric medical condition and warrants additional clinical attention, or if it persists after resolution of the nonpsychiatric medical condition.
Specific neurological, structural, or congenital disorders and conditions associated with feeding difficulties	Commonly result in feeding difficulties that are often related to problems with oral/esophageal/pharyngeal structure and function. A diagnosis of ARFID may be appropriate if the disturbance of food intake exceeds that usually associated with the medical condition and warrants additional clinical attention.
Reactive Attachment Disorder	Involves a disturbance in the caregiver-child relationship, which typically affects feeding and the child's nutritional intake. A diagnosis of ARFID may be appropriate if the feeding disturbance is a primary focus for intervention.

3.10.1 Differential Diagnosis for Avoidant/Restrictive Food Intake Disorder *(continued)*

Autism Spectrum Disorder	May be characterized by rigid eating behaviors and heightened sensory sensitivities. However, these symptoms often do not result in the level of impairment (e.g., weight loss, nutritional deficiency) that would be required for a diagnosis of ARFID. ARFID should be diagnosed only if the eating disturbance requires specific treatment.
Specific Phobia, Other Type; with a fear of vomiting/choking	Is characterized by avoidance of situations that may lead to choking or vomiting and may result in food avoidance and some restriction of food intake. If the consequences of the food avoidance (e.g., weight loss, nutritional deficiency) become the primary focus of clinical attention, a diagnosis of ARFID may be warranted.
Anorexia Nervosa	Although both ARFID and Anorexia Nervosa are characterized by food restrictions and low weight, individuals with Anorexia Nervosa also have a fear of gaining weight or becoming fat, or they may have persistent behavior that interferes with weight gain, as well as specific disturbances in their perception and experience of body weight and shape.
Major Depressive Disorder	May be characterized by appetite loss to such an extent that individuals present with significantly restricted food intake and weight loss, which usually abates with resolution of the depression. A diagnosis of ARFID may also be warranted if the eating disturbance requires specific treatment.
Schizophrenia Spectrum and Other Psychotic Disorders	May be characterized by odd eating behaviors, avoidance of specific foods due to delusional beliefs, or other manifestations of avoidant or restrictive food intake. A diagnosis of ARFID may be appropriate if the eating disturbance requires specific treatment.

3.10.2 Differential Diagnosis for Anorexia Nervosa

Anorexia Nervosa, which is characterized by a restriction of energy intake relative to requirements, leading to a significantly low body weight; an intense fear of gaining weight; and a disturbance in the way in which one's body weight or shape is experienced, must be differentiated from…

In contrast to Anorexia Nervosa…

Nonpsychiatric medical conditions	A number of other medical conditions (e.g., neoplasms, infections, metabolic or endocrine conditions) may be characterized by significant weight loss. However, in such conditions, unlike Anorexia Nervosa, there is no disturbance in the way the person's body weight or shape is experienced, there is no intense fear of weight gain, and the person does not engage in behaviors that interfere with appropriate weight gain. The weight loss is often accompanied by loss of appetite and includes signs, symptoms, or laboratory findings characteristic of the underlying medical condition.
Substance Use Disorders	May be characterized by low weight due to poor nutritional intake, but individuals abusing substances generally do not fear gaining weight and do not have disturbances in body image. Some individuals abusing stimulants for the purpose of appetite suppression may be motivated by a desire to prevent weight gain; if the other symptoms of Anorexia Nervosa are also present, the diagnosis would be warranted.

3.10.2 Differential Diagnosis for Anorexia Nervosa *(continued)*

Bulimia Nervosa	In both conditions, the person may engage in recurrent episodes of binge eating, engage in inappropriate behavior to avoid weight gain (e.g., self-induced vomiting), and be overly concerned with body shape and weight. The conditions are primarily differentiated on the basis of body weight; individuals with Bulimia Nervosa maintain body weight at or above a minimally normal level, whereas those with Anorexia Nervosa maintain a significantly low body weight.
Avoidant/Restrictive Food Intake Disorder	Is characterized by significant weight loss and nutritional deficiency and restriction of food intake, but unlike Anorexia Nervosa the weight loss and food restrictions are not motivated by a fear of gaining weight or becoming fat.
Weight loss in Depressive Disorders	Is not accompanied by a desire for excessive weight loss or an intense fear of gaining weight or getting fat, and includes the presence of characteristic features of a Depressive Disorder (e.g., depressed mood, loss of interest).
Schizophrenia	May be characterized by unusual eating behavior, but it is not accompanied by a desire for excessive weight loss or an intense fear of gaining weight or getting fat, and it is accompanied by the characteristic features of Schizophrenia (e.g., delusions, hallucinations, disorganized speech).
Obsessive-Compulsive Disorder	In both conditions, there may be repetitive intrusive thoughts and compulsive behaviors. In Anorexia Nervosa, however, these thoughts and behaviors are limited to weight, eating, or food. An additional diagnosis of Obsessive-Compulsive Disorder should be considered only if there are additional obsessions or compulsions unrelated to weight, eating, or food (e.g., related to contamination).

3.10.2 Differential Diagnosis for Anorexia Nervosa *(continued)*

Social Anxiety Disorder	In Anorexia Nervosa and Social Anxiety Disorder, individuals may feel humiliated or embarrassed to be seen eating in public. In Anorexia Nervosa, social fears are limited to eating behaviors. An additional diagnosis of Social Anxiety Disorder is warranted only if there are fears of other social situations (e.g., speaking in public).
Body Dysmorphic Disorder	In Anorexia Nervosa and Body Dysmorphic Disorder, individuals may be preoccupied with an imagined defect in bodily appearance. In Anorexia Nervosa, the preoccupation is limited to body shape and weight. An additional diagnosis of Body Dysmorphic Disorder is warranted only if there are distortions about the body that are unrelated to weight or being fat (e.g., preoccupation with the shape of one's nose).

3.10.3 Differential Diagnosis for Bulimia Nervosa

Bulimia Nervosa, which is characterized by recurrent episodes of binge eating accompanied by inappropriate compensatory behaviors to prevent weight gain, must be differentiated from...	In contrast to Bulimia Nervosa...
Vomiting or diarrhea in nonpsychiatric medical conditions or with excessive substance use	Is due to the direct physiological effects of the nonpsychiatric medical condition or substance use.
Anorexia Nervosa	May be characterized by episodes of binge eating and purging. In contrast to Bulimia Nervosa, the diagnosis of Anorexia Nervosa requires significantly low body weight (i.e., weight that is less than minimally normal). Individuals whose binge-eating behavior occurs only during episodes of Anorexia Nervosa are given the diagnosis Anorexia Nervosa, Binge-Eating/Purging Type. If the full criteria for Anorexia Nervosa, Binge-Eating/Purging Type, are no longer met because, for example, weight becomes normal, a diagnosis of Bulimia Nervosa should be given only if criteria for Bulimia Nervosa are met for at least 3 months.
Binge-Eating Disorder	Is characterized by binge eating not accompanied by the regular use of inappropriate compensatory mechanisms to counteract the effects of binge eating. In contrast, Bulimia Nervosa requires episodes of binge eating and inappropriate compensatory behaviors that occur at least once a week for 3 months.
Kleine-Levin syndrome	Is characterized by overeating, but the characteristic psychological features of Bulimia Nervosa, such as overconcern with body shape and weight, are not present.

3.10.3 Differential Diagnosis for Bulimia Nervosa *(continued)*

Major Depressive Episode, With Atypical Features, in Major Depressive Disorder or in Bipolar I or Bipolar II Disorder	May be characterized by overeating along with the other symptoms of depression, but the overeating does not necessarily occur in the form of binge eating; furthermore, individuals do not engage in inappropriate compensatory behaviors and do not exhibit the characteristic excessive concern with body shape and weight. If criteria are met for both Bulimia Nervosa and a Major Depressive Episode, With Atypical Features, then both should be diagnosed.
Borderline Personality Disorder	May be characterized by binge eating (which is one of the examples of impulsivity included in Criterion 4), along with other characteristic features of Borderline Personality Disorder (e.g., self-mutilation, pattern of unstable relationships). In contrast, the diagnosis of Bulimia Nervosa requires inappropriate compensatory behaviors after the binge eating as well as overconcern with body shape and weight. If criteria are met for Bulimia Nervosa and Borderline Personality Disorder, both can be diagnosed.

3.10.4 Differential Diagnosis for Binge-Eating Disorder

Binge-Eating Disorder, which is characterized by recurrent episodes of binge eating accompanied by marked distress, must be differentiated from…	In contrast to Binge-Eating Disorder…
Bulimia Nervosa	Both conditions are characterized by recurrent binge eating, but in Bulimia Nervosa there are recurrent inappropriate compensatory behaviors (e.g., purging, driven exercise).
Obesity	Although many individuals with Binge-Eating Disorder are obese, those with Binge-Eating Disorder are more likely to have higher levels of overvaluation of body weight and shape, have significantly higher rates of psychiatric comorbidity, and have a higher likelihood of long-term successful outcome of evidence-based psychological treatment.
Major Depressive Episode, With Atypical Features, in Major Depressive Disorder or in Bipolar I or Bipolar II Disorder	May be characterized by overeating along with the other symptoms of depression, but the overeating does not necessarily occur in the form of binge eating and the eating may or may not be associated with a loss of control. If criteria are met for Binge-Eating Disorder and a Major Depressive Episode, With Atypical Features, then both should be diagnosed.
Borderline Personality Disorder	Includes binge eating in the impulsive behavior criterion that is part of the definition of Borderline Personality Disorder. If the full criteria for Binge-Eating Disorder and Borderline Personality Disorder are met, both diagnoses can be given.

Sleep-Wake Disorders

3.11.1 Differential Diagnosis for Insomnia Disorder

Insomnia Disorder, which is characterized by dissatisfaction with sleep quantity or quality associated with difficulty initiating or maintaining sleep, or early-morning awakening with inability to return to sleep, must be differentiated from…

In contrast to Insomnia Disorder…

Short sleepers (individuals who require little sleep)	Short sleepers do not have any difficulty falling or staying asleep and lack symptoms of daytime sleepiness (e.g., fatigue, concentration problems, irritability). By attempting to sleep for a longer period of time by prolonging time in bed, some short sleepers may create an insomnia-like sleep pattern.
Sleep deprivation	Is characterized by an inadequate opportunity or circumstance for sleep and is typically temporary (e.g., professional or family obligations forcing a person to stay awake). Insomnia Disorder would not be diagnosed in such circumstances.
Circadian Rhythm Sleep-Wake Disorder, Shift Work Type and Delayed Sleep Phase Type	In Circadian Rhythm Sleep-Wake Disorder, Shift Work Type, there is a history of recent shift work with consequent disturbance in sleep. Individuals with Circadian Rhythm Sleep-Wake Disorder, Delayed Sleep Phase Type (i.e., "night owls"), report sleep-onset insomnia only when they try to sleep at socially normal times, but do not report difficulty falling asleep or staying asleep when their bedtimes and rising times are delayed and coincide with their endogenous circadian rhythm. Insomnia Disorder is not diagnosed if the difficulties initiating and maintaining sleep are better explained by, and occur exclusively during the course of, a Circadian Rhythm Sleep-Wake Disorder.

3.11.1 Differential Diagnosis for Insomnia Disorder *(continued)*

Restless Legs Syndrome	Is characterized by urges to move the legs and accompanying unpleasant leg sensations, and often produces difficulties initiating and maintaining sleep. Insomnia Disorder is not diagnosed if the difficulties initiating and maintaining sleep are better explained by, and occur exclusively during the course of, Restless Legs Syndrome.
Breathing-Related Sleep Disorders	Are characterized by loud snoring, breathing pauses during sleep, and excessive daytime sleepiness, with up to half of these individuals reporting insomnia symptoms. Insomnia Disorder is not diagnosed if the difficulties initiating and maintaining sleep are better explained by, and occur exclusively during the course of, a Breathing-Related Sleep Disorder.
Narcolepsy	Is characterized by excessive daytime sleepiness, cataplexy, sleep paralysis, and sleep-related hallucinations, along with frequent brief awakenings during nocturnal sleep. Insomnia Disorder is not diagnosed if the difficulties maintaining sleep are better explained by, and occur exclusively during the course of, Narcolepsy.
Parasomnias (i.e., Non–Rapid Eye Movement Sleep Arousal Disorders, Nightmare Disorder, Rapid Eye Movement Sleep Behavior Disorder)	Are characterized by unusual behaviors or events during sleep that may lead to intermittent awakenings and difficulty resuming sleep; however, it is these behavioral events, rather than the insomnia per se, that dominate the clinical picture. Insomnia Disorder is not diagnosed if the difficulties initiating and maintaining sleep are better explained by, and occur exclusively during the course of, the Parasomnia.

3.11.1 Differential Diagnosis for Insomnia Disorder *(continued)*

Insomnia associated with another mental disorder or nonpsychiatric medical condition	The diagnosis of Insomnia Disorder is given whether it occurs as an independent condition or occurs in association with another mental disorder (e.g., Major Depressive Disorder) or a nonpsychiatric medical condition (e.g., pain), but only if coexisting mental disorders and medical conditions do not adequately explain the predominant complaint of insomnia. In such instances, a specifier (With [Mental Disorder] or With [Medical Condition], using the name of the specific mental disorder or medical condition) can be used to indicate the association.
Substance/Medication-Induced Sleep Disorder, Insomnia Type	Is due to the direct physiological effects of a substance or medication. Insomnia Disorder is not diagnosed unless the insomnia was also present at times when the person was not using the substance or medication.

3.11.2 Differential Diagnosis for Hypersomnolence Disorder

Hypersomnolence Disorder, which is characterized by excessive sleepiness associated with lapses into sleep, unrefreshing prolonged main sleep episodes of more than 9 hours per day, or difficulty being fully awake after abrupt awakening, must be differentiated from…

In contrast to Hypersomnolence Disorder…

Normal long sleepers	Require a greater than average amount of sleep. Long sleepers do not have excessive sleepiness, sleep inertia, or automatic behavior when they obtain their required amount of nocturnal sleep, and they report their sleep to be refreshing. If social or occupational demands lead to shorter nocturnal sleep, daytime symptoms may appear. In individuals with Hypersomnolence Disorder, symptoms of excessive sleepiness occur regardless of nocturnal sleep duration.
Inadequate amount of nocturnal sleep	Can produce symptoms of daytime sleepiness very similar to those of Hypersomnolence Disorder. An average sleep duration of fewer than 7 hours per night strongly suggests inadequate nocturnal sleep, whereas an average of more than 9–10 hours of unrefreshing sleep per 24-hour period suggests a diagnosis of Hypersomnolence Disorder. Unlike Hypersomnolence Disorder, insufficient nocturnal sleep is unlikely to persist unabated for decades.
Daytime fatigue resulting from Insomnia Disorder	Is characterized by excessive sleepiness related to insufficient sleep quantity or quality. Hypersomnolence Disorder is not diagnosed if the excessive sleepiness is better explained by, and occurs exclusively during the course of, Insomnia Disorder.

3.11.2 Differential Diagnosis for Hypersomnolence Disorder *(continued)*

Narcolepsy	Is characterized by recurrent periods of irrepressible need to sleep, lapsing into sleep, or napping occurring within the same day, which are accompanied by other characteristic features such as cataplexy, hypocretin deficiency, and specific polysomnographic findings (i.e., rapid eye movement [REM] sleep latency of 15 minutes or less, or a multiple sleep latency test showing a mean sleep latency of 8 minutes or less and two or more sleep-onset REM periods). Hypersomnolence Disorder is not diagnosed if the excessive sleepiness is better explained by, and occurs exclusively during the course of, Narcolepsy.
Breathing-Related Sleep Disorders	Are characterized by daytime sleepiness accompanied by specific polysomnographic findings (e.g., a minimum number of apneas or hypopneas per hour) and often nighttime symptoms (e.g., loud snoring, breathing pauses). Hypersomnolence Disorder is not diagnosed if the excessive sleepiness is better explained by, and occurs exclusively during the course of, a Breathing-Related Sleep Disorder.
Circadian Rhythm Sleep-Wake Disorders	Are often characterized by daytime sleepiness, accompanied by a history of an abnormal sleep-wake schedule. Hypersomnolence Disorder is not diagnosed if the excessive sleepiness is better explained by, and occurs exclusively during the course of, a Circadian Rhythm Sleep-Wake Disorder.

3.11.2 Differential Diagnosis for Hypersomnolence Disorder *(continued)*

Parasomnias (i.e., Non–Rapid Eye Movement Sleep Arousal Disorders, Nightmare Disorder, Rapid Eye Movement Sleep Behavior Disorder)	May be characterized by daytime sleepiness related to nightmares, sleep terrors, sleepwalking, or episodes of arousal during REM sleep associated with vocalization and/or complex motor behaviors. Hypersomnolence Disorder is not diagnosed if the excessive sleepiness is better explained by, and occurs exclusively during the course of, a Parasomnia.
Hypersomnolence associated with another mental disorder or nonpsychiatric medical condition	The diagnosis of Hypersomnolence Disorder is given whether it occurs as an independent condition or occurs in association with another mental disorder (e.g., hypersomnia in Major Depressive Disorder) or a nonpsychiatric medical condition (e.g., Parkinson's disease), but only if coexisting mental disorders and medical conditions do not adequately explain the predominant complaint of hypersomnolence. In such instances, a specifier (With [Mental Disorder] or With [Medical Condition], using the name of the specific mental disorder or medical condition) can be used to indicate the association.
Substance/Medication-Induced Sleep Disorder, Daytime Sleepiness Type	Is due to the direct physiological effects of a substance or medication. Hypersomnolence Disorder is not diagnosed unless the hypersomnolence was also present at times when the person was not using the substance or medication.

Sexual Dysfunctions

3.12.1 Differential Diagnosis for Sexual Dysfunctions

A Sexual Dysfunction, which is characterized by the presence of sexual symptoms (i.e., hypoactive desire, arousal problems, early ejaculation, delayed orgasm, genito-pelvic pain) that are experienced in all, or almost all, occasions of sexual activity, and that cause clinically significant distress in the individual, must be differentiated from...

In contrast to a Sexual Dysfunction...

Nonpsychiatric medical condition that accounts for the sexual dysfunction	If the dysfunction is entirely attributable to the direct physiological effects of a nonpsychiatric medical condition (e.g., autonomic neuropathy), then in such cases, a DSM-5-TR Sexual Dysfunction diagnosis is not made.
Substance/Medication-Induced Sexual Dysfunction	Involves a sexual dysfunction that is better explained by the use, misuse, or discontinuation of a substance or medication. A Sexual Dysfunction diagnosis is not given if the dysfunction is entirely attributable to the direct physiological effects of a substance or medication.
Sexual problems associated with a nonsexual mental disorder (e.g., Major Depressive Disorder, Bipolar and Related Disorder, Posttraumatic Stress Disorder, Psychotic Disorder)	Are characterized by a sexual dysfunction that occurs only in the context of the symptoms of the other mental disorder (e.g., low sexual desire in the context of a Major Depressive Episode). If the sexual problems were present before the onset of the nonsexual mental disorder or persists once the nonsexual mental disorder has resolved, a separate diagnosis of Sexual Dysfunction may be warranted.

3.12.1 Differential Diagnosis for Sexual Dysfunctions *(continued)*

Sexual problems associated with severe relationship distress (e.g., partner violence) or other significant stressors	Is characterized by sexual problems that are judged to be a consequence of severe relationship distress or other significant stressors. In such cases, a Sexual Dysfunction would not be diagnosed and only the relational problem (e.g., Z63.0 Relationship Distress With Spouse or Intimate Partner) would be coded. However, if the sexual problems were present before the severe relationship distress occurred or persist after the relationship distress has resolved, an additional di-agnosis of a Sexual Dysfunction may be warranted.
Sexual problems due to inadequate or absent sexual stimuli	Are typically related to lack of knowledge about effective stimulation, which conse-quently prevents the experience of arousal or orgasm. Although there may still be a need for evaluation and/or treatment, a diagnosis of a Sexual Dys-function is not warranted.

Gender Dysphoria

3.13.1 Differential Diagnosis for Gender Dysphoria

Gender Dysphoria, which is characterized by a marked incongruence between the individual's experienced or expressed gender and their gender assigned at birth, is accompanied by a strong desire to be the experienced gender, and causes clinically significant distress or impairment, must be differentiated from…

In contrast to Gender Dysphoria…

Nonconformity of gender roles	Is characterized by nonconformity to stereotypical gender role behavior (e.g., "tomboyish" behavior in girls, occasional cross-dressing in adult men) that occurs in the absence of clinically significant distress or impairment in social, occupational, or other areas of functioning. In contrast, Gender Dysphoria is characterized by the strong desire to be of the expressed gender rather than the one assigned at birth and by the extent and pervasiveness of gender-variant activities and interests.
Transvestic Disorder	Is characterized by intense sexual arousal from dressing in women's clothing that causes distress or impairment without a marked incongruence between the individual's experienced/expressed gender and assigned gender. An individual who is sexually aroused by cross-dressing and who also has Gender Dysphoria can be given both diagnoses.
Body Dysmorphic Disorder	May be characterized by the persistent desire to alter or remove a specific body part or feature because it is perceived as abnormally formed and ugly and not because it represents a repudiated assigned gender. When an individual's presentation meets criteria for both Gender Dysphoria and Body Dysmorphic Disorder, both diagnoses can be given.

3.13.1 Differential Diagnosis for Gender Dysphoria *(continued)*

Psychotic Disorder (e.g., Schizophrenia)	May rarely be characterized by delusions of belonging to the other gender. In the absence of other symptoms characteristic of a Psychotic Disorder (e.g., hallucinations, other delusions), insistence by an individual with Gender Dysphoria that they are of the other gender is not considered a delusion.

Disruptive, Impulse-Control, and Conduct Disorders

3.14.1 Differential Diagnosis for Oppositional Defiant Disorder

Oppositional Defiant Disorder (ODD), which is characterized by a pattern of angry/irritable mood, argumentative/defiant behavior, or vindictiveness, must be differentiated from…	In contrast to Oppositional Defiant Disorder…
Nonpathological oppositional behavior typical of certain developmental stages	Is not clinically significant and/or is not a persistent pattern.
Adjustment Disorder, With Disturbance of Conduct	Is a time-limited maladaptive response to an identifiable psychosocial stressor and does not meet criteria for ODD.
Conduct Disorder	Is characterized by conduct problems that are of a more severe nature than those of ODD and include aggression toward people or animals, destruction of property, or a pattern of theft or deceit. Moreover, Conduct Disorder does not include problems of emotional dysregulation (i.e., angry and irritable mood). If criteria are met for ODD and Conduct Disorder, both may be diagnosed.
Attention-Deficit/Hyperactivity Disorder	May be characterized by oppositional behavior that occurs solely in situations related to the individual's failure to conform to requests that demand sustained effort and attention or requests to sit still. If the oppositional behavior occurs in other situations, then an additional diagnosis of ODD may be appropriate.
Disruptive Mood Dysregulation Disorder	Is characterized by temper outbursts that are much more frequent (three or more times per week), chronic (12 months or more), persistent (no periods lasting 3 or more months without symptoms), and severe (verbal rages or physical aggression toward people or property) than those in ODD. ODD is not diagnosed if criteria are met for Disruptive Mood Dysregulation Disorder.

3.14.1 Differential Diagnosis for Oppositional Defiant Disorder *(continued)*

Intermittent Explosive Disorder	Is characterized by recurrent behavioral outbursts that involve serious physical or verbal aggression toward others and that are grossly out of proportion to the provocation. Aggression in ODD is typically characterized by temper tantrums and verbal arguments with authority figures. An additional diagnosis of Intermittent Explosive Disorder can be made if the recurrent impulsive aggressive outbursts are in excess of those usually seen in ODD and warrant independent clinical attention.
Bipolar and Related Disorders, Depressive Disorders, or Psychotic Disorders	Are associated with oppositional behavior that occurs only in the context of a mood disturbance or in relation to delusions or hallucinations.
Intellectual Developmental Disorder	May be characterized by oppositional behavior that accompanies the intellectual deficits. A diagnosis of ODD is given only if the oppositional behavior is markedly greater than is commonly observed among individuals of comparable mental age and with comparable severity of Intellectual Developmental Disorder.
Language Disorder	May be associated with oppositional behavior related to a failure to follow directions that is the result of impaired language comprehension.
Selective Mutism	Is characterized by a failure to speak due to fear of negative evaluation rather than by a motivation to be oppositional.

3.14.2 Differential Diagnosis for Intermittent Explosive Disorder

Intermittent Explosive Disorder, which is characterized by recurrent behavioral outbursts that are grossly out of proportion to the provocation or any precipitating psychosocial stressors, must be differentiated from...

In contrast to Intermittent Explosive Disorder...

Substance Intoxication or Substance Withdrawal

May be characterized by aggressive behavior that is due to the direct physiological effects of intoxication with, or withdrawal from, a substance. Intermittent Explosive Disorder is not diagnosed if the aggressive outbursts occur only during episodes of Substance Intoxication or Substance Withdrawal.

Delirium Due to Another Medical Condition, Substance Intoxication Delirium, Substance Withdrawal Delirium, or Medication-Induced Delirium

Includes characteristic symptoms (e.g., impaired attention accompanied by reduced awareness of the environment, with fluctuating course) along with the aggressive outbursts and requires the presence of an etiological nonpsychiatric medical condition or substance/medication use. Intermittent Explosive Disorder should not be diagnosed if the behavioral outbursts occur only in the context of Delirium.

Major Neurocognitive Disorder Due to Another Medical Condition, With Other Behavioral or Psychological Disturbance; Mild Neurocognitive Disorder Due to Another Medical Condition, With Behavioral Disturbance; Substance/Medication-Induced Major Neurocognitive Disorder, With Other Behavioral or Psychological Disturbance; or Substance/Medication-Induced Mild Neurocognitive Disorder, With Behavioral Disturbance

Is characterized by significant cognitive decline in one or more cognitive domains (complex attention, executive function, learning and memory, language, perceptual-motor, or social cognition) that may be accompanied by clinically significant behavioral or psychological disturbances such as aggression, disinhibition, and disruptive behaviors or vocalizations. Intermittent Explosive Disorder should not be diagnosed if the aggressive behavior occurs only in the context of a Major or Mild Neurocognitive Disorder.

3.14.2 Differential Diagnosis for Intermittent Explosive Disorder *(continued)*

Personality Change Due to Another Medical Condition, Aggressive Type	The change from the person's previous characteristic personality pattern involves aggressive outbursts and requires the presence of an etiological medical condition. Nonspecific abnormalities on neurological examination (e.g., "soft signs") and nonspecific electroencephalographic changes do not constitute an etiological medical condition and instead are compatible with a diagnosis of Intermittent Explosive Disorder.
Disruptive Mood Dysregulation Disorder	Is characterized by aggressive outbursts accompanied by a persistently negative mood state (i.e., irritability, anger) most of the day, nearly every day, between the impulsive aggressive outbursts, with onset before age 10 years. Intermittent Explosive Disorder is not diagnosed if the aggressive outbursts are better explained by a diagnosis of Disruptive Mood Dysregulation Disorder.
Antisocial Personality Disorder or Borderline Personality Disorder	May be characterized by recurrent problematic impulsive aggressive outbursts occurring in the context of a long-standing Personality Disorder. Intermittent Explosive Disorder is not diagnosed if the aggressive outbursts are better explained by one of these Personality Disorders.
Attention-Deficit/Hyperactivity Disorder (ADHD), Conduct Disorder, or Oppositional Defiant Disorder	May be associated with aggressive outbursts. In ADHD, the characteristic impulsivity may be manifested by impulsive aggressive outbursts; in Conduct Disorder, aggression is characteristically proactive and predatory; in Oppositional Defiant Disorder, the aggression typically takes the form of temper tantrums and verbal arguments with authority figures. An additional diagnosis of Intermittent Explosive Disorder can be made if the recurrent impulsive aggressive outbursts are in excess of those usually seen in these disorders and warrant independent clinical attention.

3.14.2 Differential Diagnosis for Intermittent Explosive Disorder *(continued)*

Other mental disorders (e.g., Schizophrenia, Manic Episode)	May include impulsive aggression as an associated feature along with their characteristic features. Intermittent Explosive Disorder is not diagnosed if the aggressive behavior occurs only during episodes of one of these disorders (e.g., during Manic Episodes, during delusional periods).
Aggressive behavior not attributable to a mental disorder	Is motivated by a political or religious belief, revenge, monetary gain, thrill seeking, or another reason not related to a mental disorder.

3.14.3 Differential Diagnosis for Conduct Disorder

Conduct Disorder, which is characterized by a repetitive and persistent pattern of behavior in which the basic rights of others or major age-appropriate societal norms or rules are violated, must be differentiated from…	In contrast to Conduct Disorder…
Oppositional Defiant Disorder	Is characterized by disruptive behaviors that are typically of a less severe nature than those in Conduct Disorder and do not include aggression toward individuals or animals, destruction of property, or a pattern of theft or deceit. Moreover, Oppositional Defiant Disorder includes problems of emotional dysregulation (i.e., angry and irritable mood) that are not part of the definition of Conduct Disorder. If criteria are met for both conditions, both may be diagnosed.
Attention-Deficit/Hyperactivity Disorder	Is characterized by hyperactive and impulsive behavior that may be disruptive but does not by itself violate societal norms or the rights of others. If criteria are met for both disorders, both may be diagnosed.
Bipolar I or Bipolar II Disorder, Major Depressive Disorder, Persistent Depressive Disorder, or Disruptive Mood Dysregulation Disorder	May be characterized by behavioral problems associated with irritability and aggression and can be distinguished from Conduct Disorder by the absence of substantial levels of aggressive or nonaggressive conduct problems during periods in which there is no mood disturbance.
Intermittent Explosive Disorder	Is characterized by aggression that is limited to impulsive aggression, is not premeditated, and is not committed to achieve some tangible objective. If criteria for both disorders are met, the diagnosis of Intermittent Explosive Disorder should be given only when the recurrent impulsive aggressive outbursts warrant independent clinical attention.
Antisocial behavior related to a Psychotic Disorder (e.g., Schizophrenia)	Occurs only in response to delusions or hallucinations.

3.14.3 Differential Diagnosis for Conduct Disorder *(continued)*

Adjustment Disorder, With Disturbance of Conduct	Is characterized by time-limited conduct problems that do not meet criteria for Conduct Disorder and that clearly occur in response to an identifiable psychosocial stressor, as opposed to being part of a long-standing pattern.
Child or Adolescent Antisocial Behavior	Is below the severity threshold for Conduct Disorder or is not part of a long-standing pattern (i.e., isolated antisocial acts).
Antisocial Personality Disorder	Can be diagnosed only in individuals age 18 years or older. Conduct Disorder is not diagnosed if the individual is age 18 or older and criteria are met for Antisocial Personality Disorder.

Substance-Related and Addictive Disorders

3.15.1 Differential Diagnosis for Substance Use Disorders

Substance Use Disorder, which is characterized by a problematic pattern of substance use leading to clinically significant impairment or distress, must be differentiated from…	In contrast to Substance Use Disorder…
Nonpathological use of the substance	Is characterized by repeated use at relatively low doses and may involve occasional periods of intoxication not associated with clinically significant negative consequences (e.g., intoxication restricted to occasional weekends so that it does not impair work or school functioning). In contrast, Substance Use Disorders are characterized by heavy use leading to significant distress or impaired functioning. Differentiating between nonpathological substance use and a Substance Use Disorder may be complicated by the fact that denial of heavy substance use and substance-related problems is common with individuals who are referred to treatment by others (e.g., school, family, employer, criminal justice system).
Substance/Medication-Induced Mental Disorders (including Substance Intoxication and Substance Withdrawal)	Are characterized by central nervous system syndromes that develop in the context of the physiological effects of substances of abuse, medications, or toxin exposure. They are distinguished from Substance Use Disorders, which are pathological patterns of behaviors related to a pattern of use of a substance (including medication). Given that the heavy substance use characteristic of a Substance Use Disorder often leads to the development of a Substance-Induced Disorder, they commonly co-occur and both should be diagnosed (e.g., Severe Cocaine Use Disorder with comorbid Cocaine-Induced Psychotic Disorder, With Onset During Intoxication).

3.15.1 Differential Diagnosis for Substance Use Disorders *(continued)*

Conduct Disorder in childhood and Antisocial Personality Disorder in adulthood	Substance Use (including Alcohol Use) Disorders are seen in the majority of individuals with Antisocial Personality Disorder and preexisting Conduct Disorder and are associated with the early onset of the Substance Use Disorder.
Substance use during Manic Episodes	Involves episodes of characteristic symptoms (e.g., elevated mood, irritability, distractibility, decreased need for sleep, flight of ideas) that persist at times when the individual is not using substances. If substance use during a Manic Episode meets criteria for a Substance Use Disorder, both may be diagnosed.

3.15.2 Differential Diagnosis for Gambling Disorder

Gambling Disorder, which is characterized by persistent and recurrent problematic gambling behavior leading to clinically significant impairment or distress, must be differentiated from...	In contrast to Gambling Disorder...
Professional gambling	Is characterized by discipline and limited risk taking and is intended to be a source of income.
Social gambling	Usually occurs among friends and is characterized by limited time spent on gambling and limited risk taking.
Manic Episode	Is characterized by symptoms (e.g., euphoric mood, rapid speech, increased self-esteem, flight of ideas) that persist at times when the individual is not gambling. Gambling Disorder is not diagnosed if the gambling behavior is better accounted for by a Manic Episode.
Internet Gaming Disorder (in DSM-5-TR Section III)	Is characterized by a preoccupation with the use of the Internet to play games, often with other players, leading to clinically significant distress or impairment. In contrast to Gambling Disorder, the wagering of money is not involved.

Neurocognitive Disorders

3.16.1 Differential Diagnosis for Delirium

Delirium, which is characterized by a disturbance in attention (i.e., reduced ability to direct, focus, sustain, and shift attention), accompanied by reduced awareness of the environment that tends to fluctuate during the course of the day and that is due to the direct physiological effects of a substance, medication, or nonpsychiatric medical condition, must be differentiated from…

In contrast to Delirium…

Major or Mild Neurocognitive Disorder	Is characterized by a relatively stable or gradually progressive course, typically a much longer duration, and despite a number of cognitive deficits, the individual's lack of impairment of the ability to maintain attention and be aware of their environment. Episodes of Delirium, however, can occur in an individual with a preexisting Neurocognitive Disorder. Major or Mild Neurocognitive Disorder is not diagnosed if the deficits occur exclusively in the context of Delirium. When Delirium occurs in the context of a preexisting Neurocognitive Disorder, it should be separately diagnosed.
Substance Intoxication or Substance Withdrawal	May be characterized by deficits in attention and awareness of the environment, but these disturbances do not predominate in the clinical picture and are not sufficiently severe to warrant clinical attention. Substance Intoxication Delirium or Substance Withdrawal Delirium is diagnosed instead of Substance Intoxication or Substance Withdrawal if the neurocognitive disturbance meets diagnostic criteria for Delirium and warrants clinical attention.

3.16.1 Differential Diagnosis for Delirium *(continued)*

Substance/Medication-Induced Psychotic Disorder or Psychotic Disorder Due to Another Medical Condition	Is characterized by delusions or hallucinations due to the direct physiological effects of a substance/medication or nonpsychiatric medical condition, respectively, on the central nervous system, but these symptoms are not accompanied by a disturbance in attention and reduced awareness of the environment; moreover, the additional disturbances in cognition, language, or visuospatial ability characteristic of a Delirium are not present. Substance/Medication-Induced Psychotic Disorder and Psychotic Disorder Due to Another Medical Condition are not diagnosed if the psychotic symptoms occur exclusively during the course of the Delirium.
Schizophrenia Spectrum and Other Psychotic Disorders; Bipolar and Related Disorders; or Depressive Disorders	May be characterized by delusions, hallucinations, or agitation, but these are not due to the direct physiological effects of a nonpsychiatric medical condition or substance/medication use; they are accompanied neither by a disturbance in attention and awareness nor the additional disturbances in cognition, language, or visuospatial ability characteristic of a Delirium.

3.16.2 Differential Diagnosis for Major or Mild Neurocognitive Disorder[a]

Major or Mild Neurocognitive Disorder, which is characterized by evidence of cognitive decline from a previous level of performance in one or more cognitive domains (complex attention, executive function, learning and memory, language, perceptual-motor, or social cognition) that is due to a nonpsychiatric medical condition or the persisting effects of a substance or medication, must be differentiated from…	In contrast to Major or Mild Neurocognitive Disorder…
Delirium	Is characterized by a disturbance in attention (i.e., reduced ability to direct, focus, sustain, and shift attention) accompanied by reduced awareness of the environment that develops over a short period of time, usually hours to a few days, and tends to fluctuate during the course of the day. In contrast, most types of Major or Mild Neurocognitive Disorder (e.g., due to Alzheimer's disease) have a gradual onset and a gradually deteriorating course. Major or Mild Neurocognitive Disorder is not diagnosed if the cognitive deficits occur exclusively in the context of Delirium. However, periods of Delirium can be superimposed on a Major or Mild Neurocognitive Disorder and should be diagnosed if present.
Substance Intoxication or Substance Withdrawal	May be characterized by cognitive impairment that remits when the acute effects of intoxication or withdrawal subside. In contrast, Substance/Medication-Induced Major or Mild Neurocognitive Disorder is diagnosed only if the cognitive impairments persist beyond the usual duration period of intoxication and acute withdrawal.

3.16.2 Differential Diagnosis for Major or Mild Neurocognitive Disorder[a] *(continued)*

Intellectual Developmental Disorder	Is characterized by intellectual and adaptive functioning deficits in conceptual, social, and practical domains that have their onset during the developmental period. In contrast, Major or Mild Neurocognitive Disorder represents a decline in cognitive functioning. Individuals with Intellectual Developmental Disorder can also be diagnosed with a Neurocognitive Disorder if they undergo a decline in cognitive functioning due to the direct physiological effects of a comorbid nonpsychiatric medical condition on the central nervous system (e.g., an individual with Down syndrome who loses further cognitive capacity following a head injury).
Schizophrenia	May be characterized by cognitive impairment and deterioration in functioning. In contrast to Major or Mild Neurocognitive Disorder, Schizophrenia has a generally earlier age at onset, less severe cognitive impairment, and a characteristic symptom pattern (e.g., delusions and hallucinations); and it is not due to the direct physiological effects of a nonpsychiatric medical condition or substance/medication use.
Dissociative Amnesia or amnesia occurring in other Dissociative Disorders	Usually involves a circumscribed loss of memory related to traumatic events and is not due to the direct physiological effects of a nonpsychiatric medical condition or substance/medication use.
Major Depressive Disorder	May be characterized by memory deficits, difficulty concentrating, and other cognitive impairments, but in contrast to Major or Mild Neurocognitive Disorder, these deficits improve when the depression remits, are associated with other characteristic depressive symptoms, and are not due to the direct physiological effects of a nonpsychiatric medical condition or substance/medication use.

3.16.2 Differential Diagnosis for Major or Mild Neurocognitive Disorder[a] *(continued)*

Bipolar I Disorder	May be characterized by chronic cognitive impairment that impacts long-term functioning. In contrast to Major or Mild Neurocognitive Disorder, Bipolar I Disorder generally has an earlier age at onset, less severe cognitive impairment, and the presence of Manic and Major Depressive Episodes; and it is not due to the direct physiological effects of a nonpsychiatric medical condition or substance/medication use.
Age-related cognitive decline	Is characterized by cognitive impairment that is in keeping with what would be expected for the individual's age and is not due to the direct physiological effects of a nonpsychiatric medical condition or substance/medication use.

[a]The two types of Neurocognitive Disorder in DSM-5-TR, Major and Mild, are differentiated on the basis of the severity of the neurocognitive deficits and their impact on the person's functioning. Major Neurocognitive Disorder is characterized by a significant cognitive decline that is severe enough to interfere with independence in everyday activities, whereas Mild Neurocognitive Disorder is characterized by a modest cognitive decline that is not severe enough to interfere with everyday activities, although greater effort, compensatory strategies, or accommodation may be required.

Personality Disorders

3.17.1 Differential Diagnosis for Paranoid Personality Disorder

Paranoid Personality Disorder, which is characterized by pervasive distrust and suspiciousness of others such that their motives are interpreted as malevolent, must be differentiated from…	In contrast to Paranoid Personality Disorder…
Delusional Disorder, Persecutory Type; Schizophrenia; Bipolar I or Bipolar II Disorder, With Psychotic Features; and Major Depressive Disorder, With Psychotic Features	May be characterized by a period of persistent persecutory delusions. In Paranoid Personality Disorder, the paranoid beliefs (e.g., doubts about the trustworthiness of friends or associates) are not held with delusional intensity. To give an additional diagnosis of Paranoid Personality Disorder, the personality disorder must have been present before the onset of psychotic symptoms and must persist when the psychotic symptoms are in remission.
Personality Change Due to Another Medical Condition, Paranoid Type	Is characterized by a change in personality related to the direct physiological effects of a nonpsychiatric medical condition.
Social discomfort and paranoid ideation in Schizotypal Personality Disorder	Include symptoms such as magical thinking, unusual perceptual disturbances, and odd speech or behavior, in addition to paranoid ideation.
Aloof behavior toward others in Schizoid Personality Disorder	Is not characterized by concerns about the untrustworthiness of others but rather by a fundamental lack of interest in having relationships.
Stress-related paranoid ideation in Borderline Personality Disorder	Is characterized by transient paranoid ideation that develops most often in response to real or imagined abandonment.
Reluctance to confide in others in Avoidant Personality Disorder	Is due to a fear of being embarrassed or found inadequate rather than due to having mistrust and suspiciousness.
Suspiciousness or alienation in Narcissistic Personality Disorder	Is characterized by fears of having imperfections or flaws revealed.

3.17.2 Differential Diagnosis for Schizoid Personality Disorder

Schizoid Personality Disorder, which is characterized by a pervasive pattern of detachment from social relationships and a restricted range of expression of emotions in interpersonal settings, must be differentiated from…	In contrast to Schizoid Personality Disorder…
Schizophrenia	May be characterized by negative symptoms that may resemble those in Schizoid Personality Disorder (e.g., diminished emotional expression, asociality, anhedonia), as well as positive symptoms such as delusions, hallucinations, or disorganized speech. To give an additional diagnosis of Schizoid Personality Disorder, the personality disorder must have been present before the onset of Schizophrenia symptoms and must persist when the symptoms are in remission.
Autism Spectrum Disorder	Is characterized by deficits in the ability to develop social relationships that are similar to the detachment from social relationships in Schizoid Personality Disorder, but also requires restricted, repetitive patterns of behaviors, interests, or activities.
Personality Change Due to Another Medical Condition, Apathetic Type	Is characterized by a change in personality related to the direct physiological effects of a nonpsychiatric medical condition.
Schizotypal Personality Disorder	Is characterized by cognitive and perceptual disturbances (e.g., ideas of reference, odd beliefs, bodily illusions, paranoid ideation) in addition to the social isolation.
Avoidant Personality Disorder	Is characterized by an active desire for relationships that is constrained by a fear of embarrassment or rejection, as opposed to the lack of desire for relationships in Schizoid Personality Disorder.
Obsessive-Compulsive Personality Disorder	May be characterized by social detachment related to devotion to work and discomfort with emotions, as opposed to a lack of capacity to form intimate relationships in Schizoid Personality Disorder.

3.17.3 Differential Diagnosis for Schizotypal Personality Disorder

Schizotypal Personality Disorder, which is characterized by a pervasive pattern of social and interpersonal deficits marked by acute discomfort with, and reduced capacity for, close relationships as well as by cognitive or perceptual distortions and eccentricities of behavior, must be differentiated from…	In contrast to Schizotypal Personality Disorder…
Delusional Disorder; Schizophrenia; Bipolar I or Bipolar II Disorder, With Psychotic Features; or Major Depressive Disorder, With Psychotic Features	Is characterized by periods of psychotic symptoms, in contrast to the subthreshold psychotic-like symptoms (ideas of reference, odd beliefs or magical thinking, unusual perceptual experiences, odd thinking and speech, suspiciousness or paranoid ideation) characteristic of Schizotypal Personality Disorder. To give an additional diagnosis of Schizotypal Personality Disorder, the personality disorder must have been present before the onset of psychotic symptoms and must persist when the psychotic symptoms are in remission.
Autism Spectrum Disorder	Is characterized by deficits in the ability to develop social relationships, which may result in a lack of close friends or confidants, a feature of Schizotypal Personality Disorder. However, Autism Spectrum Disorder also requires the presence of restricted, repetitive patterns of behaviors, interests, or activities, which are not characteristic of Schizotypal Personality Disorder.
Personality Change Due to Another Medical Condition, Paranoid Type	Is characterized by the development of paranoia and suspiciousness related to the direct physiological effects of a nonpsychiatric medical condition.
Paranoid Personality Disorder	Is characterized by paranoid ideation and suspiciousness but lacks the other features of Schizotypal Personality Disorder (e.g., perceptual distortions; eccentricities of behavior and appearance; vague, circumstantial, metaphorical, or overelaborate thinking and speech).

3.17.3 Differential Diagnosis for Schizotypal Personality Disorder *(continued)*

Schizoid Personality Disorder	Is characterized by detachment from social relationships and a restricted range of expression of emotions but lacks the other features of Schizotypal Personality Disorder (e.g., perceptual distortions; eccentricities of behavior and appearance; vague, circumstantial, metaphorical, or overelaborate thinking and speech).
Avoidant Personality Disorder	Is also characterized by a lack of close friends or confidants, but unlike Schizotypal Personality Disorder (in which there is a decreased desire for intimate contacts and persistent detachment), an active desire for relationships is constrained by a fear of embarrassment or rejection.
Suspiciousness, social withdrawal, or alienation in Narcissistic Personality Disorder	Is derived from fears of having imperfections revealed.
Transient psychotic symptoms in Borderline Personality Disorder	When these occur, they are usually closely related to shifts in affect in response to stress (e.g., intense anger, anxiety, disappointment) and are usually more dissociative (e.g., derealization, depersonalization) then those in Schizotypal Personality Disorder. In contrast, individuals with Schizotypal Personality Disorder have enduring psychotic-like symptoms that may worsen under stress and are not associated with shifts in affect.
Transient schizotypal traits in adolescents	Reflect transient emotional turmoil rather than an enduring personality disorder.

3.17.4 Differential Diagnosis for Antisocial Personality Disorder

Antisocial Personality Disorder, which is characterized by a pervasive pattern of disregard for and violation of the rights of others occurring since age 15 years, must be differentiated from…	In contrast to Antisocial Personality Disorder…
Antisocial behavior in the context of substance use	Is exclusively related to drug taking (e.g., stealing, prostitution) and is not part of an overall pattern of antisocial behavior that began in childhood.
Antisocial behavior occurring in a Manic Episode	Is a consequence of the impulsivity and poor judgment characteristic of a Manic Episode (i.e., the behavior is not associated with preexisting Conduct Disorder). Antisocial Personality Disorder should not be diagnosed if the antisocial behavior occurs exclusively during the course of a Manic Episode.
Conduct Disorder	Can be diagnosed at any age and is characterized by a repetitive and persistent pattern of behavior in which the basic rights of others or major age-appropriate societal norms or rules are violated. In contrast, the diagnosis of Antisocial Personality Disorder is not given to individuals under age 18 years and is given only if there is a history of some symptoms of Conduct Disorder before age 15 years. For individuals over age 18 years, a diagnosis of Conduct Disorder is given only if the criteria for Antisocial Personality Disorder are not met.
Glibness, exploitativeness, or lack of empathy in Narcissistic Personality Disorder	Is not accompanied by symptoms such as impulsivity and aggressiveness, and there is no history of Conduct Disorder before age 15.
Superficial emotionality in Histrionic Personality Disorder	Is not accompanied by symptoms such as deceitfulness, reckless disregard for the safety of self, and lack of remorse, and there is no history of Conduct Disorder before age 15.

3.17.4 Differential Diagnosis for Antisocial Personality Disorder *(continued)*

Manipulative behavior in Borderline Personality Disorder	Is not accompanied by symptoms such as criminality, reckless disregard for the safety of self, and lack of remorse, and there is no history of Conduct Disorder before age 15.
Antisocial behavior in Paranoid Personality Disorder	Is motivated by revenge against others who are perceived to have insulted, injured, or slighted the individual, rather than by desire for gain.
Criminal behavior not associated with a mental disorder	Is undertaken for gain and is not part of a persistent pattern of disregard for and violation of the rights of others, and there is no history of Conduct Disorder before age 15.

3.17.5 Differential Diagnosis for Borderline Personality Disorder

Borderline Personality Disorder, which is characterized by a pervasive pattern of instability of interpersonal relationships, self-image, and affects, as well as marked impulsivity, must be differentiated from…	In contrast to Borderline Personality Disorder…
Histrionic Personality Disorder	May also be characterized by attention seeking, manipulative behavior, and rapidly shifting emotions, but not by self-destructiveness, angry disruptions in close relationships, and chronic feelings of deep emptiness and loneliness.
Schizotypal Personality Disorder	May be characterized by paranoid ideation that is less interpersonally reactive and less amenable to the provision of external structure and support than in Borderline Personality Disorder.
Paranoid ideation or angry reactions to minor stimuli in Paranoid Personality Disorder or Narcissistic Personality Disorder	Occur in the context of relative stability of self-image and relative lack of impulsivity, and abandonment concerns.
Manipulative behavior in Antisocial Personality Disorder	Is motivated by a desire for power, profit, or material gain rather than a desire for nurturance.
Abandonment concerns in Dependent Personality Disorder	Are characterized by a reaction to the threat of abandonment with increasing appeasement and submission and attempts to seek a replacement relationship to provide caregiving and support.
Personality Change Due to Another Medical Condition, Labile Type	Is characterized by a change in personality related to the direct physiological effects of a nonpsychiatric medical condition.

3.17.6 Differential Diagnosis for Histrionic Personality Disorder

Histrionic Personality Disorder, which is characterized by a pervasive pattern of excessive emotionality and attention seeking, must be differentiated from...	In contrast to Histrionic Personality Disorder...
Borderline Personality Disorder	Is characterized by self-destructiveness, angry disruptions in close relationships, and identity disturbance.
Manipulative behavior in Antisocial Personality Disorder	Is motivated by a desire for profit, power, or material gain rather than a desire for attention and approval.
Attention seeking in Narcissistic Personality Disorder	Is characterized by a need for praise for being superior, as opposed to a need to be the center of attention.
Dependent Personality Disorder	Is characterized by excessive dependence on others for praise and guidance without the flamboyant emotions characteristic of Histrionic Personality Disorder.
Personality Change Due to Another Medical Condition, Disinhibited Type	Is characterized by a change in personality related to the direct physiological effects of a nonpsychiatric medical condition.

3.17.7 Differential Diagnosis for Narcissistic Personality Disorder

Narcissistic Personality Disorder, which is characterized by a pervasive pattern of grandiosity (in fantasy or behavior), need for admiration, and lack of empathy, must be differentiated from…	In contrast to Narcissistic Personality Disorder…
Need for attention in Histrionic Personality Disorder	Is related to a need for approval, as opposed to a need for admiration.
Lack of empathy in Antisocial Personality Disorder	Is characterized by impulsivity, aggression, and deceit, and is less characterized by a need for admiration by others.
Need for attention in Borderline Personality Disorder	Is characterized by instability in self-image, impulsivity, and abandonment concerns.
Perfectionism in Obsessive-Compulsive Personality Disorder	Is characterized by striving to attain perfection and a belief that others cannot do things as well, as opposed to a belief that perfection has already been achieved.
Suspiciousness and social withdrawal in Schizotypal Personality Disorder and Paranoid Personality Disorder	Are related to paranoid ideation, as opposed to fears that imperfections or flaws will be revealed.
Grandiosity in Manic or Hypomanic Episodes	Occurs only during episodes of elevated or irritable mood.
Personality Change Due to Another Medical Condition, Labile Type	Is characterized by a change in personality related to the direct physiological effects of a nonpsychiatric medical condition.

3.17.8 Differential Diagnosis for Avoidant Personality Disorder

Avoidant Personality Disorder, which is characterized by a pervasive pattern of social inhibition, feelings of inadequacy, and hypersensitivity to negative evaluation, must be differentiated from…	In contrast to Avoidant Personality Disorder…
Avoidance in Agoraphobia	Is characterized by avoiding situations where escape might be difficult or help might not be available in the event of developing panic-like symptoms or other incapacitating or embarrassing symptoms, as opposed to a more generalized pattern of avoidance.
Feelings of inadequacy, hypersensitivity to criticism, and need for reassurance in Dependent Personality Disorder	Are characterized by concerns about being taken care of, as opposed to avoidance of humiliation or rejection.
Social isolation in Schizoid Personality Disorder and Schizotypal Personality Disorder	Is characterized by contentment with (or even a preference for) the social isolation.
Reluctance to confide in others in Paranoid Personality Disorder	Is motivated by fears that personal information will be used with malicious intent, as opposed to fears of being embarrassed.
Personality Change Due to Another Medical Condition	Is characterized by a change in personality related to the direct physiological effects of a nonpsychiatric medical condition.

3.17.9 Differential Diagnosis for Dependent Personality Disorder

Dependent Personality Disorder, which is characterized by a pervasive and excessive need to be taken care of that leads to submissive and clinging behavior and fears of separation, must be differentiated from…	In contrast to Dependent Personality Disorder…
Separation Anxiety Disorder	Is characterized by a persistent and excessive fear or anxiety concerning being physically separated from major attachment figures. In Dependent Personality Disorder, the focus of concern is specifically on the need to be taken care of, rather than separated per se. If criteria are met for both disorders, both can be diagnosed.
Dependency arising as a consequence of another mental disorder or a nonpsychiatric medical condition	Emanates from the impairment related to the mental disorder or nonpsychiatric medical condition and the consequent need to rely on others.
Fear of abandonment in Borderline Personality Disorder	Is characterized by a reaction to anticipated abandonment with feelings of emotional emptiness, rage, and demands, as opposed to the individual's fears of being unable to take care of themself in Dependent Personality Disorder.
Need for reassurance and approval in Histrionic Personality Disorder	Is characterized by gregarious flamboyance with active demands for attention, as opposed to an extreme need to be taken care of.
Avoidant Personality Disorder	Is characterized by such a strong fear of humiliation and rejection that there is social withdrawal until the person is certain of being accepted.
Personality Change Due to Another Medical Condition	Is characterized by a change in personality related to the direct physiological effects of a nonpsychiatric medical condition.

3.17.10 Differential Diagnosis for Obsessive-Compulsive Personality Disorder

Obsessive-Compulsive Personality Disorder, which is characterized by a pervasive pattern of preoccupation with orderliness, perfectionism, and mental and interpersonal control, at the expense of flexibility, openness, and efficiency, must be differentiated from…	In contrast to Obsessive-Compulsive Personality Disorder…
Obsessive-Compulsive Disorder	Is characterized by the presence of true obsessions and/or compulsions, as described in Criterion A. About 20% of individuals with Obsessive-Compulsive Disorder also have Obsessive-Compulsive Personality Disorder. If criteria are met for both, both should be diagnosed.
Hoarding Disorder	Is characterized by persistent difficulty discarding or parting with possessions regardless of their actual value, which is only one of the criteria for Obsessive-Compulsive Personality Disorder. In Hoarding Disorder, in contrast to Obsessive-Compulsive Personality Disorder, this symptom predominates in the clinical picture and results in the accumulation of possessions that clutter active living areas and substantially compromise their intended use. If criteria are met for both conditions, both can be diagnosed.
Perfectionism in Narcissistic Personality Disorder	Is characterized by a belief that perfection has already been achieved, as opposed to striving for perfectionism.
Lack of generosity in Antisocial Personality Disorder	Is characterized by an indulgence of self, as opposed to a miserly spending style toward both self and others.
Social detachment in Schizoid Personality Disorder	Occurs in the context of a lack of capacity for intimacy, as opposed to discomfort with emotion and excessive devotion to work.
Personality Change Due to Another Medical Condition	Is characterized by a change in personality related to the direct physiological effects of a nonpsychiatric medical condition.

3.17.11 Differential Diagnosis for Personality Change Due to Another Medical Condition

Personality Change Due to Another Medical Condition, which is characterized by persistent personality disturbance due to the direct physiological effects of a nonpsychiatric medical condition that represents a change from the individual's characteristic personality pattern, must be differentiated from…	In contrast to Personality Change Due to Another Medical Condition…
Personality change in Major or Mild Neurocognitive Disorder Due to Another Medical Condition	Is accompanied by cognitive decline in one or more cognitive domains (complex attention, executive function, learning and memory, language, perceptual-motor, or social cognition). Personality Change Due to Another Medical Condition may be diagnosed in addition to the Major or Mild Neurocognitive Disorder if the personality disturbance is a prominent feature of the presentation.
Personality change associated with another Mental Disorder Due to Another Medical Condition (e.g., disinhibited behavior in Bipolar and Related Disorder Due to Another Medical Condition)	Includes additional prominent psychiatric symptoms due to the direct physiological effects of a nonpsychiatric medical condition (e.g., irritable mood). Personality Change Due to Another Medical Condition is not diagnosed if the disturbance is better accounted for by the other Mental Disorder Due to Another Medical Condition.
Personality change as a result of a Substance Use Disorder (e.g., emotional lability)	Is not due to the direct physiological effects of a nonpsychiatric medical condition and abates when the Substance Use Disorder is in remission.
Personality change associated with another mental disorder (e.g., social withdrawal in Schizophrenia, persistent feelings of insecurity in Posttraumatic Stress Disorder)	Is not due to the direct physiological effects of a nonpsychiatric medical condition.
Personality Disorders	Have a different age at onset (i.e., by adolescence or early adulthood), course, and characteristic features and are not due to the direct physiological effects of a nonpsychiatric medical condition.

Paraphilic Disorders

3.18.1 Differential Diagnosis for Paraphilic Disorders

Paraphilic Disorders—characterized by the individual's intense and persistent sexual interest in any of the following or for which sexual urges or fantasies cause clinically significant distress or impairment: spying on others in private activities without their consent (Voyeuristic Disorder); exposing their own genitals to others without their consent (Exhibitionistic Disorder); touching or rubbing against a nonconsenting person (Frotteuristic Disorder); acting on sexual urges with a prepubescent child (Pedophilic Disorder); inflicting humiliation, bondage, or physical or psychological suffering on a nonconsenting person (Sexual Sadism Disorder); intense and persistent sexual arousal from undergoing humiliation, bondage, or suffering (Sexual Masochism Disorder); focusing on nonliving objects or a highly specific body part (Fetishistic Disorder); or cross-dressing (Transvestic Disorder)—must be differentiated from...	In contrast to a Paraphilic Disorder...
Nonpathological use of sexual fantasies, behaviors, or objects to enhance sexual arousal	Does not cause clinically significant distress or impairment, is typically not obligatory for sexual functioning, and involves only consenting partners.
Sexual behavior resulting from a decrease in judgment, social skills, or impulse control related to another mental disorder (e.g., Manic Episode, Major or Mild Neurocognitive Disorder, Schizophrenia)	Is typically not an individual's preferred or obligatory pattern, occurs exclusively during the course of the mental disorder, often has a later age at onset, and is accompanied by the characteristic features of the mental disorder (e.g., cognitive impairment, delusions).

3.18.1 Differential Diagnosis for Paraphilic Disorders *(continued)*

Spying on others engaged in private activities in Conduct Disorder or Antisocial Personality Disorder (as distinguished from Voyeuristic Disorder)	Is part of a pattern of disregard for, and violation of, the rights of others. Such behavior is differentiated from "peeping" in Voyeuristic Disorder by the lack of the specific sexual interest in and arousal from secretly watching unsuspecting others who are naked or engaging in sexual activity.
Opportunistic child molestation in Conduct Disorder or Antisocial Personality Disorder (as distinguished from Pedophilic Disorder)	Is part of a pattern of lack of empathy and disregard for the rights of others, which may include opportunistic child molestation. This is differentiated from Pedophilic Disorder, in which there is a persistent pattern of sexual arousal to children that is acted on or that causes marked distress or interpersonal difficulty.
Substance Intoxication	Is characterized by the individual's disinhibited behaviors that might involve committing certain sexual offenses (e.g., "peeping," exhibiting their genitals, rubbing against an unsuspecting person). This is differentiated from such behaviors occurring in the context of a Paraphilic Disorder by the absence of a persistent pattern of sexual interest in spying on nonconsenting others, exposing genitals to nonconsenting others, or rubbing against a nonconsenting person.
Medication side effect (e.g., dopamine agonist medication)	Is characterized by paraphilia-like sexual behavior that occurs as a side effect of a medication (particularly dopamine agonist medications used to treat Parkinson's disease) and is uncharacteristic of the individual's sexual behavior when not taking the medication.
Sexual thoughts or images in Obsessive-Compulsive Disorder (as distinguished from Pedophilic Disorder)	Are experienced as ego-dystonic and involve distressing worries about possibly being attracted to children. In contrast to Pedophilic Disorder, there is an absence of sexual thoughts about children during high states of sexual arousal (e.g., approaching orgasm during masturbation).

Appendix

DSM-5-TR Classification

Before each disorder name, ICD-10-CM codes are provided. Blank lines indicate that the ICD-10-CM code depends on the applicable subtype, specifier, or class of substance. For periodic DSM-5-TR coding and other updates, see www.dsm5.org.

Note for all mental disorders due to another medical condition: Insert the name of the etiological medical condition within the name of the mental disorder due to [the medical condition]. The code and name for the etiological medical condition should be listed first immediately before the mental disorder due to the medical condition.

Neurodevelopmental Disorders

Intellectual Developmental Disorders

___.__   Intellectual Developmental Disorder (Intellectual Disability)
        Specify current severity:

F70   Mild

F71   Moderate

F72   Severe

F73   Profound

F88   Global Developmental Delay

F79   Unspecified Intellectual Developmental Disorder (Intellectual Disability)

Communication Disorders

F80.2   Language Disorder

F80.0   Speech Sound Disorder

F80.81   Childhood-Onset Fluency Disorder (Stuttering)
        Note: Later-onset cases are diagnosed as F98.5 adult-onset fluency disorder.

F80.82   Social (Pragmatic) Communication Disorder

F80.9   Unspecified Communication Disorder

Autism Spectrum Disorder

F84.0   Autism Spectrum Disorder

Specify current severity: Requiring very substantial support, Requiring substantial support, Requiring support

Specify if: With or without accompanying intellectual impairment, With or without accompanying language impairment

Specify if: Associated with a known genetic or other medical condition or environmental factor (**Coding note:** Use additional code to identify the associated genetic or other medical condition); Associated with a neurodevelopmental, mental, or behavioral problem

Specify if: With catatonia (use additional code F06.1)

Attention-Deficit/Hyperactivity Disorder

___.__   Attention-Deficit/Hyperactivity Disorder

Specify if: In partial remission

Specify current severity: Mild, Moderate, Severe

Specify whether:

F90.2   Combined presentation

F90.0   Predominantly inattentive presentation

F90.1   Predominantly hyperactive/impulsive presentation

F90.8   Other Specified Attention-Deficit/Hyperactivity Disorder

F90.9   Unspecified Attention-Deficit/Hyperactivity Disorder

Specific Learning Disorder

___.__   Specific Learning Disorder

Specify current severity: Mild, Moderate, Severe

Specify if:

F81.0   With impairment in reading (specify if with word reading accuracy, reading rate or fluency, reading comprehension)

F81.81   With impairment in written expression (specify if with spelling accuracy, grammar and punctuation accuracy, clarity or organization of written expression)

F81.2   With impairment in mathematics (specify if with number sense, memorization of arithmetic facts, accurate or fluent calculation, accurate math reasoning)

Motor Disorders

F82   Developmental Coordination Disorder

F98.4   Stereotypic Movement Disorder

Specify if: With self-injurious behavior, Without self-injurious behavior

Specify if: Associated with a known genetic or other medical condition, neurodevelopmental disorder, or environmental factor

Specify current severity: Mild, Moderate, Severe

Tic Disorders

F95.2   Tourette's Disorder

F95.1   Persistent (Chronic) Motor or Vocal Tic Disorder
Specify if: With motor tics only, With vocal tics only

F95.0   Provisional Tic Disorder

F95.8   Other Specified Tic Disorder

F95.9   Unspecified Tic Disorder

Other Neurodevelopmental Disorders

F88   Other Specified Neurodevelopmental Disorder

F89   Unspecified Neurodevelopmental Disorder

Schizophrenia Spectrum and Other Psychotic Disorders

The following specifiers apply to Schizophrenia Spectrum and Other Psychotic Disorders where indicated:

[a]*Specify* if: The following course specifiers are only to be used after a 1-year duration of the disorder: First episode, currently in acute episode; First episode, currently in partial remission; First episode, currently in full remission; Multiple episodes, currently in acute episode; Multiple episodes, currently in partial remission; Multiple episodes, currently in full remission; Continuous; Unspecified

[b]*Specify* if: With catatonia (use additional code F06.1)

[c]*Specify* current severity of delusions, hallucinations, disorganized speech, abnormal psychomotor behavior, negative symptoms, impaired cognition, depression, and mania symptoms

F21   Schizotypal (Personality) Disorder

F22   Delusional Disorder[a,c]
Specify whether: Erotomanic type, Grandiose type, Jealous type, Persecutory type, Somatic type, Mixed type, Unspecified type
Specify if: With bizarre content

F23   Brief Psychotic Disorder[b,c]
Specify if: With marked stressor(s), Without marked stressor(s), With peripartum onset

F20.81   Schizophreniform Disorder[b,c]
Specify if: With good prognostic features, Without good prognostic features

F20.9   Schizophrenia[a,b,c]

___.___   Schizoaffective Disorder[a,b,c]
Specify whether:

F25.0   Bipolar type

F25.1   Depressive type

___.___   Substance/Medication-Induced Psychotic Disorder[c]
Note: For applicable ICD-10-CM codes, refer to the substance classes under Substance-Related and Addictive Disorders for the specific substance/medication-induced

psychotic disorder. See also the criteria set and corresponding recording procedures in the manual for more information.

Coding note: The ICD-10-CM code depends on whether or not there is a comorbid substance use disorder present for the same class of substance. In any case, an additional separate diagnosis of a substance use disorder is not given.

Specify if: With onset during intoxication, With onset during withdrawal, With onset after medication use

___.___   Psychotic Disorder Due to Another Medical Condition[c]
              Specify whether:

F06.2   With delusions

F06.0   With hallucinations

F06.1   Catatonia Associated With Another Mental Disorder (Catatonia Specifier)

F06.1   Catatonic Disorder Due to Another Medical Condition

F06.1   Unspecified Catatonia
         Note: Code first **R29.818** other symptoms involving nervous and musculoskeletal systems.

F28   Other Specified Schizophrenia Spectrum and Other Psychotic Disorder

F29   Unspecified Schizophrenia Spectrum and Other Psychotic Disorder

Bipolar and Related Disorders

The following specifiers apply to Bipolar and Related Disorders where indicated:

[a]*Specify:* With anxious distress (*specify* current severity: mild, moderate, moderate-severe, severe); With mixed features; With rapid cycling; With melancholic features; With atypical features; With mood-congruent psychotic features; With mood-incongruent psychotic features; With catatonia (use additional code F06.1); With peripartum onset; With seasonal pattern

[b]*Specify:* With anxious distress (*specify* current severity: mild, moderate, moderate-severe, severe); With mixed features; With rapid cycling; With peripartum onset; With seasonal pattern

___.___   Bipolar I Disorder[a]

___.___   Current or most recent episode manic

F31.11   Mild

F31.12   Moderate

F31.13   Severe

F31.2   With psychotic features

F31.73   In partial remission

F31.74   In full remission

F31.9   Unspecified

F31.0   Current or most recent episode hypomanic

F31.71   In partial remission

F31.72   In full remission

F31.9   Unspecified

___.___   Current or most recent episode depressed

F31.31   Mild

F31.32   Moderate

F31.4   Severe

F31.5	With psychotic features
F31.75	In partial remission
F31.76	In full remission
F31.9	Unspecified
F31.9	Current or most recent episode unspecified

F31.81 Bipolar II Disorder
Specify current or most recent episode: Hypomanic[b], Depressed[a]
Specify course if full criteria for a mood episode are not currently met: In partial remission, In full remission
Specify severity if full criteria for a major depressive episode are currently met: Mild, Moderate, Severe

F34.0 Cyclothymic Disorder
Specify if: With anxious distress (*specify* current severity: mild, moderate, moderate-severe, severe)

___.__ Substance/Medication-Induced Bipolar and Related Disorder
Note: For applicable ICD-10-CM codes, refer to the substance classes under Substance-Related and Addictive Disorders for the specific substance/medication-induced bipolar and related disorder. See also the criteria set and corresponding recording procedures in the manual for more information.
Coding note: The ICD-10-CM code depends on whether or not there is a comorbid substance use disorder present for the same class of substance. In any case, an additional separate diagnosis of a substance use disorder is not given.
Specify if: With onset during intoxication, With onset during withdrawal, With onset after medication use

___.__ Bipolar and Related Disorder Due to Another Medical Condition
Specify if:

F06.33	With manic features
F06.33	With manic- or hypomanic-like episode
F06.34	With mixed features

F31.89 Other Specified Bipolar and Related Disorder

F31.9 Unspecified Bipolar and Related Disorder

F39 Unspecified Mood Disorder

Depressive Disorders

F34.81 Disruptive Mood Dysregulation Disorder

___.__ Major Depressive Disorder
Specify: With anxious distress (*specify* current severity: mild, moderate, moderate-severe, severe); With mixed features; With melancholic features; With atypical features; With mood-congruent psychotic features; With mood-incongruent psychotic features; With catatonia (use additional code F06.1); With peripartum onset; With seasonal pattern

___.__	Single episode
F32.0	Mild
F32.1	Moderate
F32.2	Severe
F32.3	With psychotic features

F32.4	In partial remission
F32.5	In full remission
F32.9	Unspecified
___.__	Recurrent episode
F33.0	Mild
F33.1	Moderate
F33.2	Severe
F33.3	With psychotic features
F33.41	In partial remission
F33.42	In full remission
F33.9	Unspecified

F34.1   Persistent Depressive Disorder

Specify: With anxious distress (*specify* current severity: mild, moderate, moderate-severe, severe); With atypical features

Specify if: In partial remission, In full remission

Specify if: Early onset, Late onset

Specify if: With pure dysthymic syndrome; With persistent major depressive episode; With intermittent major depressive episodes, with current episode; With intermittent major depressive episodes, without current episode

Specify current severity: Mild, Moderate, Severe

F32.81   Premenstrual Dysphoric Disorder

___.__   Substance/Medication-Induced Depressive Disorder

Note: For applicable ICD-10-CM codes, refer to the substance classes under Substance-Related and Addictive Disorders for the specific substance/medication-induced depressive disorder. See also the criteria set and corresponding recording procedures in the manual for more information.

Coding note: The ICD-10-CM code depends on whether or not there is a comorbid substance use disorder present for the same class of substance. In any case, an additional separate diagnosis of a substance use disorder is not given.

Specify if: With onset during intoxication, With onset during withdrawal, With onset after medication use

___.__   Depressive Disorder Due to Another Medical Condition

Specify if:

F06.31	With depressive features
F06.32	With major depressive–like episode
F06.34	With mixed features

F32.89   Other Specified Depressive Disorder

F32.A   Unspecified Depressive Disorder

F39   Unspecified Mood Disorder

Anxiety Disorders

F93.0	Separation Anxiety Disorder
F94.0	Selective Mutism

___.__	Specific Phobia
	Specify if:
F40.218	Animal
F40.228	Natural environment
___.__	Blood-injection-injury
F40.230	Fear of blood
F40.231	Fear of injections and transfusions
F40.232	Fear of other medical care
F40.233	Fear of injury
F40.248	Situational
F40.298	Other
F40.10	Social Anxiety Disorder
	Specify if: Performance only
F41.0	Panic Disorder
___.__	Panic Attack Specifier
F40.00	Agoraphobia
F41.1	Generalized Anxiety Disorder
___.__	Substance/Medication-Induced Anxiety Disorder

Note: For applicable ICD-10-CM codes, refer to the substance classes under Substance-Related and Addictive Disorders for the specific substance/medication-induced anxiety disorder. See also the criteria set and corresponding recording procedures in the manual for more information.

Coding note: The ICD-10-CM code depends on whether or not there is a comorbid substance use disorder present for the same class of substance. In any case, an additional separate diagnosis of a substance use disorder is not given.

Specify if: With onset during intoxication, With onset during withdrawal, With onset after medication use

F06.4	Anxiety Disorder Due to Another Medical Condition
F41.8	Other Specified Anxiety Disorder
F41.9	Unspecified Anxiety Disorder

Obsessive-Compulsive and Related Disorders

The following specifier applies to Obsessive-Compulsive and Related Disorders where indicated:
[a]*Specify* if: With good or fair insight, With poor insight, With absent insight/delusional beliefs

F42.2	Obsessive-Compulsive Disorder[a]
	Specify if: Tic-related
F45.22	Body Dysmorphic Disorder[a]
	Specify if: With muscle dysmorphia
F42.3	Hoarding Disorder[a]
	Specify if: With excessive acquisition
F63.3	Trichotillomania (Hair-Pulling Disorder)
F42.4	Excoriation (Skin-Picking) Disorder

___.__   Substance/Medication-Induced Obsessive-Compulsive and Related
               Disorder
               Note: For applicable ICD-10-CM codes, refer to the substance classes under Substance-
               Related and Addictive Disorders for the specific substance/medication-induced
               obsessive-compulsive and related disorder. See also the criteria set and correspond-
               ing recording procedures in the manual for more information.
               Coding note: The ICD-10-CM code depends on whether or not there is a comorbid
               substance use disorder present for the same class of substance. In any case, an ad-
               ditional separate diagnosis of a substance use disorder is not given.
               Specify if: With onset during intoxication, With onset during withdrawal, With onset
               after medication use

F06.8   Obsessive-Compulsive and Related Disorder Due to Another Medical
               Condition
               Specify if: With obsessive-compulsive disorder–like symptoms, With appearance pre-
               occupations, With hoarding symptoms, With hair-pulling symptoms, With skin-
               picking symptoms

F42.8   Other Specified Obsessive-Compulsive and Related Disorder

F42.9   Unspecified Obsessive-Compulsive and Related Disorder

---

Trauma- and Stressor-Related Disorders

F94.1   Reactive Attachment Disorder
               Specify if: Persistent
               Specify current severity: Severe

F94.2   Disinhibited Social Engagement Disorder
               Specify if: Persistent
               Specify current severity: Severe

F43.10   Posttraumatic Stress Disorder
               Specify whether: With dissociative symptoms
               Specify if: With delayed expression
___.__   Posttraumatic Stress Disorder in Individuals Older Than 6 Years
___.__   Posttraumatic Stress Disorder in Children 6 Years and Younger

F43.0   Acute Stress Disorder

___.__   Adjustment Disorders
               Specify if: Acute, Persistent (chronic)
               Specify whether:
F43.21   With depressed mood
F43.22   With anxiety
F43.23   With mixed anxiety and depressed mood
F43.24   With disturbance of conduct
F43.25   With mixed disturbance of emotions and conduct
F43.20   Unspecified

F43.81   Prolonged Grief Disorder

F43.89   Other Specified Trauma- and Stressor-Related Disorder

F43.9   Unspecified Trauma- and Stressor-Related Disorder

Dissociative Disorders

F44.81 Dissociative Identity Disorder

F44.0 Dissociative Amnesia
Specify if:
F44.1   With dissociative fugue

F48.1 Depersonalization/Derealization Disorder

F44.89 Other Specified Dissociative Disorder

F44.9 Unspecified Dissociative Disorder

Somatic Symptom and Related Disorders

F45.1 Somatic Symptom Disorder
Specify if: With predominant pain
Specify if: Persistent
Specify current severity: Mild, Moderate, Severe

F45.21 Illness Anxiety Disorder
Specify whether: Care-seeking type, Care-avoidant type

___.__ Functional Neurological Symptom Disorder (Conversion Disorder)
Specify if: Acute episode, Persistent
Specify if: With psychological stressor (specify stressor), Without psychological stressor
Specify symptom type:
F44.4   With weakness or paralysis
F44.4   With abnormal movement
F44.4   With swallowing symptoms
F44.4   With speech symptom
F44.5   With attacks or seizures
F44.6   With anesthesia or sensory loss
F44.6   With special sensory symptom
F44.7   With mixed symptoms

F54 Psychological Factors Affecting Other Medical Conditions
Specify current severity: Mild, Moderate, Severe, Extreme

___.__ Factitious Disorder
Specify: Single episode, Recurrent episodes
F68.10   Factitious Disorder Imposed on Self
F68.A   Factitious Disorder Imposed on Another

F45.8 Other Specified Somatic Symptom and Related Disorder

F45.9 Unspecified Somatic Symptom and Related Disorder

Feeding and Eating Disorders

The following specifiers apply to Feeding and Eating Disorders where indicated:
[a]*Specify* if: In remission
[b]*Specify* if: In partial remission, In full remission
[c]*Specify* current severity: Mild, Moderate, Severe, Extreme

___.__	Pica[a]
F98.3	In children
F50.89	In adults
F98.21	Rumination Disorder[a]
F50.82	Avoidant/Restrictive Food Intake Disorder[a]
___.__	Anorexia Nervosa[b,c]
	Specify whether:
F50.01	Restricting type
F50.02	Binge-eating/purging type
F50.2	Bulimia Nervosa[b,c]
F50.81	Binge-Eating Disorder[b,c]
F50.89	Other Specified Feeding or Eating Disorder
F50.9	Unspecified Feeding or Eating Disorder

Elimination Disorders

F98.0	Enuresis
	Specify whether: Nocturnal only, Diurnal only, Nocturnal and diurnal
F98.1	Encopresis
	Specify whether: With constipation and overflow incontinence, Without constipation and overflow incontinence
___.__	Other Specified Elimination Disorder
N39.498	With urinary symptoms
R15.9	With fecal symptoms
___.__	Unspecified Elimination Disorder
R32	With urinary symptoms
R15.9	With fecal symptoms

Sleep-Wake Disorders

The following specifiers apply to Sleep-Wake Disorders where indicated:
[a]*Specify* if: Episodic, Persistent, Recurrent
[b]*Specify* if: Acute, Subacute, Persistent
[c]*Specify* current severity: Mild, Moderate, Severe

F51.01	Insomnia Disorder[a]
	Specify if: With mental disorder, With medical condition, With another sleep disorder

F51.11	Hypersomnolence Disorder[b,c]
	Specify if: With mental disorder, With medical condition, With another sleep disorder
__.__	Narcolepsy[c]
	Specify whether:
G47.411	Narcolepsy with cataplexy or hypocretin deficiency (type 1)
G47.419	Narcolepsy without cataplexy and either without hypocretin deficiency or hypocretin unmeasured (type 2)
G47.421	Narcolepsy with cataplexy or hypocretin deficiency due to a medical condition
G47.429	Narcolepsy without cataplexy and without hypocretin deficiency due to a medical condition

Breathing-Related Sleep Disorders

G47.33	Obstructive Sleep Apnea Hypopnea[c]
__.__	Central Sleep Apnea
	Specify current severity
	Specify whether:
G47.31	Idiopathic central sleep apnea
R06.3	Cheyne-Stokes breathing
G47.37	Central sleep apnea comorbid with opioid use
	Note: First code opioid use disorder, if present.
__.__	Sleep-Related Hypoventilation
	Specify current severity
	Specify whether:
G47.34	Idiopathic hypoventilation
G47.35	Congenital central alveolar hypoventilation
G47.36	Comorbid sleep-related hypoventilation

__.__	Circadian Rhythm Sleep-Wake Disorders[a]
	Specify whether:
G47.21	Delayed sleep phase type
	Specify if: Familial, Overlapping with non-24-hour sleep-wake type
G47.22	Advanced sleep phase type
	Specify if: Familial
G47.23	Irregular sleep-wake type
G47.24	Non-24-hour sleep-wake type
G47.26	Shift work type
G47.20	Unspecified type

Parasomnias

__.__	Non–Rapid Eye Movement Sleep Arousal Disorders
	Specify whether:
F51.3	Sleepwalking type
	Specify if: With sleep-related eating, With sleep-related sexual behavior (sexsomnia)
F51.4	Sleep terror type

F51.5   Nightmare Disorder[b,c]
              Specify if: During sleep onset
              Specify if: With mental disorder, With medical condition, With another sleep
                disorder

G47.52   Rapid Eye Movement Sleep Behavior Disorder

G25.81   Restless Legs Syndrome

___.__   Substance/Medication-Induced Sleep Disorder
              Note: For applicable ICD-10-CM codes, refer to the substance classes under Substance-
                Related and Addictive Disorders for the specific substance/medication-induced
                sleep disorder. See also the criteria set and corresponding recording procedures in
                the manual for more information.
              Coding note: The ICD-10-CM code depends on whether or not there is a comorbid
                substance use disorder present for the same class of substance. In any case, an ad-
                ditional separate diagnosis of a substance use disorder is not given.
              Specify whether: Insomnia type, Daytime sleepiness type, Parasomnia type, Mixed
                type
              Specify if: With onset during intoxication, With onset during withdrawal, With onset
                after medication use

G47.09   Other Specified Insomnia Disorder

G47.00   Unspecified Insomnia Disorder

G47.19   Other Specified Hypersomnolence Disorder

G47.10   Unspecified Hypersomnolence Disorder

G47.8   Other Specified Sleep-Wake Disorder

G47.9   Unspecified Sleep-Wake Disorder

Sexual Dysfunctions

The following specifiers apply to Sexual Dysfunctions where indicated:
[a]*Specify* whether: Lifelong, Acquired
[b]*Specify* whether: Generalized, Situational
[c]*Specify* current severity: Mild, Moderate, Severe

F52.32   Delayed Ejaculation[a,b,c]

F52.21   Erectile Disorder[a,b,c]

F52.31   Female Orgasmic Disorder[a,b,c]
              Specify if: Never experienced an orgasm under any situation

F52.22   Female Sexual Interest/Arousal Disorder[a,b,c]

F52.6   Genito-Pelvic Pain/Penetration Disorder[a,c]

F52.0   Male Hypoactive Sexual Desire Disorder[a,b,c]

F52.4   Premature (Early) Ejaculation[a,b,c]

___.__   Substance/Medication-Induced Sexual Dysfunction[c]
              Note: For applicable ICD-10-CM codes, refer to the substance classes under Substance-
                Related and Addictive Disorders for the specific substance/medication-induced

sexual dysfunction. See also the criteria set and corresponding recording procedures in the manual for more information.

Coding note: The ICD-10-CM code depends on whether or not there is a comorbid substance use disorder present for the same class of substance. In any case, an additional separate diagnosis of a substance use disorder is not given.

Specify if: With onset during intoxication, With onset during withdrawal, With onset after medication use

F52.8   Other Specified Sexual Dysfunction

F52.9   Unspecified Sexual Dysfunction

Gender Dysphoria

The following specifier and note apply to Gender Dysphoria where indicated:
[a]*Specify* if: With a disorder/difference of sex development
[b]**Note:** Code the disorder/difference of sex development if present, in addition to gender dysphoria.

__.__   Gender Dysphoria

F64.2   Gender Dysphoria in Children[a,b]

F64.0   Gender Dysphoria in Adolescents and Adults[a,b]
                Specify if: Posttransition

F64.8   Other Specified Gender Dysphoria

F64.9   Unspecified Gender Dysphoria

Disruptive, Impulse-Control, and Conduct Disorders

F91.3   Oppositional Defiant Disorder
            Specify current severity: Mild, Moderate, Severe

F63.81   Intermittent Explosive Disorder

__.__   Conduct Disorder
            Specify if: With limited prosocial emotions
            Specify current severity: Mild, Moderate, Severe
            Specify whether:

F91.1   Childhood-onset type

F91.2   Adolescent-onset type

F91.9   Unspecified onset

F60.2   Antisocial Personality Disorder

F63.1   Pyromania

F63.2   Kleptomania

F91.8   Other Specified Disruptive, Impulse-Control, and Conduct Disorder

F91.9   Unspecified Disruptive, Impulse-Control, and Conduct Disorder

Substance-Related and Addictive Disorders

Substance-Related Disorders

Alcohol-Related Disorders

___.__	Alcohol Use Disorder
	Specify if: In a controlled environment
	Specify current severity/remission:
F10.10	Mild
F10.11	In early remission
F10.11	In sustained remission
F10.20	Moderate
F10.21	In early remission
F10.21	In sustained remission
F10.20	Severe
F10.21	In early remission
F10.21	In sustained remission
___.__	Alcohol Intoxication
F10.120	With mild use disorder
F10.220	With moderate or severe use disorder
F10.920	Without use disorder
___.__	Alcohol Withdrawal
	Without perceptual disturbances
F10.130	With mild use disorder
F10.230	With moderate or severe use disorder
F10.930	Without use disorder
	With perceptual disturbances
F10.132	With mild use disorder
F10.232	With moderate or severe use disorder
F10.932	Without use disorder
___.__	Alcohol-Induced Mental Disorders

Note: Disorders are listed in their order of appearance in the manual.
[a]*Specify* With onset during intoxication, With onset during withdrawal
[b]*Specify* if: Acute, Persistent
[c]*Specify* if: Hyperactive, Hypoactive, Mixed level of activity

___.__	Alcohol-Induced Psychotic Disorder[a]
F10.159	With mild use disorder
F10.259	With moderate or severe use disorder
F10.959	Without use disorder
___.__	Alcohol-Induced Bipolar and Related Disorder[a]
F10.14	With mild use disorder
F10.24	With moderate or severe use disorder
F10.94	Without use disorder

__.__	Alcohol-Induced Depressive Disorder[a]
F10.14	With mild use disorder
F10.24	With moderate or severe use disorder
F10.94	Without use disorder
__.__	Alcohol-Induced Anxiety Disorder[a]
F10.180	With mild use disorder
F10.280	With moderate or severe use disorder
F10.980	Without use disorder
__.__	Alcohol-Induced Sleep Disorder[a]
	Specify whether Insomnia type
F10.182	With mild use disorder
F10.282	With moderate or severe use disorder
F10.982	Without use disorder
__.__	Alcohol-Induced Sexual Dysfunction[a]
	Specify if: Mild, Moderate, Severe
F10.181	With mild use disorder
F10.281	With moderate or severe use disorder
F10.981	Without use disorder
__.__	Alcohol Intoxication Delirium[b,c]
F10.121	With mild use disorder
F10.221	With moderate or severe use disorder
F10.921	Without use disorder
__.__	Alcohol Withdrawal Delirium[b,c]
F10.131	With mild use disorder
F10.231	With moderate or severe use disorder
F10.931	Without use disorder
__.__	Alcohol-Induced Major Neurocognitive Disorder
	Specify if: Persistent
__.__	Amnestic-confabulatory type
F10.26	With moderate or severe use disorder
F10.96	Without use disorder
__.__	Nonamnestic-confabulatory type
F10.27	With moderate or severe use disorder
F10.97	Without use disorder
__.__	Alcohol-Induced Mild Neurocognitive Disorder
	Specify if: Persistent
F10.188	With mild use disorder
F10.288	With moderate or severe use disorder
F10.988	Without use disorder
F10.99	Unspecified Alcohol-Related Disorder

Caffeine-Related Disorders

F15.920	Caffeine Intoxication
F15.93	Caffeine Withdrawal

___.___   Caffeine-Induced Mental Disorders

Note: Disorders are listed in their order of appearance in the manual.

Specify With onset during intoxication, With onset during withdrawal, With onset after medication use. **Note:** When taken over the counter, substances in this class can also induce the relevant substance-induced mental disorder.

F15.980   Caffeine-Induced Anxiety Disorder

F15.982   Caffeine-Induced Sleep Disorder

Specify whether Insomnia type, Daytime sleepiness type, Mixed type

F15.99   Unspecified Caffeine-Related Disorder

Cannabis-Related Disorders

___.___   Cannabis Use Disorder

Specify if: In a controlled environment
Specify current severity/remission:

F12.10   Mild
F12.11   In early remission
F12.11   In sustained remission

F12.20   Moderate
F12.21   In early remission
F12.21   In sustained remission

F12.20   Severe
F12.21   In early remission
F12.21   In sustained remission

___.___   Cannabis Intoxication

Without perceptual disturbances
F12.120   With mild use disorder
F12.220   With moderate or severe use disorder
F12.920   Without use disorder

With perceptual disturbances
F12.122   With mild use disorder
F12.222   With moderate or severe use disorder
F12.922   Without use disorder

___.___   Cannabis Withdrawal

F12.13   With mild use disorder

F12.23   With moderate or severe use disorder

F12.93   Without use disorder

___.___   Cannabis-Induced Mental Disorders

Note: Disorders are listed in their order of appearance in the manual.

[a]*Specify* With onset during intoxication, With onset during withdrawal, With onset after medication use. **Note:** When prescribed as medication, substances in this class can also induce the relevant substance-induced mental disorder.

[b]*Specify* if: Acute, Persistent

[c]*Specify* if: Hyperactive, Hypoactive, Mixed level of activity

___.___   Cannabis-Induced Psychotic Disorder[a]
F12.159   With mild use disorder

F12.259	With moderate or severe use disorder
F12.959	Without use disorder
___.__	Cannabis-Induced Anxiety Disorder[a]
F12.180	With mild use disorder
F12.280	With moderate or severe use disorder
F12.980	Without use disorder
___.__	Cannabis-Induced Sleep Disorder[a]
	Specify whether Insomnia type, Daytime sleepiness type, Mixed type
F12.188	With mild use disorder
F12.288	With moderate or severe use disorder
F12.988	Without use disorder
___.__	Cannabis Intoxication Delirium[b,c]
F12.121	With mild use disorder
F12.221	With moderate or severe use disorder
F12.921	Without use disorder
F12.921	Pharmaceutical Cannabis Receptor Agonist–Induced Delirium[b,c]
	Note: When pharmaceutical cannabis receptor agonist medication taken as prescribed. The designation "taken as prescribed" is used to differentiate medication-induced delirium from substance intoxication delirium.
F12.99	Unspecified Cannabis-Related Disorder

Hallucinogen-Related Disorders

___.__	Phencyclidine Use Disorder
	Specify if: In a controlled environment
	Specify current severity/remission:
F16.10	Mild
F16.11	In early remission
F16.11	In sustained remission
F16.20	Moderate
F16.21	In early remission
F16.21	In sustained remission
F16.20	Severe
F16.21	In early remission
F16.21	In sustained remission
___.__	Other Hallucinogen Use Disorder
	Specify the particular hallucinogen
	Specify if: In a controlled environment
	Specify current severity/remission:
F16.10	Mild
F16.11	In early remission
F16.11	In sustained remission
F16.20	Moderate
F16.21	In early remission
F16.21	In sustained remission
F16.20	Severe

F16.21	In early remission
F16.21	In sustained remission

___.__	Phencyclidine Intoxication
F16.120	With mild use disorder
F16.220	With moderate or severe use disorder
F16.920	Without use disorder

___.__	Other Hallucinogen Intoxication
F16.120	With mild use disorder
F16.220	With moderate or severe use disorder
F16.920	Without use disorder

F16.983	Hallucinogen Persisting Perception Disorder

___.__ Phencyclidine-Induced Mental Disorders

Note: Disorders are listed in their order of appearance in the manual.

[a]*Specify* With onset during intoxication, With onset after medication use. **Note:** When prescribed as medication, substances in this class can also induce the relevant substance-induced mental disorder.

___.__	Phencyclidine-Induced Psychotic Disorder[a]
F16.159	With mild use disorder
F16.259	With moderate or severe use disorder
F16.959	Without use disorder

___.__	Phencyclidine-Induced Bipolar and Related Disorder[a]
F16.14	With mild use disorder
F16.24	With moderate or severe use disorder
F16.94	Without use disorder

___.__	Phencyclidine-Induced Depressive Disorder[a]
F16.14	With mild use disorder
F16.24	With moderate or severe use disorder
F16.94	Without use disorder

___.__	Phencyclidine-Induced Anxiety Disorder[a]
F16.180	With mild use disorder
F16.280	With moderate or severe use disorder
F16.980	Without use disorder

___.__ Phencyclidine Intoxication Delirium

Specify if: Acute, Persistent
Specify if: Hyperactive, Hypoactive, Mixed level of activity

F16.121	With mild use disorder
F16.221	With moderate or severe use disorder
F16.921	Without use disorder

___.__ Hallucinogen-Induced Mental Disorders

Note: Disorders are listed in their order of appearance in the manual.

[a]*Specify* With onset during intoxication, With onset after medication use. **Note:** When prescribed as medication, substances in this class can also induce the relevant substance-induced mental disorder.

[b]*Specify* if: Acute, Persistent
[c]*Specify* if: Hyperactive, Hypoactive, Mixed level of activity

___.__	Other Hallucinogen–Induced Psychotic Disorder[a]
F16.159	With mild use disorder
F16.259	With moderate or severe use disorder
F16.959	Without use disorder
___.__	Other Hallucinogen–Induced Bipolar and Related Disorder[a]
F16.14	With mild use disorder
F16.24	With moderate or severe use disorder
F16.94	Without use disorder
___.__	Other Hallucinogen–Induced Depressive Disorder[a]
F16.14	With mild use disorder
F16.24	With moderate or severe use disorder
F16.94	Without use disorder
___.__	Other Hallucinogen-Induced Anxiety Disorder[a]
F16.180	With mild use disorder
F16.280	With moderate or severe use disorder
F16.980	Without use disorder
___.__	Other Hallucinogen Intoxication Delirium[b,c]
F16.121	With mild use disorder
F16.221	With moderate or severe use disorder
F16.921	Without use disorder
F16.921	Ketamine or Other Hallucinogen–Induced Delirium[b,c]

Note: When ketamine or other hallucinogen medication taken as prescribed. The designation "taken as prescribed" is used to differentiate medication-induced delirium from substance intoxication delirium.

F16.99   Unspecified Phencyclidine-Related Disorder

F16.99   Unspecified Hallucinogen-Related Disorder

Inhalant-Related Disorders

___.__	Inhalant Use Disorder

Specify the particular inhalant
Specify if: In a controlled environment
Specify current severity/remission:

F18.10	Mild
F18.11	In early remission
F18.11	In sustained remission
F18.20	Moderate
F18.21	In early remission
F18.21	In sustained remission
F18.20	Severe
F18.21	In early remission
F18.21	In sustained remission
___.__	Inhalant Intoxication
F18.120	With mild use disorder
F18.220	With moderate or severe use disorder
F18.920	Without use disorder

___.___	Inhalant-Induced Mental Disorders

Note: Disorders are listed in their order of appearance in the manual.
[a]*Specify* With onset during intoxication

___.___	Inhalant-Induced Psychotic Disorder[a]
F18.159	With mild use disorder
F18.259	With moderate or severe use disorder
F18.959	Without use disorder
___.___	Inhalant-Induced Depressive Disorder[a]
F18.14	With mild use disorder
F18.24	With moderate or severe use disorder
F18.94	Without use disorder
___.___	Inhalant-Induced Anxiety Disorder[a]
F18.180	With mild use disorder
F18.280	With moderate or severe use disorder
F18.980	Without use disorder
___.___	Inhalant Intoxication Delirium

Specify if: Acute, Persistent
Specify if: Hyperactive, Hypoactive, Mixed level of activity

F18.121	With mild use disorder
F18.221	With moderate or severe use disorder
F18.921	Without use disorder
___.___	Inhalant-Induced Major Neurocognitive Disorder

Specify if: Persistent

F18.17	With mild use disorder
F18.27	With moderate or severe use disorder
F18.97	Without use disorder
___.___	Inhalant-Induced Mild Neurocognitive Disorder

Specify if: Persistent

F18.188	With mild use disorder
F18.288	With moderate or severe use disorder
F18.988	Without use disorder
F18.99	Unspecified Inhalant-Related Disorder

Opioid-Related Disorders

___.___	Opioid Use Disorder

Specify if: On maintenance therapy, In a controlled environment
Specify current severity/remission:

F11.10	Mild
F11.11	In early remission
F11.11	In sustained remission
F11.20	Moderate
F11.21	In early remission
F11.21	In sustained remission
F11.20	Severe

F11.21	In early remission
F11.21	In sustained remission
___.__	Opioid Intoxication

Without perceptual disturbances

F11.120	With mild use disorder
F11.220	With moderate or severe use disorder
F11.920	Without use disorder

With perceptual disturbances

F11.122	With mild use disorder
F11.222	With moderate or severe use disorder
F11.922	Without use disorder

___.__	Opioid Withdrawal
F11.13	With mild use disorder
F11.23	With moderate or severe use disorder
F11.93	Without use disorder

___.__ Opioid-Induced Mental Disorders

Note: Disorders are listed in their order of appearance in the manual.

[a]*Specify* With onset during intoxication, With onset during withdrawal, With onset after medication use. **Note:** When prescribed as medication, substances in this class can also induce the relevant substance-induced mental disorder.

[b]*Specify* if: Acute, Persistent

[c]*Specify* if: Hyperactive, Hypoactive, Mixed level of activity

___.__	Opioid-Induced Depressive Disorder[a]
F11.14	With mild use disorder
F11.24	With moderate or severe use disorder
F11.94	Without use disorder

___.__	Opioid-Induced Anxiety Disorder[a]
F11.188	With mild use disorder
F11.288	With moderate or severe use disorder
F11.988	Without use disorder

___.__ Opioid-Induced Sleep Disorder[a]

Specify whether Insomnia type, Daytime sleepiness type, Mixed type

F11.182	With mild use disorder
F11.282	With moderate or severe use disorder
F11.982	Without use disorder

___.__ Opioid-Induced Sexual Dysfunction[a]

Specify if: Mild, Moderate, Severe

F11.181	With mild use disorder
F11.281	With moderate or severe use disorder
F11.981	Without use disorder

___.__	Opioid Intoxication Delirium[b,c]
F11.121	With mild use disorder
F11.221	With moderate or severe use disorder
F11.921	Without use disorder

___.___   Opioid Withdrawal Delirium[b,c]
F11.188   With mild use disorder
F11.288   With moderate or severe use disorder
F11.988   Without use disorder

___.___   Opioid-Induced Delirium[b,c]
     Note: The designation "taken as prescribed" is used to differentiate medication-induced delirium from substance intoxication delirium and substance withdrawal delirium.
F11.921   When opioid medication taken as prescribed
F11.988   During withdrawal from opioid medication taken as prescribed

F11.99   Unspecified Opioid-Related Disorder

Sedative-, Hypnotic-, or Anxiolytic-Related Disorders

___.___   Sedative, Hypnotic, or Anxiolytic Use Disorder
     Specify if: In a controlled environment
     Specify current severity/remission:
F13.10   Mild
F13.11   In early remission
F13.11   In sustained remission
F13.20   Moderate
F13.21   In early remission
F13.21   In sustained remission
F13.20   Severe
F13.21   In early remission
F13.21   In sustained remission

___.___   Sedative, Hypnotic, or Anxiolytic Intoxication
F13.120   With mild use disorder
F13.220   With moderate or severe use disorder
F13.920   Without use disorder

___.___   Sedative, Hypnotic, or Anxiolytic Withdrawal
     Without perceptual disturbances
F13.130   With mild use disorder
F13.230   With moderate or severe use disorder
F13.930   Without use disorder
     With perceptual disturbances
F13.132   With mild use disorder
F13.232   With moderate or severe use disorder
F13.932   Without use disorder

___.___   Sedative-, Hypnotic-, or Anxiolytic-Induced Mental Disorders
     Note: Disorders are listed in their order of appearance in the manual.
     [a]*Specify* With onset during intoxication, With onset during withdrawal, With onset after medication use. **Note:** When prescribed as medication, substances in this class can also induce the relevant substance-induced mental disorder.

^b*Specify* if: Acute, Persistent
^c*Specify* if: Hyperactive, Hypoactive, Mixed level of activity

	Sedative-, Hypnotic-, or Anxiolytic-Induced Psychotic Disorder[a]
___.__	
F13.159	With mild use disorder
F13.259	With moderate or severe use disorder
F13.959	Without use disorder

	Sedative-, Hypnotic-, or Anxiolytic-Induced Bipolar and Related Disorder[a]
___.__	
F13.14	With mild use disorder
F13.24	With moderate or severe use disorder
F13.94	Without use disorder

	Sedative-, Hypnotic-, or Anxiolytic-Induced Depressive Disorder[a]
___.__	
F13.14	With mild use disorder
F13.24	With moderate or severe use disorder
F13.94	Without use disorder

	Sedative-, Hypnotic-, or Anxiolytic-Induced Anxiety Disorder[a]
___.__	
F13.180	With mild use disorder
F13.280	With moderate or severe use disorder
F13.980	Without use disorder

___.__ Sedative-, Hypnotic-, or Anxiolytic-Induced Sleep Disorder[a]

Specify whether Insomnia type, Daytime sleepiness type, Parasomnia type, Mixed type

F13.182 With mild use disorder

F13.282 With moderate or severe use disorder

F13.982 Without use disorder

___.__ Sedative-, Hypnotic-, or Anxiolytic-Induced Sexual Dysfunction[a]

Specify if: Mild, Moderate, Severe

F13.181 With mild use disorder

F13.281 With moderate or severe use disorder

F13.981 Without use disorder

	Sedative-, Hypnotic-, or Anxiolytic Intoxication Delirium[b,c]
___.__	
F13.121	With mild use disorder
F13.221	With moderate or severe use disorder
F13.921	Without use disorder

	Sedative-, Hypnotic-, or Anxiolytic Withdrawal Delirium[b,c]
___.__	
F13.131	With mild use disorder
F13.231	With moderate or severe use disorder
F13.931	Without use disorder

___.__ Sedative-, Hypnotic-, or Anxiolytic-Induced Delirium[b,c]

Note: The designation "taken as prescribed" is used to differentiate medication-induced delirium from substance intoxication delirium and substance withdrawal delirium.

F13.921 When sedative, hypnotic, or anxiolytic medication taken as prescribed

F13.931 During withdrawal from sedative, hypnotic, or anxiolytic medication taken as prescribed

___.__	Sedative-, Hypnotic-, or Anxiolytic-Induced Major Neurocognitive Disorder
	Specify if: Persistent
F13.27	With moderate or severe use disorder
F13.97	Without use disorder
___.__	Sedative-, Hypnotic-, or Anxiolytic-Induced Mild Neurocognitive Disorder
	Specify if: Persistent
F13.188	With mild use disorder
F13.288	With moderate or severe use disorder
F13.988	Without use disorder
F13.99	Unspecified Sedative-, Hypnotic-, or Anxiolytic-Related Disorder

Stimulant-Related Disorders

___.__	Stimulant Use Disorder
	Specify if: In a controlled environment
	Specify current severity/remission:
___.__	Mild
F15.10	Amphetamine-type substance
F14.10	Cocaine
F15.10	Other or unspecified stimulant
___.__	Mild, In early remission
F15.11	Amphetamine-type substance
F14.11	Cocaine
F15.11	Other or unspecified stimulant
___.__	Mild, In sustained remission
F15.11	Amphetamine-type substance
F14.11	Cocaine
F15.11	Other or unspecified stimulant
___.__	Moderate
F15.20	Amphetamine-type substance
F14.20	Cocaine
F15.20	Other or unspecified stimulant
___.__	Moderate, In early remission
F15.21	Amphetamine-type substance
F14.21	Cocaine
F15.21	Other or unspecified stimulant
___.__	Moderate, In sustained remission
F15.21	Amphetamine-type substance
F14.21	Cocaine
F15.21	Other or unspecified stimulant
___.__	Severe
F15.20	Amphetamine-type substance
F14.20	Cocaine
F15.20	Other or unspecified stimulant

___.___	Severe, In early remission
F15.21	Amphetamine-type substance
F14.21	Cocaine
F15.21	Other or unspecified stimulant
___.___	Severe, In sustained remission
F15.21	Amphetamine-type substance
F14.21	Cocaine
F15.21	Other or unspecified stimulant

___.___ Stimulant Intoxication

Specify the particular intoxicant

Without perceptual disturbances

___.___	Amphetamine-type substance or other stimulant intoxication
F15.120	With mild use disorder
F15.220	With moderate or severe use disorder
F15.920	Without use disorder
___.___	Cocaine intoxication
F14.120	With mild use disorder
F14.220	With moderate or severe use disorder
F14.920	Without use disorder

With perceptual disturbances

___.___	Amphetamine-type substance or other stimulant intoxication
F15.122	With mild use disorder
F15.222	With moderate or severe use disorder
F15.922	Without use disorder
___.___	Cocaine intoxication
F14.122	With mild use disorder
F14.222	With moderate or severe use disorder
F14.922	Without use disorder

___.___ Stimulant Withdrawal

Specify the particular substance that causes the withdrawal syndrome

___.___	Amphetamine-type substance or other stimulant withdrawal
F15.13	With mild use disorder
F15.23	With moderate or severe use disorder
F15.93	Without use disorder
___.___	Cocaine withdrawal
F14.13	With mild use disorder
F14.23	With moderate or severe use disorder
F14.93	Without use disorder

___.___ Stimulant-Induced Mental Disorders

Note: Disorders are listed in their order of appearance in the manual.

[a]*Specify* With onset during intoxication, With onset during withdrawal, With onset after medication use. **Note:** When prescribed as medication, amphetamine-type substances and other stimulants can also induce the relevant substance-induced mental disorder.

[b]*Specify* if: Acute, Persistent
[c]*Specify* if: Hyperactive, Hypoactive, Mixed level of activity

	Amphetamine-Type Substance (or Other Stimulant)–Induced Psychotic Disorder[a]
F15.159	With mild use disorder
F15.259	With moderate or severe use disorder
F15.959	Without use disorder
	Cocaine-Induced Psychotic Disorder[a]
F14.159	With mild use disorder
F14.259	With moderate or severe use disorder
F14.959	Without use disorder
	Amphetamine-Type Substance (or Other Stimulant)–Induced Bipolar and Related Disorder[a]
F15.14	With mild use disorder
F15.24	With moderate or severe use disorder
F15.94	Without use disorder
	Cocaine-Induced Bipolar and Related Disorder[a]
F14.14	With mild use disorder
F14.24	With moderate or severe use disorder
F14.94	Without use disorder
	Amphetamine-Type Substance (or Other Stimulant)–Induced Depressive Disorder[a]
F15.14	With mild use disorder
F15.24	With moderate or severe use disorder
F15.94	Without use disorder
	Cocaine-Induced Depressive Disorder[a]
F14.14	With mild use disorder
F14.24	With moderate or severe use disorder
F14.94	Without use disorder
	Amphetamine-Type Substance (or Other Stimulant)–Induced Anxiety Disorder[a]
F15.180	With mild use disorder
F15.280	With moderate or severe use disorder
F15.980	Without use disorder
	Cocaine-Induced Anxiety Disorder[a]
F14.180	With mild use disorder
F14.280	With moderate or severe use disorder
F14.980	Without use disorder
	Amphetamine-Type Substance (or Other Stimulant)–Induced Obsessive-Compulsive and Related Disorder[a]
F15.188	With mild use disorder
F15.288	With moderate or severe use disorder
F15.988	Without use disorder
	Cocaine-Induced Obsessive-Compulsive and Related Disorder[a]
F14.188	With mild use disorder
F14.288	With moderate or severe use disorder
F14.988	Without use disorder

___.__	Amphetamine-Type Substance (or Other Stimulant)–Induced Sleep Disorder[a]
	Specify whether Insomnia type, Daytime sleepiness type, Mixed type
F15.182	With mild use disorder
F15.282	With moderate or severe use disorder
F15.982	Without use disorder
___.__	Cocaine-Induced Sleep Disorder[a]
	Specify whether Insomnia type, Daytime sleepiness type, Mixed type
F14.182	With mild use disorder
F14.282	With moderate or severe use disorder
F14.982	Without use disorder
___.__	Amphetamine-Type Substance (or Other Stimulant)–Induced Sexual Dysfunction[a]
	Specify if: Mild, Moderate, Severe
F15.181	With mild use disorder
F15.281	With moderate or severe use disorder
F15.981	Without use disorder
___.__	Cocaine-Induced Sexual Dysfunction[a]
	Specify if: Mild, Moderate, Severe
F14.181	With mild use disorder
F14.281	With moderate or severe use disorder
F14.981	Without use disorder
___.__	Amphetamine-Type Substance (or Other Stimulant) Intoxication Delirium[b,c]
F15.121	With mild use disorder
F15.221	With moderate or severe use disorder
F15.921	Without use disorder
___.__	Cocaine Intoxication Delirium[b,c]
F14.121	With mild use disorder
F14.221	With moderate or severe use disorder
F14.921	Without use disorder
F15.921	Amphetamine-Type (or Other Stimulant) Medication–Induced Delirium[b,c]
	Note: When amphetamine-type or other stimulant medication taken as prescribed. The designation "taken as prescribed" is used to differentiate medication-induced delirium from substance intoxication delirium.
___.__	Amphetamine-Type Substance (or Other Stimulant)–Induced Mild Neurocognitive Disorder
	Specify if: Persistent
F15.188	With mild use disorder
F15.288	With moderate or severe use disorder
F15.988	Without use disorder
___.__	Cocaine-Induced Mild Neurocognitive Disorder
	Specify if: Persistent
F14.188	With mild use disorder
F14.288	With moderate or severe use disorder
F14.988	Without use disorder

___.__	Unspecified Stimulant-Related Disorder
F15.99	Amphetamine-type substance or other stimulant
F14.99	Cocaine

Tobacco-Related Disorders

___.__   Tobacco Use Disorder
    Specify if: On maintenance therapy, In a controlled environment
    Specify current severity/remission:

Z72.0	Mild
F17.200	Moderate
F17.201	In early remission
F17.201	In sustained remission
F17.200	Severe
F17.201	In early remission
F17.201	In sustained remission

F17.203   Tobacco Withdrawal
    Note: The ICD-10-CM code indicates the comorbid presence of a moderate or severe tobacco use disorder, which must be present in order to apply the code for tobacco withdrawal.

___.__   Tobacco-Induced Mental Disorders

F17.208   Tobacco-Induced Sleep Disorder, With moderate or severe use disorder
    Specify whether Insomnia type, Daytime sleepiness type, Mixed type
    Specify With onset during withdrawal, With onset after medication use

F17.209   Unspecified Tobacco-Related Disorder

Other (or Unknown) Substance–Related Disorders

___.__   Other (or Unknown) Substance Use Disorder
    Specify if: In a controlled environment
    Specify current severity/remission:

F19.10	Mild
F19.11	In early remission
F19.11	In sustained remission
F19.20	Moderate
F19.21	In early remission
F19.21	In sustained remission
F19.20	Severe
F19.21	In early remission
F19.21	In sustained remission

___.__   Other (or Unknown) Substance Intoxication
    Without perceptual disturbances

F19.120	With mild use disorder
F19.220	With moderate or severe use disorder
F19.920	Without use disorder

    With perceptual disturbances

F19.122	With mild use disorder

F19.222	With moderate or severe use disorder
F19.922	Without use disorder

___.___   Other (or Unknown) Substance Withdrawal

    Without perceptual disturbances

F19.130	With mild use disorder
F19.230	With moderate or severe use disorder
F19.930	Without use disorder

    With perceptual disturbances

F19.132	With mild use disorder
F19.232	With moderate or severe use disorder
F19.932	Without use disorder

___.___   Other (or Unknown) Substance–Induced Mental Disorders

Note: Disorders are listed in their order of appearance in the manual.

[a]*Specify* With onset during intoxication, With onset during withdrawal, With onset after medication use. **Note:** When prescribed as medication or taken over the counter, substances in this class can also induce the relevant substance-induced mental disorder.

[b]*Specify* if: Acute, Persistent

[c]*Specify* if: Hyperactive, Hypoactive, Mixed level of activity

    Other (or Unknown) Substance–Induced Psychotic Disorder[a]

F19.159	With mild use disorder
F19.259	With moderate or severe use disorder
F19.959	Without use disorder

    Other (or Unknown) Substance–Induced Bipolar and Related Disorder[a]

F19.14	With mild use disorder
F19.24	With moderate or severe use disorder
F19.94	Without use disorder

    Other (or Unknown) Substance–Induced Depressive Disorder[a]

F19.14	With mild use disorder
F19.24	With moderate or severe use disorder
F19.94	Without use disorder

    Other (or Unknown) Substance–Induced Anxiety Disorder[a]

F19.180	With mild use disorder
F19.280	With moderate or severe use disorder
F19.980	Without use disorder

    Other (or Unknown) Substance–Induced Obsessive-Compulsive and Related Disorder[a]

F19.188	With mild use disorder
F19.288	With moderate or severe use disorder
F19.988	Without use disorder

    Other (or Unknown) Substance–Induced Sleep Disorder[a]

Specify whether Insomnia type, Daytime sleepiness type, Parasomnia type, Mixed type

F19.182	With mild use disorder
F19.282	With moderate or severe use disorder
F19.982	Without use disorder

___.__	Other (or Unknown) Substance–Induced Sexual Dysfunction[a]
	Specify if: Mild, Moderate, Severe
F19.181	With mild use disorder
F19.281	With moderate or severe use disorder
F19.981	Without use disorder
___.__	Other (or Unknown) Substance Intoxication Delirium[b,c]
F19.121	With mild use disorder
F19.221	With moderate or severe use disorder
F19.921	Without use disorder
___.__	Other (or Unknown) Substance Withdrawal Delirium[b,c]
F19.131	With mild use disorder
F19.231	With moderate or severe use disorder
F19.931	Without use disorder
___.__	Other (or Unknown) Medication–Induced Delirium[b,c]
	Note: The designation "taken as prescribed" is used to differentiate medication-induced delirium from substance intoxication delirium and substance withdrawal delirium.
F19.921	When other (or unknown) medication taken as prescribed
F19.931	During withdrawal from other (or unknown) medication taken as prescribed
___.__	Other (or Unknown) Substance–Induced Major Neurocognitive Disorder
	Specify if: Persistent
F19.17	With mild use disorder
F19.27	With moderate or severe use disorder
F19.97	Without use disorder
___.__	Other (or Unknown) Substance–Induced Mild Neurocognitive Disorder
	Specify if: Persistent
F19.188	With mild use disorder
F19.288	With moderate or severe use disorder
F19.988	Without use disorder
F19.99	Unspecified Other (or Unknown) Substance–Related Disorder

Non-Substance-Related Disorders

F63.0	Gambling Disorder
	Specify if: Episodic, Persistent
	Specify if: In early remission, In sustained remission
	Specify current severity: Mild, Moderate, Severe

Neurocognitive Disorders

___.__	Delirium
	Specify if: Acute, Persistent
	Specify if: Hyperactive, Hypoactive, Mixed level of activity
	[a]**Note:** For applicable ICD-10-CM codes, refer to the substance classes under Substance-Related and Addictive Disorders for the specific substance/medication-induced delirium. See also the criteria set and corresponding recording procedures in the manual for more information.

Specify whether:

___.___	Substance intoxication delirium[a]
___.___	Substance withdrawal delirium[a]
___.___	Medication-induced delirium[a]
F05	Delirium due to another medical condition
F05	Delirium due to multiple etiologies
F05	Other Specified Delirium
F05	Unspecified Delirium

Major and Mild Neurocognitive Disorders

Refer to the following sequence for coding and recording major and mild neurocognitive disorders (NCDs) in context with specific diagnoses listed, exceptions as noted:

Major and mild NCDs: *Specify* whether due to *[any of the following medical etiologies]*: Alzheimer's disease, Frontotemporal degeneration, Lewy body disease, Vascular disease, Traumatic brain injury, Substance/medication use, HIV infection, Prion disease, Parkinson's disease, Huntington's disease, Another medical condition, Multiple etiologies, Unknown etiology.

Major and mild NCDs: Code first the *specific medical etiology* for the major or mild NCD. **Note:** No etiological medical code is used for major vascular NCD, major NCDs due to possible etiologies, substance/medication-induced major or mild NCD, or major or mild NCD due to unknown etiology.

[a]**Major NCD only:** Next code *severity* (placeholder "x" in 4th character of diagnostic codes below) as follows: .Ay mild, .By moderate, .Cy severe. **Note:** Not applicable to any substance/medication-induced NCD.

[b]**Major NCD only:** Then code any *accompanying behavioral or psychological disturbance* (placeholder "y" in 5th and 6th characters of diagnostic codes below): .x11 with agitation; .x4 with anxiety; .x3 with mood symptoms; .x2 with psychotic disturbance; .x18 with other behavioral or psychological disturbance (e.g., apathy); .x0 without accompanying behavioral or psychological disturbance. **Note:** In cases where there is more than one type of associated behavioral or psychological disturbance, each is coded separately. See coding table in DSM-5-TR, pp. 682–683, for more information.

[c]**Mild NCD only** *(exceptions: see note d below)*: Code either **F06.70** without behavioral disturbance or **F06.71** with behavioral disturbance (e.g., apathy, agitation, anxiety, mood symptoms, psychotic disturbance, or other behavioral symptoms). **Coding note for mild NCDs only:** Use additional disorder code(s) to indicate clinically significant psychiatric symptoms due to the same medical condition causing the mild NCD (e.g., **F06.2** psychotic disorder due to Alzheimer's disease with delusions; **F06.32** depressive disorder due to Parkinson's disease, with major depressive-like episode). *Note:* The additional codes for mental disorders due to another medical condition are included with disorders with which they share phenomenology (e.g., for depressive disorders due to another medical condition, see "Depressive Disorders").

[d]**Mild NCD due to possible or unknown etiology:** Code only **G31.84.** No additional medical code is used. **Note:** "With behavioral disturbance" and "Without behavioral disturbance" cannot be coded but should still be recorded.

Major or Mild Neurocognitive Disorder Due to Alzheimer's Disease

F02.[xy] Major Neurocognitive Disorder Due to Probable Alzheimer's Disease[a,b]
Note: Code first **G30.9** Alzheimer's disease.

F03.[xy] Major Neurocognitive Disorder Due to Possible Alzheimer's Disease[a,b]
Note: No additional medical code.

___.___   Mild Neurocognitive Disorder Due to Probable Alzheimer's Disease[c]
Note: Code first **G30.9** Alzheimer's disease.

F06.71   With behavioral disturbance

F06.70   Without behavioral disturbance

G31.84   Mild Neurocognitive Disorder Due to Possible Alzheimer's Disease[d]

Major or Mild Frontotemporal Neurocognitive Disorder

F02.[xy]   Major Neurocognitive Disorder Due to Probable Frontotemporal Degeneration[a,b]
Note: Code first **G31.09** frontotemporal degeneration.

F03.[xy]   Major Neurocognitive Disorder Due to Possible Frontotemporal Degeneration[a,b]
Note: No additional medical code.

___.___   Mild Neurocognitive Disorder Due to Probable Frontotemporal Degeneration[c]
Note: Code first **G31.09** frontotemporal degeneration.

F06.71   With behavioral disturbance

F06.70   Without behavioral disturbance

G31.84   Mild Neurocognitive Disorder Due to Possible Frontotemporal Degeneration[d]

Major or Mild Neurocognitive Disorder With Lewy Bodies

F02.[xy]   Major Neurocognitive Disorder With Probable Lewy Bodies[a,b]
Note: Code first **G31.83** Lewy body disease.

F03.[xy]   Major Neurocognitive Disorder With Possible Lewy Bodies[a,b]
Note: No additional medical code.

___.___   Mild Neurocognitive Disorder With Probable Lewy Bodies[c]
Note: Code first **G31.83** Lewy body disease.

F06.71   With behavioral disturbance

F06.70   Without behavioral disturbance

G31.84   Mild Neurocognitive Disorder With Possible Lewy Bodies[d]

Major or Mild Vascular Neurocognitive Disorder

F01.[xy]   Major Neurocognitive Disorder Probably Due to Vascular Disease[a,b]
Note: No additional medical code.

F03.[xy]   Major Neurocognitive Disorder Possibly Due to Vascular Disease[a,b]
Note: No additional medical code.

___.___   Mild Neurocognitive Disorder Probably Due to Vascular Disease[c]
Note: Code first **I67.9** cerebrovascular disease.

F06.71   With behavioral disturbance

F06.70   Without behavioral disturbance

G31.84   Mild Neurocognitive Disorder Possibly Due to Vascular Disease[d]

Major or Mild Neurocognitive Disorder Due to Traumatic Brain Injury
Note: Code first **S06.2XAS** diffuse traumatic brain injury with loss of consciousness of unspecified duration, sequela.

F02.[xy]   Major Neurocognitive Disorder Due to Traumatic Brain Injury[a,b]

___.___   Mild Neurocognitive Disorder Due to Traumatic Brain Injury[c]
F06.71   With behavioral disturbance
F06.70   Without behavioral disturbance

Substance/Medication-Induced Major or Mild Neurocognitive Disorder
Note: No additional medical code is used. For applicable ICD-10-CM codes, refer to the substance classes under Substance-Related and Addictive Disorders for the specific substance/medication-induced major or mild NCD. See also the criteria set and corresponding recording procedures in the manual for more information.

Coding note: The ICD-10-CM code depends on whether or not there is a comorbid substance use disorder present for the same class of substance. In any case, an additional separate diagnosis of a substance use disorder is not given. *Note:* The symptom specifiers "With agitation," "With anxiety," "With mood symptoms," "With psychotic disturbance," "With other behavioral or psychological disturbance," "Without accompanying behavioral or psychological disturbance" cannot be coded but should still be recorded.

Specify if: Persistent

___.___   Substance/Medication-Induced Major Neurocognitive Disorder
Specify current NCD severity: Mild, Moderate, Severe
___.___   Substance/Medication-Induced Mild Neurocognitive Disorder

Major or Mild Neurocognitive Disorder Due to HIV Infection
Note: Code first **B20** HIV infection.

F02.[xy]   Major Neurocognitive Disorder Due to HIV Infection[a,b]

___.___   Mild Neurocognitive Disorder Due to HIV Infection[c]
F06.71   With behavioral disturbance
F06.70   Without behavioral disturbance

Major or Mild Neurocognitive Disorder Due to Prion Disease
Note: Code first **A81.9** prion disease.

F02.[xy]   Major Neurocognitive Disorder Due to Prion Disease[a,b]

___.___   Mild Neurocognitive Disorder Due to Prion Disease[c]
F06.71   With behavioral disturbance
F06.70   Without behavioral disturbance

Major or Mild Neurocognitive Disorder Due to Parkinson's Disease

F02.[xy]   Major Neurocognitive Disorder Probably Due to Parkinson's Disease[a,b]
Note: Code first **G20.C** Parkinson's disease.

F03.[xy]   Major Neurocognitive Disorder Possibly Due to Parkinson's Disease[a,b]
Note: No additional medical code.

___.___   Mild Neurocognitive Disorder Probably Due to Parkinson's Disease[c]
Note: Code first **G20.C** Parkinson's disease.
F06.71   With behavioral disturbance
F06.70   Without behavioral disturbance

G31.84 Mild Neurocognitive Disorder Possibly Due to Parkinson's Disease[d]

Major or Mild Neurocognitive Disorder Due to Huntington's Disease
Note: Code first **G10** Huntington's disease.

F02.[xy] Major Neurocognitive Disorder Due to Huntington's Disease[a,b]

___.__ Mild Neurocognitive Disorder Due to Huntington's Disease[c]

F06.71 With behavioral disturbance

F06.70 Without behavioral disturbance

Major or Mild Neurocognitive Disorder Due to Another Medical Condition
Note: Code first the other medical condition.

F02.[xy] Major Neurocognitive Disorder Due to Another Medical Condition[a,b]

___.__ Mild Neurocognitive Disorder Due to Another Medical Condition[c]

F06.71 With behavioral disturbance

F06.70 Without behavioral disturbance

Major or Mild Neurocognitive Disorder Due to Multiple Etiologies

F02.[xy] Major Neurocognitive Disorder Due to Multiple Etiologies[a,b]

Note: Code first all the etiological medical conditions (with the exception of cerebrovascular disease, which is not coded). Then code **F02.[xy]**[a,b] once for major NCD due to all etiologies that apply. Code also **F01.[xy]**[a,b] for major NCD probably due to vascular disease, if present. Code also the relevant substance/medication-induced major NCDs if substances or medications play a role in the etiology.

___.__ Mild Neurocognitive Disorder Due to Multiple Etiologies[c]

Note: Code first all the etiological medical conditions, including **I67.9** cerebrovascular disease, if present. Then code **F06.70** or **F06.71** once (see below for 5th character) for mild NCD due to all etiologies that apply, including mild NCD probably due to vascular disease, if present. Code also the relevant substance/medication-induced mild NCDs if substances or medications play a role in the etiology.

F06.71 With behavioral disturbance

F06.70 Without behavioral disturbance

Major or Mild Neurocognitive Disorder Due to Unknown Etiology
Note: No additional medical code.

F03.[xy] Major Neurocognitive Disorder Due to Unknown Etiology[a,b]

G31.84 Mild Neurocognitive Disorder Due to Unknown Etiology[d]

R41.9 Unspecified Neurocognitive Disorder
Note: No additional medical code.

Personality Disorders

Cluster A Personality Disorders

F60.0.   Paranoid Personality Disorder

F60.1.   Schizoid Personality Disorder

F21.   Schizotypal Personality Disorder

Cluster B Personality Disorders

F60.2.   Antisocial Personality Disorder

F60.3.   Borderline Personality Disorder

F60.4.   Histrionic Personality Disorder

F60.81.   Narcissistic Personality Disorder

Cluster C Personality Disorders

F60.6.   Avoidant Personality Disorder

F60.7.   Dependent Personality Disorder

F60.5.   Obsessive-Compulsive Personality Disorder

Other Personality Disorders

F07.0.   Personality Change Due to Another Medical Condition
Specify whether: Labile type, Disinhibited type, Aggressive type, Apathetic type, Paranoid type, Other type, Combined type, Unspecified type

F60.89.   Other Specified Personality Disorder

F60.9.   Unspecified Personality Disorder

Paraphilic Disorders

The following specifier applies to Paraphilic Disorders where indicated:
[a]*Specify* if: In a controlled environment, In full remission

F65.3   Voyeuristic Disorder[a]

F65.2   Exhibitionistic Disorder[a]
Specify whether: Sexually aroused by exposing genitals to prepubertal children, Sexually aroused by exposing genitals to physically mature individuals, Sexually aroused by exposing genitals to prepubertal children and to physically mature individuals

F65.81   Frotteuristic Disorder[a]

F65.51   Sexual Masochism Disorder[a]
Specify if: With asphyxiophilia

F65.52   Sexual Sadism Disorder[a]

F65.4   Pedophilic Disorder
Specify whether: Exclusive type, Nonexclusive type
Specify if: Sexually attracted to males, Sexually attracted to females, Sexually attracted to both
Specify if: Limited to incest

F65.0   Fetishistic Disorder[a]
             Specify: Body part(s), Nonliving object(s), Other
F65.1   Transvestic Disorder[a]
             Specify if: With fetishism, With autogynephilia
F65.89   Other Specified Paraphilic Disorder
F65.9   Unspecified Paraphilic Disorder

Other Mental Disorders and Additional Codes

F06.8   Other Specified Mental Disorder Due to Another Medical Condition
F09   Unspecified Mental Disorder Due to Another Medical Condition
F99   Other Specified Mental Disorder
F99   Unspecified Mental Disorder
Z03.89   No Diagnosis or Condition

Medication-Induced Movement Disorders and Other Adverse Effects of Medication

___.__   Medication-Induced Parkinsonism
G21.11   Antipsychotic Medication– and Other Dopamine Receptor Blocking
                 Agent–Induced Parkinsonism
G21.19   Other Medication-Induced Parkinsonism
G21.0   Neuroleptic Malignant Syndrome
G24.02   Medication-Induced Acute Dystonia
G25.71   Medication-Induced Acute Akathisia
G24.01   Tardive Dyskinesia
G24.09   Tardive Dystonia
G25.71   Tardive Akathisia
G25.1   Medication-Induced Postural Tremor
G25.79   Other Medication-Induced Movement Disorder
___.__   Antidepressant Discontinuation Syndrome
T43.205A   Initial encounter
T43.205D   Subsequent encounter
T43.205S   Sequelae
___.__   Other Adverse Effect of Medication
T50.905A   Initial encounter
T50.905D   Subsequent encounter
T50.905S   Sequelae

Other Conditions That May Be a Focus of Clinical Attention

Suicidal Behavior and Nonsuicidal Self-Injury

Suicidal Behavior

___.__ Current Suicidal Behavior

T14.91XA Initial encounter

T14.91XD Subsequent encounter

Z91.51 History of Suicidal Behavior

Nonsuicidal Self-Injury

R45.88 Current Nonsuicidal Self-Injury

Z91.52 History of Nonsuicidal Self-Injury

Abuse and Neglect

Child Maltreatment and Neglect Problems

Child Physical Abuse

___.__ Child Physical Abuse, Confirmed

T74.12XA Initial encounter

T74.12XD Subsequent encounter

___.__ Child Physical Abuse, Suspected

T76.12XA Initial encounter

T76.12XD Subsequent encounter

___.__ Other Circumstances Related to Child Physical Abuse

Z69.010 Encounter for mental health services for victim of child physical abuse by parent

Z69.020 Encounter for mental health services for victim of nonparental child physical abuse

Z62.810 Personal history (past history) of physical abuse in childhood

Z69.011 Encounter for mental health services for perpetrator of parental child physical abuse

Z69.021 Encounter for mental health services for perpetrator of nonparental child physical abuse

Child Sexual Abuse

___.__ Child Sexual Abuse, Confirmed

T74.22XA Initial encounter

T74.22XD Subsequent encounter

___.__ Child Sexual Abuse, Suspected

T76.22XA Initial encounter

T76.22XD   Subsequent encounter

___.__   Other Circumstances Related to Child Sexual Abuse

Z69.010   Encounter for mental health services for victim of child sexual abuse by
              parent

Z69.020   Encounter for mental health services for victim of nonparental child sexual
              abuse

Z62.810   Personal history (past history) of sexual abuse in childhood

Z69.011   Encounter for mental health services for perpetrator of parental child
              sexual abuse

Z69.021   Encounter for mental health services for perpetrator of nonparental child
              sexual abuse

Child Neglect

___.__   Child Neglect, Confirmed

T74.02XA   Initial encounter

T74.02XD   Subsequent encounter

___.__   Child Neglect, Suspected

T76.02XA   Initial encounter

T76.02XD   Subsequent encounter

___.__   Other Circumstances Related to Child Neglect

Z69.010   Encounter for mental health services for victim of child neglect by parent

Z69.020   Encounter for mental health services for victim of nonparental child
              neglect

Z62.812   Personal history (past history) of neglect in childhood

Z69.011   Encounter for mental health services for perpetrator of parental child
              neglect

Z69.021   Encounter for mental health services for perpetrator of nonparental child
              neglect

Child Psychological Abuse

___.__   Child Psychological Abuse, Confirmed

T74.32XA   Initial encounter

T74.32XD   Subsequent encounter

___.__   Child Psychological Abuse, Suspected

T76.32XA   Initial encounter

T76.32XD   Subsequent encounter

___.__   Other Circumstances Related to Child Psychological Abuse

Z69.010   Encounter for mental health services for victim of child psychological
              abuse by parent

Z69.020   Encounter for mental health services for victim of nonparental child
              psychological abuse

Z62.811   Personal history (past history) of psychological abuse in childhood

Z69.011   Encounter for mental health services for perpetrator of parental child psychological abuse

Z69.021   Encounter for mental health services for perpetrator of nonparental child psychological abuse

Adult Maltreatment and Neglect Problems

Spouse or Partner Violence, Physical

___.__   Spouse or Partner Violence, Physical, Confirmed

T74.11XA   Initial encounter

T74.11XD   Subsequent encounter

___.__   Spouse or Partner Violence, Physical, Suspected

T76.11XA   Initial encounter

T76.11XD   Subsequent encounter

___.__   Other Circumstances Related to Spouse or Partner Violence, Physical

Z69.11   Encounter for mental health services for victim of spouse or partner violence, physical

Z91.410   Personal history (past history) of spouse or partner violence, physical

Z69.12   Encounter for mental health services for perpetrator of spouse or partner violence, physical

Spouse or Partner Violence, Sexual

___.__   Spouse or Partner Violence, Sexual, Confirmed

T74.21XA   Initial encounter

T74.21XD   Subsequent encounter

___.__   Spouse or Partner Violence, Sexual, Suspected

T76.21XA   Initial encounter

T76.21XD   Subsequent encounter

___.__   Other Circumstances Related to Spouse or Partner Violence, Sexual

Z69.81   Encounter for mental health services for victim of spouse or partner violence, sexual

Z91.410   Personal history (past history) of spouse or partner violence, sexual

Z69.12   Encounter for mental health services for perpetrator of spouse or partner violence, sexual

Spouse or Partner Neglect

___.__   Spouse or Partner Neglect, Confirmed

T74.01XA   Initial encounter

T74.01XD   Subsequent encounter

___.__   Spouse or Partner Neglect, Suspected

T76.01XA   Initial encounter

T76.01XD   Subsequent encounter

__.__   Other Circumstances Related to Spouse or Partner Neglect

Z69.11   Encounter for mental health services for victim of spouse or partner neglect

Z91.412   Personal history (past history) of spouse or partner neglect

Z69.12   Encounter for mental health services for perpetrator of spouse or partner neglect

Spouse or Partner Abuse, Psychological

__.__   Spouse or Partner Abuse, Psychological, Confirmed

T74.31XA   Initial encounter

T74.31XD   Subsequent encounter

__.__   Spouse or Partner Abuse, Psychological, Suspected

T76.31XA   Initial encounter

T76.31XD   Subsequent encounter

__.__   Other Circumstances Related to Spouse or Partner Abuse, Psychological

Z69.11   Encounter for mental health services for victim of spouse or partner psychological abuse

Z91.411   Personal history (past history) of spouse or partner psychological abuse

Z69.12   Encounter for mental health services for perpetrator of spouse or partner psychological abuse

Adult Abuse by Nonspouse or Nonpartner

__.__   Adult Physical Abuse by Nonspouse or Nonpartner, Confirmed

T74.11XA   Initial encounter

T74.11XD   Subsequent encounter

__.__   Adult Physical Abuse by Nonspouse or Nonpartner, Suspected

T76.11XA   Initial encounter

T76.11XD   Subsequent encounter

__.__   Adult Sexual Abuse by Nonspouse or Nonpartner, Confirmed

T74.21XA   Initial encounter

T74.21XD   Subsequent encounter

__.__   Adult Sexual Abuse by Nonspouse or Nonpartner, Suspected

T76.21XA   Initial encounter

T76.21XD   Subsequent encounter

__.__   Adult Psychological Abuse by Nonspouse or Nonpartner, Confirmed

T74.31XA   Initial encounter

T74.31XD   Subsequent encounter

__.__   Adult Psychological Abuse by Nonspouse or Nonpartner, Suspected

T76.31XA   Initial encounter

T76.31XD   Subsequent encounter

___.___	Other Circumstances Related to Adult Abuse by Nonspouse or Nonpartner
Z69.81	Encounter for mental health services for victim of nonspousal or nonpartner adult abuse
Z69.82	Encounter for mental health services for perpetrator of nonspousal or nonpartner adult abuse

Relational Problems

___.___	Parent-Child Relational Problem
Z62.820	Parent–Biological Child
Z62.821	Parent–Adopted Child
Z62.822	Parent–Foster Child
Z62.898	Other Caregiver–Child
Z62.891	Sibling Relational Problem
Z63.0	Relationship Distress With Spouse or Intimate Partner

Problems Related to the Family Environment

Z62.29.	Upbringing Away From Parents
Z62.898.	Child Affected by Parental Relationship Distress
Z63.5.	Disruption of Family by Separation or Divorce
Z63.8.	High Expressed Emotion Level Within Family

Educational Problems

Z55.0	Illiteracy and Low-Level Literacy
Z55.1	Schooling Unavailable and Unattainable
Z55.2	Failed School Examinations
Z55.3	Underachievement in School
Z55.4	Educational Maladjustment and Discord With Teachers and Classmates
Z55.8	Problems Related to Inadequate Teaching
Z55.9	Other Problems Related to Education and Literacy

Occupational Problems

Z56.82	Problem Related to Current Military Deployment Status
Z56.0	Unemployment
Z56.1	Change of Job
Z56.2	Threat of Job Loss
Z56.3	Stressful Work Schedule
Z56.4	Discord With Boss and Workmates
Z56.5	Uncongenial Work Environment
Z56.6	Other Physical and Mental Strain Related to Work
Z56.81	Sexual Harassment on the Job
Z56.9	Other Problem Related to Employment

Housing Problems

Z59.01   Sheltered Homelessness

Z59.02   Unsheltered Homelessness

Z59.10   Inadequate Housing

Z59.2   Discord With Neighbor, Lodger, or Landlord

Z59.3   Problem Related to Living in a Residential Institution

Z59.9   Other Housing Problem

Economic Problems

Z59.41   Food Insecurity

Z58.6   Lack of Safe Drinking Water

Z59.5   Extreme Poverty

Z59.6   Low Income

Z59.7   Insufficient Social or Health Insurance or Welfare Support

Z59.9   Other Economic Problem

Problems Related to the Social Environment

Z60.2   Problem Related to Living Alone

Z60.3   Acculturation Difficulty

Z60.4   Social Exclusion or Rejection

Z60.5   Target of (Perceived) Adverse Discrimination or Persecution

Z60.9   Other Problem Related to Social Environment

Problems Related to Interaction With the Legal System

Z65.0   Conviction in Criminal Proceedings Without Imprisonment

Z65.1   Imprisonment or Other Incarceration

Z65.2   Problems Related to Release From Prison

Z65.3   Problems Related to Other Legal Circumstances

Problems Related to Other Psychosocial, Personal, and Environmental Circumstances

Z72.9   Problem Related to Lifestyle

Z64.0   Problems Related to Unwanted Pregnancy

Z64.1   Problems Related to Multiparity

Z64.4   Discord With Social Service Provider, Including Probation Officer, Case Manager, or Social Services Worker

Z65.4   Victim of Crime

Z65.4   Victim of Terrorism or Torture

Z65.5   Exposure to Disaster, War, or Other Hostilities

Problems Related to Access to Medical and Other Health Care

Z75.3   Unavailability or Inaccessibility of Health Care Facilities

Z75.4   Unavailability or Inaccessibility of Other Helping Agencies

Circumstances of Personal History

Z91.49   Personal History of Psychological Trauma

Z91.82   Personal History of Military Deployment

Other Health Service Encounters for Counseling and Medical Advice

Z31.5   Genetic Counseling

Z70.9   Sex Counseling

Z71.3   Dietary Counseling

Z71.9   Other Counseling or Consultation

Additional Conditions or Problems That May Be a Focus of Clinical Attention

Z91.83   Wandering Associated With a Mental Disorder

Z63.4   Uncomplicated Bereavement

Z60.0   Phase of Life Problem

Z65.8   Religious or Spiritual Problem

Z72.811   Adult Antisocial Behavior

Z72.810   Child or Adolescent Antisocial Behavior

Z91.199   Nonadherence to Medical Treatment

E66.9   Overweight or Obesity

Z76.5   Malingering

R41.81   Age-Related Cognitive Decline

R41.83   Borderline Intellectual Functioning

R45.89   Impairing Emotional Outbursts

Alphabetical Index of Decision Trees

Alphabetical Index of Differential Diagnosis Tables